Churchill Livingstone

Commissioning Editor: Andrew Miller/Fiona Conn
Project Development Editor: Joan Morrison
Project Manager: Frances Affleck
Designer: Erik Bigland

POCKETBOOK OF
Orthopaedics
and Fractures

POCKETBOOK OF
Orthopaedics and Fractures

Ronald McRae FRCS (Eng, Glas) AIMBI

With original drawings by the author

SECOND EDITION

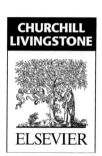

CHURCHILL LIVINGSTONE

ELSEVIER

EDINBURGH LONDON NEW YORK OXFORD PHILADELPHIA ST LOUIS SYDNEY TORONTO 2006

CHURCHILL
LIVINGSTONE
ELSEVIER

First edition 1999
Second edition 2006

ISBN: 978-0-443-10272-1
  Reprinted 2007, 2008, 2009, 2010

International Student Edition ISBN: 978-0-443-10273-8
  Reprinted 2007, 2008, 2009 (twice), 2010

British Library Cataloguing in Publication Data
A catalogue record for this book is available from the British Library

Library of Congress Cataloging in Publication Data
A catalog record for this book is available from the Library of Congress

Note
Knowledge and best practice in this field are constantly changing. As new research and
experience broaden our knowledge, changes in practice, treatment and drug therapy may
become necessary or appropriate. Readers are advised to check the most current information provided (i) on procedures featured or (ii) by the manufacturer of each product to be
administered, to verify the recommended dose or formula, the method and duration of
administration, and contraindications. It is the responsibility of the practitioner, relying on
their own experience and knowledge of the patient, to make diagnoses, to determine
dosages and the best treatment for each individual patient, and to take all appropriate safety
precautions. To the fullest extent of the law, neither the publisher nor the author assumes any
liability for any injury and/or damage to persons or property arising out of or related to any
use of the material contained in this book. Neither the publishers nor the author will be liable
for any loss or damage of any nature occasioned to or suffered by any person acting or
refraining from acting as a result of reliance on the material contained in this publication.
The Publisher

The
Publisher's
policy is to use
**paper manufactured
from sustainable forests**

Typeset by IMH(Cartrif), Loanhead, Scotland
Printed in China

CONTENTS

ORTHOPAEDIC EXAMINATION   1

1. General principles   3
2. Segmental and peripheral nerves   9
3. The cervical spine   27
4. The shoulder   39
5. The elbow   53
6. The wrist   61
7. The hand   71
8. The thoracic and lumbar spine   83
9. The hip   111
10. The knee   137
11. The tibia   169
12. The ankle   175
13. The foot   185

FRACTURES AND DISLOCATIONS   209

14. Fractures: basic terminology   211
15. The diagnosis of fractures and the principles of treatment   223
16. Closed reduction and fixation of fractures   237
17. Open fractures/gunshot wounds/internal fixation   249
18. Fracture healing/complications/pathological fractures   253
19. Regional injuries: the shoulder girdle and humerus   269
20. Regional injuries: the elbow   295

21. Regional injuries: the forearm bones 315
22. Regional injuries: the wrist and hand 327
23. Regional injuries: the spine 367
24. Regional injuries: fractures of the pelvis, hip and femoral neck 399
25. Regional injuries: fractures of the femur and injuries about the knee 433
26. Regional injuries: fractures of the tibia 465
27. Regional injuries: the ankle 479
28. Regional injuries: the foot 497
29. The fracture clinic 519

Biochemical values 525
Index 529

PREFACE

In this small text I have tried to include in a convenient pocket book form as much information as possible, firstly as a guide to the examination of the orthopaedic patient in the ward and clinic, and secondly to the immediate treatment of fracture cases.

Although it is not intended to replace *Clinical Orthopaedic Examination*[1] and *Practical Fracture Treatment*[2] (which may be referred to for more detail), the content and much of the material is based on those two volumes.

Dictates of space have obliged condensation and the discarding of more specialised text and illustrations (such as some anatomical descriptions, orthopaedic treatment details, refinements of the AO classification, surgical descriptions, secondary treatment, self-tests etc.).

In the important matter of selecting what to include, and what to leave out, I am greatly indebted to the many helpful suggestions made by Dr Matthew Henderson and Dr Jonathan Wyatt.

In this *second edition* I have taken the opportunity of bringing the text into line with current practice, and giving more detail in certain areas where I felt this would be helpful and of interest.

Gourock 2005   R.M.

[1] Clinical Orthopaedic Examination, 5Ed. Ronald McRae: 2004 Elsevier Ltd.
[2] Practical Fracture Treatment, 4Ed. Ronald McRae, Max Esser: 2003 Elsevier Ltd.

Conventions

As a rule the limb being examined or treated is tinted in a light grey, and the hands of the examiner, surgeon and assistant are in a darker grey. Where two limbs are shown, the right illustrates the pathology. Some of the following keys have been used where it was thought that there was some risk of confusion:

N = Normal
L&M = Lateral and Medial
L&R = Left and Right

ORTHOPAEDIC EXAMINATION

1

General principles

Inspection 4
Palpation 4
Movements 4
Conduction of special tests
    5
Examination of radiographs
    6
Arranging further
    investigations 6
Additional imaging
    techniques 6
Functional imaging
    techniques 7

In practice, orthopaedic surgery is concerned primarily with the joints of the limbs and spine, and how well they function. The major part of most orthopaedic examinations is therefore centred on the joints that trouble the patient; but the examination must often be extended to include the nerves and muscles which are responsible for their movements, and the state of the bones themselves: and some of the patient's other joints may have to be checked to see if they are also affected. The examination may be broken down into six distinct steps:

1. Inspection
2. Palpation
3. Examination of movements
4. Conduction of special tests
5. Examination of radiographs
6. Arranging further investigations.

It is not always necessary to keep strictly to this order or indeed to carry out all of these procedures.

STEP 1: INSPECTION
Look carefully at the joint, paying particular attention to the following points:

1. *Is there swelling?* If so, is the swelling *diffuse* or *localised*? If it is confined to the joint it may be due to excess synovial fluid (effusion), blood within the joint cavity (haemarthrosis), or pus (pyarthrosis). Swelling extending beyond the confines of the joint may occur in major infections in a limb, tumours and problems of lymphatic and venous drainage.
2. *Is there bruising?* Is this due to trauma, or an abnormality of the vessels or the clotting mechanisms?
3. *Is there any other discoloration, or oedema?*
4. *Is there muscle wasting?* If so, is this due to inactivity from pain or incapacity, or from denervation?
5. *Is there any alteration in shape or posture, or is there evidence of shortening?* This will require careful examination to establish the cause.

STEP 2: PALPATION
Some of the points to note include the following:

1. *Is the joint warm?* If so, note whether the temperature increase is diffuse or localised, always bearing in mind the false impression which may be caused by the effects of local bandaging. A *diffuse* increase in heat occurs when a substantial tissue mass is involved, and is seen most commonly in pyogenic and non-pyogenic inflammatory processes, vascular abnormalities and tumours. A *localised* increase in temperature generally pin-points an inflammatory process to an isolated structure.
2. *Is there tenderness?* The causes of diffuse and localised tenderness are similar to the causes of increased joint temperature.

STEP 3: MOVEMENTS
Estimation of the *range of movements in the joint* is an essential part of any orthopaedic examination. To assess any deviation from normal, the good side may be compared with the bad. Where this is not suitable (e.g. when both sides are involved), resort must be made to published figures of calculated average ranges.

Complete loss of movements follows surgical ablation of a joint (arthrodesis), or may occur in the course of some pathological process (ankylosis). In many conditions there is loss of some extension, giving rise to a *fixed flexion deformity.* This may result from joint capsule or other soft tissue contractures, deformities of the articular surfaces of the bone forming the joint, or the interposition of loose bodies or torn menisci.

Estimation of the *range of movements in the joint* is an essential part of any orthopaedic examination, as any restriction is nearly always due to a mechanical cause and is a sure indicator of pathology. If the muscles controlling a joint are paralysed, then a full range of *passive movements* may be retained. Occasionally, pain or other factors may restrict the *active range of movements* to a range less than the passive.

In many joints it is also mandatory to look for evidence of *movements in an abnormal plane,* the commonest cause being ligamentous laxity. Other accompaniments of movement may require assessment. Rough articular surfaces will produce grating sensations (crepitus) when the joint is moved. Clicks coming from the joint on movement may he produced by soft tissues moving over bony prominences, from meniscal abnormalities or from disturbances in bony contours (e.g. from previous fracture).

The strength of the muscles controlling the joint must be carefully assessed, and if found reduced, recorded on the MRC scale:

M0— No active contraction can be detected.
M1— A flicker of muscle contraction can be seen or found by palpation, but the activity is insufficient to cause any joint movement.
M2— Contraction is very weak, but can just produce movement so long as the weight of the part can be countered by careful positioning of the limb.
M3— Contraction is still very weak, but can produce movement against gravitational resistance.
M4— Strength is not full, but can produce movement against gravity and some added resistance.
M5—Normal power is present.

Muscle strength may be impaired by pain, wasting from disuse, disease or denervation.

Finally, attention should be paid to any impairment of overall function in the affected limb as a result of disturbance of movement or muscle power: in the case of the legs, this implies an assessment of the gait.

STEP 4: CONDUCTION OF SPECIAL TESTS

In most joints there are a number of tests which may be used to assess particular functions; the commonest check the supporting ligaments. Also of particular importance is an appropriate neurological examination. In the case of sensory testing, the MRC gradings may be used:

S0— Absence of all modalities of sensation in the area exclusively supplied by the affected nerve.
S1— Recovery of deep pain sensation.
S2— Recovery of protective sensation (skin touch, pain and thermal sensation).
S3— Recovery of protective sensation, with accurate localisation. Sensitivity (and hypersensitivity) to cold are usual.

S3+— Recovery of ability to recognise objects and texture; any residual cold sensitivity and hypersensitivity should now be minimal. In the case of the hand, recovery of two point discrimination to less than 8 mm.

S4— Normal sensation.

STEP 5: EXAMINATION OF RADIOGRAPHS

Check the following:

1. Are the bones of normal shape, size and contour, or are they thicker or thinner than normal, shorter or longer than usual or abnormally curved or angled?
2. At the joints themselves, are the bony components in correct alignment, or are they displaced or angled?
3. Is the bone texture normal?
4. Are there are any areas of new bone formation, such as exostoses or subperiosteal new bone formation, or is their evidence of bone destruction?
5. Is there any evidence of congenital abnormality, infection or inflammation, rheumatoid or osteoarthritis?

STEP 6: ARRANGING FURTHER INVESTIGATIONS

These may not be required, but the commonest screening tests include the following:

1. Erythrocyte sedimentation rate (ESR) (and in certain cases, C-reactive protein).
2. Full blood count with differential.
3. Latex fixation test.
4. Serum calcium, phosphate, and alkaline phosphatase.
5. Serum uric acid.
6. X-ray of chest.

ADDITIONAL IMAGING TECHNIQUES

CAT (CT) scans. These can show tissue slices in any plane, but characteristically in median sagittal, parasagittal, coronal, and most importantly, the transverse planes. In the CAT scan there is a better range of grey scale separation than in plain radiographs, allowing a greater differentiation of tissue types.

AP and lateral tomography. In this X-ray technique the tube and film are rotated (or slid) in opposite directions during the exposure. Their position relative to one another and to the part being examined determines the tissue slice being clearly visualised. The results are inferior to those obtained by CAT scanning, but may be helpful if the latter is not available.

MRI scans. These avoid any exposure to X-radiation and produce image cuts as in CAT scans, but with a greater ability to distinguish between different soft tissues. They are of particular value in assessing neurological structures within the skull and spinal canal, and meniscal and ligamentous structures about the knee and shoulder.

Ultrasound. Ultrasound imaging, which is generally regarded as being hazard free, is readily available and inexpensive; it is of great sensitivity and of value in assessing the presence of fluid (e.g. blood) within and around joints, and discontinuities in soft tissue structures. It is frequently used in evaluating cases of developmental dysplasia of the hip.

Arthroscopy. Methods for the examination of all the major joints have been developed, and allow direct visualisation of the articular surfaces, the joint capsule, many associated ligaments, and in the case of the knee, the menisci. At the same session, biopsy samples may be taken if required, and sometimes treatment procedures may be carried out.

FUNCTIONAL IMAGING TECHNIQUES

Technetium bone scans. Bone scans may be performed after the injection of technetium tagged methylene diphosphonate ($^{99}Tc^m$-methylene diphosphonate [MDP]). The facility is widely available, inexpensive and gives rapid results. In the trauma field, such scans may assist in the diagnosis of hairline fractures (e.g. of the scaphoid, shin or neck of femur). They may assist in gauging the age of a fracture, and in detecting avascular necrosis of bone. They are of value in the investigation of unexplained pain in the long bones and the spine, infections in bone and in the region of prostheses, and in assessing Sudeck's atrophy (complex regional pain syndrome).

SPECT (single-photon emission controlled tomography). This technique may be used to give better localisation and assessment of an active area discovered by a technetium bone scan. It is of particular value in the investigation of back pain.

PET (fluorodeoxyglucose [FDG]-positron emission tomography). This may be of value in localising infection within a bone. Leucocyte labelling is of particular value in the evaluation of infection round implants, but requires special facilities.

Segmental and peripheral nerves

Segmental distribution 10
Myotomes and dermatomes
    10
The brachial plexus 11
Types of plexus lesion 12
Long-standing plexus lesions
    12
Acute traumatic lesions of the
    brachial plexus 13
Examination of the
    peripheral nerves of the
    upper limb 15
Peripheral nerves of the
    lower limb 23

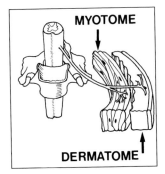

1. SEGMENTAL DISTRIBUTION

Where you suspect involvement of *spinal* rather than *peripheral* nerves (e.g. after disc prolapses or spinal injuries) your examination should concentrate on *myotomes* and *dermatomes*. These are the muscle masses and areas of skin supplied by single spinal nerves, and in this case it does not matter how the nerve fibres are finally distributed via the limb plexuses and peripheral nerves. It is necessary to know which movements are controlled by each spinal segment, and the area of skin exclusively supplied by each spinal nerve.

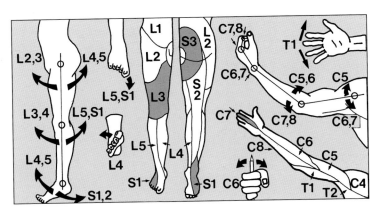

2. MYOTOMES AND DERMATOMES

The key to understanding myotomes is that each joint is typically supplied by four spinal nerves, with a difference of one segment only between adjacent joints. *In the lower limb* this simple plan is perfectly maintained: **hip** flexion and extension: L2, 3 and L4, 5; **knee** extension (including the knee jerk) and knee flexion: L3, 4 and L5, S1; **ankle** dorsiflexion and plantar flexion (including the ankle jerk): L4, 5 and S1, S2. (Movements of **inversion and eversion** are supplied by L4 and L5, S1 respectively.)

In the upper limb the same simple plan holds at the **elbow** where flexion (including the biceps jerk) and extension (including the triceps jerk) are supplied by C5, 6 and C6, 7 respectively. At the **shoulder**, C4 has been suppressed, with the result that abduction is controlled by C5 alone (but adduction is still by C6, 7). Flexion *and* extension of the **wrist** and the **fingers** are supplied by just two segments, namely C6, 7 for the wrist and C7, 8 for the fingers. Pronation and supination are mediated by C6, and the small muscles of the hand by T1.

As far as dermatomes are concerned, in the *upper limb* there is a regular progression round the axial line, with the middle 1–3 fingers being supplied by C7. In the *lower limb* it may be helpful to remember that we kneel on L3, stand on S1 and sit on S3.

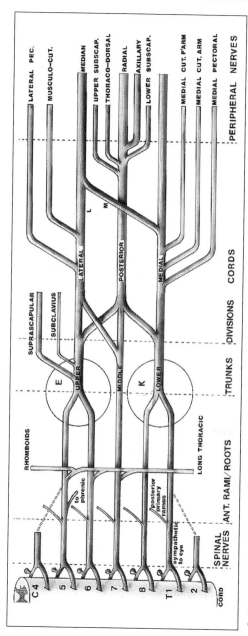

3. THE BRACHIAL PLEXUS

The plexus is generally injured as a result of being stretched. This may follow the application of severe traction to the arm, from depression of the shoulder, from lateral flexion of the neck, or from a combination of these. Such damage may occur at birth: in *Erb's* (*upper obstetrical*) *palsy* (**E**) the C5–6 roots are affected, but the nerve to rhomboids and the long thoracic nerve are spared. In *Klumpke's* (*lower obstetrical*) *palsy* (**K**), the C8–T1 roots are affected. Involvement of the T1 root may cause a Horner's syndrome through sympathetic nerve disturbance (with pseudo-ptosis, contraction of the pupil and decreased sweating in the hand). *In traumatic plexus lesions in adults*, the commonest patterns of injury are: C5–6 (Erb type); C5, 6, 7; C5–T1 inclusive. Penetrating injuries of the plexus (e.g. from stab wounds) are rare.

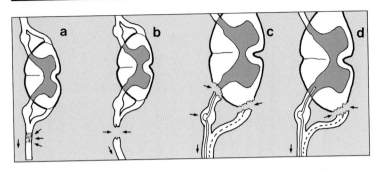

4. TYPES OF PLEXUS LESION

(a) Lesions in continuity. More than half of plexus injuries are of this pattern, with the nerve roots being affected between the intervertebral foramina and the clavipectoral fascia. The lesions may be transient (neurapraxia): if the axons degenerate (axonotmesis), regeneration occurs at the rate of 1 mm per day, provided the axons can penetrate the intraneural scar. **(b) Lesions with ruptured nerve roots.** In more severe injuries the nerves are disrupted at the same level. Only surgical intervention can offer any hope of recovery. **(c) Complete avulsion lesions.** The nerve is avulsed from the cord, and surgical repair is impossible. Motor axons degenerate, and the paralysed muscles show denervation fibrillation potentials on the EMG. The cells of the sensory nerves in the dorsal root ganglion remain intact; although sensation is lost, conduction within the distal nerve remains and may be detected through externally applied electrodes. **(d) Partial avulsion lesions.** Rarely, the posterior roots are spared so that there may be the paradox of muscle paralysis accompanied by preservation of sensation.

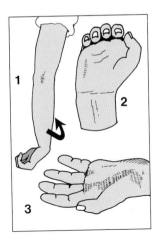

5. LONG-STANDING PLEXUS LESIONS

(1) In Erb's palsy the shoulder is internally rotated, the elbow extended, the forearm pronated, and the wrist and fingers flexed (waiter's tip deformity). The nerve to rhomboids and the long thoracic nerve are usually spared. **(2)** In *Klumpké's paralysis* there is generally wasting of the intrinsic muscles and a claw hand deformity, with sensory loss on the medial side of the forearm and wrist. In many cases there is an associated Horner syndrome. **(3)** In milder cases the T1 root alone may be involved, the sole signs being wasting of the small muscles of the hand, with sensory loss being confined to its medial side. Lesions of this type are also seen in cervical spondylosis, cervical rib syndrome, neurofibromatosis, and apical and metastatic carcinoma.

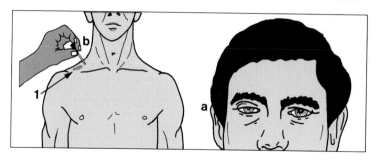

6. ACUTE TRAUMATIC LESIONS OF THE BRACHIAL PLEXUS

The commonest mechanisms of injury involve depression of the shoulder combined with lateral flexion of the neck to the opposite side or traction on the arm. Motorcycle accidents are the single commonest cause.

Assessment

(1) Look for tell-tale bruising over the shoulder or at the root of the neck. In the more severe cases the arm hangs flatly at the side. (2) Using your knowledge of myotomes and dermatomes, determine which roots are involved. (3) Attempt to determine the type of injury; the more evidence there is of proximal damage, the greater the chance of cord avulsion and a poor prognosis. In particular, is there (a) a Horner's syndrome? (This occurs when the T1 root is involved close to the canal and is characterised by pseudo-ptosis, smallness of the pupil on the affected side and dryness of the hand from absence of sweating.) (b) Is there sensory loss above the clavicle? If this area (C3, 4) is affected it indicates that the injury has been severe enough to involve not only the plexus but the roots above, and that the lesion is proximal with a poor prognosis. Deep bruising in the posterior triangle is also strongly suggestive of a preganglionic lesion. (c) Are the first nerves which come off the plexus spared or involved? (i) **Nerve to**

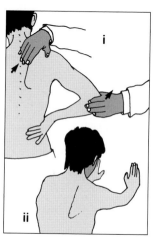

rhomboids (C5): Ask the patient to place the hand on the hip and to resist the elbow being pushed forwards; feel for contraction in the rhomboid muscles. *Absence* of activity is indicative of a lesion proximal to the formation of the upper trunk of the plexus (and suggestive of cord avulsion). *Presence* of activity means a lesion distal to the intervertebral foramen. (ii) **Nerve to serratus anterior (C5, 6, 7).** Damage to this nerve produces winging of the scapula, which is normally demonstrated by asking the patient to lean with both hands against a wall; but this test may have to be abandoned in the presence of an extensive plexus lesion. Note that the nerve to serratus anterior may be damaged in isolation through lifting very heavy weights.

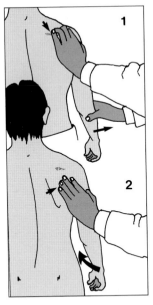

(iii) **The suprascapular nerve (C5, 6).** This nerve arises from the upper trunk of the plexus and supplies both the supraspinatus and the infraspinatus. To test the *supraspinatus* (1), palpate the scapula and identify its spine. Place the fingers above the spine and over the supraspinatus. Steady the forearm with the other hand, and ask the patient to attempt to abduct the arm against this resistance. If the suprascapular nerve is intact, the contraction of the supraspinatus should be easily felt.

Further confirmation of the state of the suprascapular nerve may be made (2) by testing for contraction in the *infraspinatus* muscle which it also supplies. Place the fingers below the spine of the scapula and over the infraspinatus. Ask the patient to externally rotate the arm, applying counter pressure if required, and note any muscle activity.

Other tests and investigations

Tinel's sign. Tap vigorously at the side of the neck, working from above downwards in the line of the nerve roots as they emerge from the spine. The test is positive if there is marked, painful paraesthesia in the corresponding dermatomes (e.g. if tapping over the C6 root produces severe pain and tingling in the thumb). A positive test generally indicates a ruptured nerve root (but the test may also be positive in the presence of an avulsed posterior root ganglion).

X-ray examination.   Plain films of the cervical spine should be obtained. These may occasionally reveal a transverse process fracture, indicative of a severe and probably irrecoverable injury. A plain PA radiograph of the chest may show paralysis of a hemidiaphragm, indicating a proximal lesion.

MRI scanning (and/or myelography). This may give valuable information regarding the presence or absence of nerve root avulsion from the cord.

Electromyography.   To test *motor activity,* at least two muscles supplied by each root should be examined by the insertion of needle electrodes: the presence of action potentials indicates some continuity in that root. *Sensory conduction* may be assessed in two ways: (i) by electrically stimulating (say) the median nerve at the wrist, and by means of separate electrodes attempting to pick up resultant potentials over the plexus or in the neck (evoked potentials); or (ii) stimulating (say) the median nerve at the wrist and attempting to pick up potentials *distally* by means of ring electrodes round the index finger (sensory action [antidromic] potentials). The latter method appears preferable. One side is compared with the other. If the sides are the same, this suggests a severe or complete preganglionic lesion (avulsion of nerve roots from the cord). No sensory action potentials suggest a postganglionic lesion; and if diminished action potentials are present, a mixed lesion is likely.

Histamine test. A drop of 1% histamine is placed over the centre of each affected dermatome, and the skin is pricked through it. The normal side is used as a control, and it should show the usual triple response, with the flare fully developed within ten minutes. Absence of a flare on the injured side suggests postganglionic damage.

Summary of signs indicative of a poor prognosis in traumatic lesion of the plexus

1. A complete lesion involving all five roots.
2. Severe pain in an anaesthetic arm.
3. Sensory loss above the clavicle.
4. Fracture of a transverse process.
5. Horner's syndrome.
6. Paralysis of rhomboids and serratus anterior.
7. Retention of sensory conduction in the presence of sensory loss.

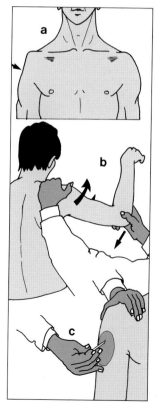

7. EXAMINATION OF THE PERIPHERAL NERVES OF THE UPPER LIMB

The axillary (circumflex) nerve (posterior cord) C5, 6

This nerve is most commonly damaged during shoulder dislocations and in displaced fractures of the proximal humerus (humeral neck). Denervation of the deltoid muscle leads to wasting which at its height produces conspicuous flattening over the lateral aspect of the shoulder (**a**). (Note that spontaneous recovery is the commonest outcome.)

With or without clinical evidence of wasting, test deltoid power (**b**). Ask the patient to attempt to move the arm from the side (pain permitting) while you resist any movement. Look for and feel for deltoid contraction. Sometimes this is difficult to assess, and the two sides should be carefully compared if there is any doubt.

The axillary nerve exclusively supplies sensation to an area of skin on the lateral aspect of the upper arm, often referred to as the 'regimental badge' area because of its position (**c**). Where the shoulder is too painful to move (e.g. if dislocated), loss of sensation in this sharply localised area is enough to diagnose axillary nerve involvement without testing muscle power.

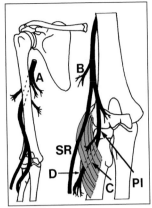

The radial nerve (posterior cord) C5, 6, 7, 8 (T1)

Motor distribution. (A) In the upper arm, the radial nerve supplies triceps. (B) In front of the elbow it supplies brachialis, brachioradialis and extensor carpi radialis longus before dividing into its superficial radial (SR) and posterior interosseous (PI) branches. The latter supplies extensor carpi radialis brevis and part of supinator before it enters the supinator tunnel. Within the tunnel (C) it supplies the rest of supinator. On leaving supinator (D) it supplies extensor digitorum communis, extensors digiti minimi and indicis, extensor carpi ulnaris, abductor pollicis longus, and extensors pollicis longus and brevis.

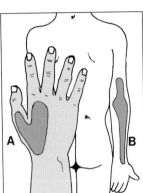

Sensory distribution. (A) The terminal part (superficial radial) supplies the radial side of the back of the hand. (B) The posterior cutaneous branch of the radial, given off in the upper part of the arm, supplies a variable area on the back of the arm and forearm. The distribution of any sensory loss gives useful information on the possible site of the causal pathology.

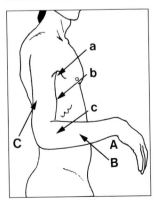

Common sites affected. (a) In the axilla (e.g. from crutches, or the back of a chair in the so-called 'Saturday night' palsy); (b) at mid-humeral level, e.g. from fractures of the humeral shaft or from a tourniquet applied at too high a pressure or for too long (tourniquet palsy); or (c) at or below the elbow, e.g. after dislocations of the elbow, Monteggia fractures, ganglions and sometimes surgical trauma following exposures in this region.

On inspection. Note in particular the following: (A) Is there an obvious wrist drop? (B) Is there wasting of the forearm muscles? (C) Is there wasting of the triceps, suggesting a high (proximal) lesion?

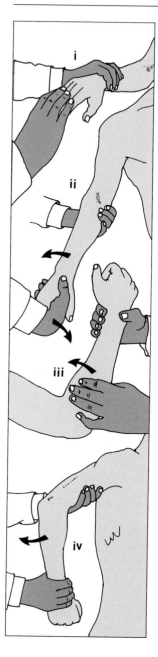

Testing the motor distribution of the radial nerve. **(i)** Working proximally from the most distally innervated sites, begin by testing the extensors of the wrist and fingers. The elbow should be flexed and the hand placed in pronation. Support the wrist, and ask the patient first to try and straighten the fingers, and then to pull the wrist back. If there is any activity, assess its strength by applying counter-pressure on the fingers or hand.

(ii) Now test the supinator muscle. The elbow must be extended to eliminate the supinating action of biceps. Ask the patient to turn his hand while you apply counter force. Loss of supination suggests a lesion proximal to the point where the posterior interosseous nerve exits the supinator tunnel.

(iii) Test the brachioradialis. Ask the patient to try to flex the elbow against resistance while in the mid-prone position. Feel and look for contraction in the muscle. Loss of power suggests a lesion above (i.e. proximal to) the supinator tunnel.

(iv) Now test the triceps. Extend the shoulder and ask the patient to extend the elbow—first against gravity and then resistance. Weakness of triceps suggests a lesion at mid-humeral level, or an incomplete high lesion; loss of all triceps activity suggests a high (e.g. brachial plexus) lesion.

Sensory distribution. Test for sensory impairment in the area supplied by the nerve. Careful analysis of both the motor and sensory deficits should allow accurate localisation of the lesion.

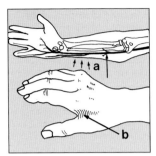

The ulnar nerve (medial cord) C8, T1

Motor distribution. In the forearm it supplies flexor carpi ulnaris and half of flexor digitorum profundus; their loss leads to wasting on the medial side (a). In the hand, it supplies the hypothenar muscles, the interossei, the two medial lumbricals, and adductor pollicis. The first sign of loss in the hand is usually wasting of the first dorsal interosseous muscle, with hollowing in the first web space (b).

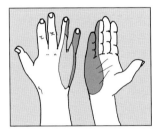

Sensory distribution. Note that there are variations in the areas supplied by the median and ulnar nerves in the hand: the commonest pattern of ulnar distribution is illustrated. The areas supplied by branches arising from the nerve in the hand are highlighted in dark grey. The area on the dorsum shown in light grey is supplied by a branch of the ulnar nerve arising in the forearm; loss here indicates a lesion *proximal to the wrist.*

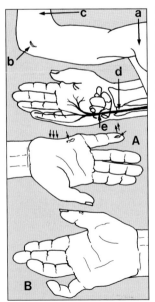

Common sites affected. (a) In the brachial plexus (e.g. from trauma or tumour); (b) at the medial epicondyle, e.g. in ulnar neuritis from local friction, pressure or stretching—such as may occur in cubitus valgus (which should be sought); (c) distal to the elbow, by compression, as it passes between the two heads of flexor carpi ulnaris; (d) at the wrist, especially from lacerations, occupational trauma and ganglions; (e) in the ulnar tunnel syndrome, where the nerve passes between the pisiform and the hook of the hamate (e.g. from a ganglion, or a hook of hamate fracture). The most distal lesions affect the deep palmar nerve and are entirely motor.

Associated deformities. Note (A) if there is abduction of the little finger, hypothenar wasting, skin ulceration, nail brittleness or other trophic changes, or (B) an ulnar claw hand, with flexion of the ring and little fingers at the PIP joints. If the DIP joints are flexed as well, this suggests that the flexor digitorum profundus is intact, and the lesion is *distally* (sic) placed.

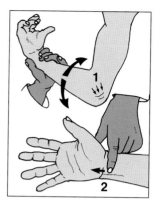

Inspection and palpation of the ulnar nerve. (1) Flex and extend the elbow, looking for abnormal mobility where it passes behind the medial epicondyle. If the nerve is seen to snap over the medial epicondyle, there may be an associated traumatic ulnar neuritis. Palpate it above, behind and distal to the epicondyle, looking for confirmatory tenderness, local thickening or undue paraesthesia. (2) At the wrist, palpate the nerve as it lies just lateral to the tendon of flexor carpi ulnaris. Follow it down to the region of the ulnar tunnel, again looking for undue tenderness and paraesthesia on pressure.

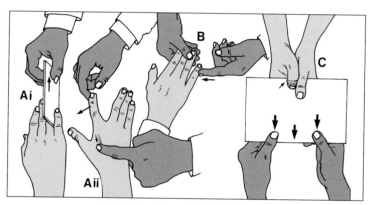

Testing for motor function

(A) The interossei. (i) Ask the patient to hold a sheet of paper between the ring and little fingers. The fingers must be fully extended. Withdraw the paper, noting the resistance offered. In a complete palsy, the patient will not be able to grip the paper at all. (ii) Place the patient's hand in a palm down position, and ask him to resist while you attempt to adduct the index. Look and feel for contraction in the first dorsal interosseous.

(B) Abductor digiti minimi. Ask the patient to resist as you adduct the extended little finger with your index. Note the resistance offered, and compare one hand with the other.

(C) Adductor pollicis. (i) Ask the patient to grasp a sheet of paper between the thumbs and sides of the index fingers while you attempt to withdraw it. If the adductor of the thumb is paralysed, the thumb will flex at the interphalangeal joint (Froment's test).

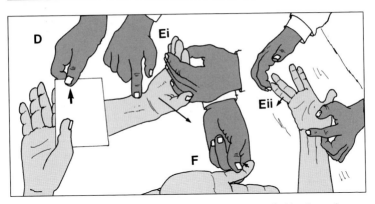

(D) Adductor pollicis. (ii) Ask the patient to attempt to hold a sheet of paper between the thumb and the *anterior* aspect of the index metacarpal. Assess the resistance offered.

(E) Flexor carpi ulnaris. (i) Ask the patient to resist while you attempt to extend the flexed wrist. Feel for the tendon tightening at the wrist while you note the resistance offered. (ii) Place the hand on a flat surface and ask the patient to resist while you attempt to adduct the little finger. Again feel for contraction in the tendon. Loss of activity indicates a lesion proximal to the wrist.

(F) Flexor digitorum profundus. The ulnar half only of this muscle is supplied by the ulnar nerve. Support the middle phalanx of the little finger, and ask the patient to try to flex the distal joint. Apply counter pressure to the finger tip, and note the resistance. Loss of power indicates a lesion near, or above, the elbow.

Testing sensory function. Test in the areas previously indicated.

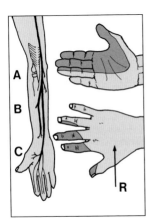

The median nerve (lateral and medial cords) C(5), 6, 7, 8, T1
Motor distribution. (A) near the elbow: flexor digitorum superficialis, flexor carpi radialis, palmaris longus, pronator teres; (B) in the forearm (through its anterior interosseous branch), flexor pollicis longus, half of flexor digitorum profundus, pronator quadratus; (C) in the hand, the thenar muscles and the lateral two lumbricals.

Sensory distribution. The distribution is related to that of the ulnar nerve and varies; the commonest pattern is shown in dark grey (left). Note that on the back of the hand, the area corresponding to thenar area is supplied by the superficial radial (R).

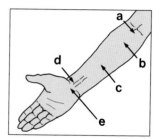

Common sites affected. (a) At the elbow (e.g. after elbow dislocations in children); (b) just distal to the elbow, in the pronator teres (nerve) entrapment syndrome; (c) in the forearm (anterior interosseous nerve), from forearm bone fractures; (d) at the wrist (e.g. from lacerations, including suicide attempts); (e) in the carpal tunnel (e.g. in the carpal tunnel syndrome, or after fractures and dislocations about the wrist).

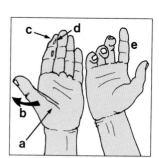

Inspection. Note (a) if there is any thenar wasting; (b) in long-standing cases the thumb may come to lie in the plane of the palm (Simian thumb); (c) atrophy of the pulp of the index, cracking of the nails and other trophic changes; (d) cigarette burns and other signs of local sensory deprivation; (e) in proximal lesions of the nerve or its anterior interosseous branch, there may be wasting of the lateral aspect of the forearm, and the index is held in a position of extension (Benediction attitude).

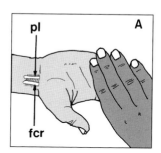

Testing for motor function
(A) Flexor carpi radialis. Place the patient's hand on a flat surface, palm uppermost. Restrain his fingers with one hand, and ask him to attempt to flex his wrist. Normally this should render prominent the tendon of flexor carpi radialis (**fcr**), and if present, that of palmaris longus (**pl**). (Note that the nerve lies between these two tendons, or medial to flexor carpi radialis longus if palmaris longus is absent.)

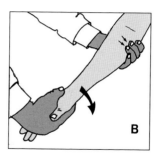

(B) Pronator teres. Extend the patient's elbow, and feel for contraction in the muscle as he attempts to pronate the arm against resistance. Loss indicates a lesion at or above the elbow. Accompanying pain and tenderness over pronator teres is found in the pronator teres entrapment syndrome.

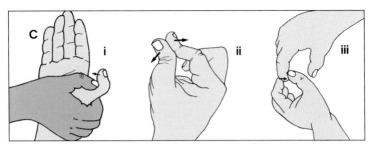

(C) Flexor pollicis longus and flexor digitorum profundus in the index. (i) Ask the patient to try to flex the distal joint of the thumb while you support the phalanx proximal to it. Repeat with the index finger. Loss of power indicates a lesion proximal to the wrist, either of the median nerve itself or of its anterior interosseous branch. (ii) Anterior interosseous nerve screening in adults: ask the patient to form a circle with his index and thumb, and to press the tips tightly together. In an isolated anterior nerve palsy the terminal phalanges of the index and thumb will hyperextend but the thenar muscles will not be affected. (iii) Anterior interosseous nerve screening in children: ask the child to bend the end joint of the index finger. If there is an anterior nerve palsy he will use his other hand to do this. This shows that he understands the question, that movement of the finger is not painful (as in a compartment syndrome) and that it is unlikely that he is able to undertake the movement actively.

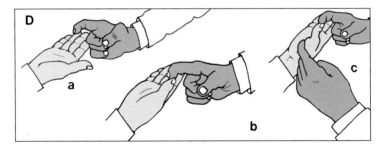

(D) Abductor pollicis brevis. This muscle is invariably and exclusively supplied by the median nerve. Begin by placing the patient's hand, palm upwards, on a flat surface (**a**). Hold your index finger above his palm, and ask him to try to touch it with his thumb (**b**). Steady his hand if he tends to move it. Assess his ability to carry out the movement (he may not be able to do it); look for contraction in the muscle. Then ask him to resist while you attempt to force the thumb back to the starting position (**c**). Note the resistance offered; palpate the muscle to confirm its tone and bulk; compare the power on the affected side with that of the other.

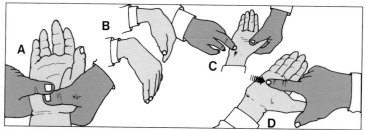

Special tests for median nerve impairment in suspected carpal tunnel syndrome. (A) Pressure test: apply firm pressure over the nerve for 30 seconds, using both thumbs. If positive, the onset of numbness, pain or paraesthesia occurs on average in about 16 seconds. This is the single most reliable test. (B) Phalen's test: ask the patient to hold the hands in a fully flexed position for 1–2 minutes. If positive, paraesthesia in the median distribution appears or is exacerbated. (C) Tinels's sign: this is positive if gentle, repeated percussion over the nerve causes paraesthesia in the median distribution. (D) Sweating test: slide the tip of the index across the palm. Impaired median function leads to an increase in frictional resistance and temperature (from lack of sweating) in the thenar area. **Tourniquet test:** inflate to just above the systolic and hold for 1–2 minutes; the onset of symptoms should be interpreted with caution. **Cast test:** symptomatic relief normally occurs after 10 days in a scaphoid cast, with a relapse on its removal. **Nerve conduction studies:** impaired conduction in the nerve at the wrist is virtually diagnostic.

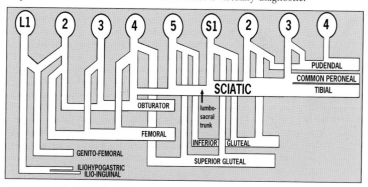

PERIPHERAL NERVES OF THE LOWER LIMB

The most important nerves are: **1.** the *femoral* (L2, 3, 4); **2.** the *obturator* (L2, 3, 4); **3.** the *superior gluteal* (L4, 5 S1); **4.** the *inferior gluteal* (L5 S1, 2); **5.** the *sciatic* (L4, 5 S1, 2, 3) and its two divisions, the *tibial* (L4, 5 S1, 3) and the *common peroneal* (L4, 5 S1, 2, 3). Other branches include the *pudendal* (S2, 3, 4), the *iliohypogastric* and *ilioinguinal* (L1), and the *genitofemoral* (L1, 2). The *lumbosacral trunk* (L4, 5) crosses the triangle of Marcille (bounded medially by L5, inferiorly by the sacrum and laterally by the medial border of psoas) where it is vulnerable to pressure, possibly accounting for some cases of drop foot in pregnancy (rather than disc prolapse). Nerves not shown include the *lateral cutaneous of thigh* (L2, 3) and the *nerves to levator ani* and the *external sphincter* (L4).

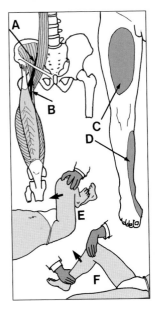

The femoral nerve L2, 3, 4

Motor distribution. (**A**) Above the inguinal ligament the femoral nerve supplies iliopsoas. (**B**) Below the inguinal ligament it supplies the quadriceps, sartorius and pectineus.

Sensory distribution. On emerging below the inguinal ligament it supplies the front of the thigh (**C**) through its femoral cutaneous branches. The terminal part of the femoral nerve (the saphenous nerve) supplies the medial side of the leg and the foot (**D**).

Sites of involvement. Closed lesions of the femoral nerve are rare. Damage may occur if a haematoma forms in the iliacus causing local pressure. This is seen in haemophilia and in extension injuries of the hip.

Testing. (**E**) Iliopsoas—test hip flexion against resistance. (**F**) Quadriceps—ask the patient to extend the knee against resistance. In doubtful cases try to elicit the knee jerk. Observe any quadriceps wasting, and test for loss of sensation to pin-prick in the area supplied by the nerve.

Common peroneal nerve (lateral popliteal) L4, 5, S1

Motor distribution. (**A**) Muscles of the anterior compartment (tibialis anterior, ext. hallucis longus, ext. dig. longus, peroneus tertius). (**B**) Muscles of peroneal compartment (peroneus brevis and longus). (**C**) On the foot, extensor dig. brevis.

Sensory distribution. (**D**) First web space (deep peroneal contribution). (**E**) Dorsum of foot and front and side of leg (superficial peroneal contribution).

Common sites of involvement. (a) At the fibular neck it may be affected by direct pressure, e.g. from blows in the area, pressure from casts or the side irons of a Thomas splint, or ganglions. It may be affected by ischaemia (e.g. from a tourniquet), or the nerve may be stretched in lateral ligament injuries of the knee. It may be affected in many neurological disorders: (b) in the anterior compartment syndrome (deep peroneal branch).

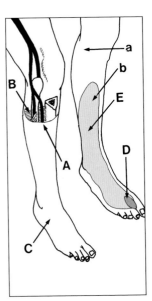

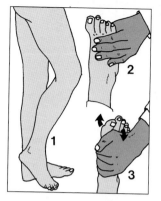

Common peroneal nerve assessment.

Note the patient's gait (**1**). In common peroneal nerve palsy there will be a drop foot and a drop foot gait: either the leg will be lifted high to allow the plantar flexed foot to clear the ground, or the foot will be slid along the ground, with rapid wear of the shoe. Test for motor function. Ask the patient to dorsiflex the foot (**2**) (deep peroneal branch) and to evert the foot (**3**) (superficial peroneal branch). Test for sensation in the area of distribution of the nerve. Note any wasting at the front or side of the leg.

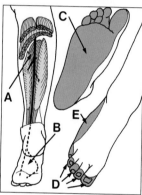

The tibial nerve (medial popliteal) L4, 5, S1, 2

Motor distribution. (**A**) Soleus and deep muscles of the posterior compartment (tibialis posterior, flexor hallucis longus, flexor digitorum longus); (**B**) all the muscles of the sole of the foot through the medial and lateral plantar nerves.

Sensory distribution. (**C**) Sole of foot through the medial and lateral plantar nerves whose territory includes (**D**) the nail beds and distal phalanges. Note (**E**) that the side of the foot is supplied by the sural nerve derived from the tibial and the common peroneal nerves.

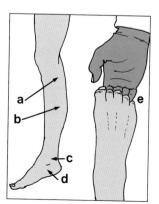

Common sites of involvement.

(a) Under the soleal arch, from tibial fractures; (**b**) in the calf, from ischaemia (e.g. tight plasters, posterior compartment syndrome) and diabetic neuropathy; (**c**) behind the medial malleolus (lacerations and fractures); (**d**) in the tarsal tunnel, in the tarsal tunnel syndrome.

Assessment. Note any muscle wasting in the sole of the foot, clawing of the toes and trophic ulceration. Test the power of toe flexion (**e**). Look for sensory loss in the area supplied by the nerve. High divisions of the nerve are rare but check by looking for calf wasting and loss of power of plantar flexion (from paralysis of gastrocnemius as well as soleus).

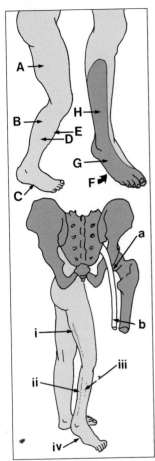

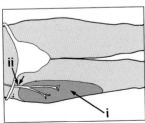

Sciatic nerve: L4, 5, S1, 2, 3
Motor distribution. (A) The hamstrings in the thigh; (B) the superficial and deep muscles of the calf (tibial nerve); (C) the muscles of the foot (medial and lateral plantar nerves); (D) the peroneal muscles (superficial peroneal); (E) the muscles of the anterior compartment (deep peroneal).

Sensory distribution. (F) All of the sole of the foot; (G) the dorsum of the foot; (H) the lateral aspect of the leg and lateral half of the calf. The medial side of the calf and foot are spared. If the posterior cutaneous nerve of the thigh is involved, there is loss of sensation at the back of the thigh.

Common sites involved. (a) Behind the hip (e.g. in some cases of posterior dislocation of the hip, pelvic fracture (rare) and hip surgery); (b) uncommonly, after deep wounds in the back of the thigh. Do not confuse with root involvement in lumbar disc prolapses.

Assessment. Note typically extensive wasting of (i) the thigh, (ii) calf, (iii) peronei and (iv) sole of the foot. Note the presence of a drop foot. Observe any trophic ulceration. Note loss of power in the hamstrings and all three muscle compartments below the knee, an absent ankle jerk and extensive sensory loss in the area indicated.

Lateral cutaneous nerve of thigh (L2, 3)
The nerve pierces the lateral portion of the inguinal ligament and supplies the lateral aspect of the thigh. It may become compressed as it passes through the ligament, giving pain and paraesthesia in the leg (*meralgia paraesthetica*).

Assessment. (i) Look for sensory impairment in the area of distribution of the nerve. (ii) Apply pressure over the nerve at the level of the inguinal ligament and see if this produces paraesthesia in the upper lateral thigh.

3

The cervical spine

Common syndromes 28
Assessment 29
Neurological examination 32
Radiographs 33

COMMON SYNDROMES

Postural neck pain. In this condition, pain in the neck and shoulders occurs in association with some abnormality of neck posture. It is seen most frequently in sedentary female workers under the age of 40. The head and neck may be held in a somewhat protracted position, but there is usually a full range of neck movements, with normal radiographs.

Acute neck pain in the young adult. In the 20 to 35 age group, a sudden movement of the neck may produce severe neck and arm pain accompanied by striking protective muscle spasm and limitation of cervical movements which usually resolve spontaneously. This may on occasion be due to a disc prolapse, but in most cases investigation fails to clarify the nature of the pathology.

Cervical spondylosis. Cervical spondylosis is the commonest condition affecting the neck, with the C5/6 space most often involved. It may remain symptomless, but pain may occur spontaneously or follow minor trauma. This may be felt in the midline, to the sides or over the trapezius muscles. There may be radiation to the head, arms or upper back, but positive neurological signs are rare. In some cases the cervical canal may be narrowed, leading to cervical myelopathy which may cause difficulty in walking, loss of manual dexterity, and bladder dysfunction. Vertebral artery involvement may cause drop attacks precipitated by extension of the neck. Anterior osteophytes may lead to dysphagia.

Thoracic outlet syndrome. This results from involvement of the brachial plexus and axillary artery. These structures may be kinked by a cervical rib, fibrous bands in the scalene attachments at the root of the neck, or a retrosternal dislocation of the clavicle. It often causes paraesthesia and increased sweating in the hand, hypothenar and thenar wasting, and a disturbed radial pulse. Complete vascular occlusion may lead to gangrene of the finger tips. When signs of vascular involvement predominate, arteriography and exploration may be required.

Cord compression and cervical myelopathy. This may be due to developmental malformations of the cervical spine, but more commonly occurs as a complication of cervical spondylosis. There is muscle weakness which is greater in the upper than the lower limbs. In the arms, lower motor signs predominate, while in the legs the reflexes may be exaggerated, with an extensor plantar response, clonus and a broad-based ataxic gait. The sensory loss is not dermatomal. Multiple sclerosis, amyotrophic lateral sclerosis, syringomyelia, subacute combined degeneration of the cord, hydrocephalus and cerebral or cord tumours must be excluded.

Rheumatoid arthritis in the cervical spine. Rheumatoid arthritis frequently involves the neck, and there may be progressive vertebral subluxation, particularly at the atlantoaxial and mid-cervical levels. With progressive root and cord involvement, pain worsens, the gait tends to become ataxic, and there may be progressive paralysis, often with bladder involvement.

Klippel–Feil syndrome. This congenital abnormality is characterised by a failure of the cervical vertebrae to differentiate. It may be associated with congenital elevation of the shoulder (Sprengel's shoulder).

Neoplasms in the cervical region. Tumours of the cervical spine are rare; secondary deposits are the most common. They may cause vertebral body erosion or collapse, affect issuing nerve roots, or give rise to cord involvement.

Osteitis of the cervical spine. Cervical spinal osteitis is rare in the UK. Tuberculosis when it occurs is seen most frequently in children, and may produce widespread bone destruction, vertebral collapse and cord involvement.

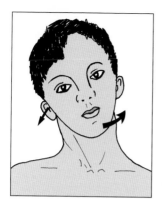

ASSESSMENT
Inspection

Is there a *torticollis*, where the head is pulled to the affected side and the chin often tilted to the other? In *congenital torticollis*, there may be a small tumour in the sternomastoid muscle and (later) some facial asymmetry. Note that in about a third of cases the cause is *ocular muscle weakness*, and a specialist ocular assessment is mandatory. *Acquired torticollis* may result from tonsillitic or upper respiratory infection, vertebral body disease or mal-alignment, trauma or the Klippel–Feil syndrome. In advanced infections and tumours, the head may be supported by the hands.

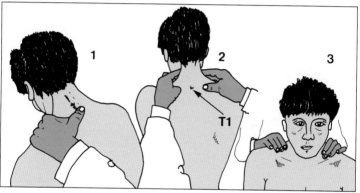

Palpation

- Begin by looking for tenderness in the midline, working from the occiput downwards (**1**). Tenderness localised to one intervertebral space is common in cervical spondylosis, and in the very much rarer infections of the cervical spine.
- Now palpate the lateral aspects of the vertebrae (**2**), looking for masses and tenderness. Note that the most prominent spinous process is that of **T1**, and *not* the vertebra prominens (C7).
- Continue palpation into the supraclavicular fossae (**3**), looking particularly for the prominence of a cervical rib with local tenderness; look also for tumour masses and enlarged cervical lymph nodes. If there is any asymmetry in the supraclavicular fossae (e.g. from a Pancoast tumour), further investigation will be required.
- Examine the anterior structures, including the thyroid gland.
- Note any crepitus (a common finding in cervical spondylosis) as the patient flexes and extends the neck. If in doubt, confirm by auscultation.

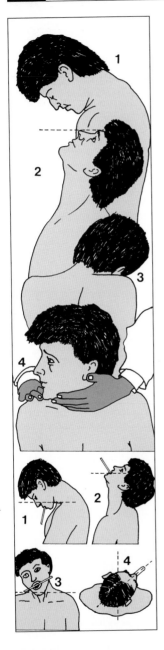

Movements

(1) Flexion (normal = 80°). Ask the patient to bend the head forwards. Normally the chin can be made to touch the region of the sternoclavicular joints. The chin–chest distance may be used for record purposes.

(2) Extension (normal = 50°). Ask the patient to tilt the head backwards. The patient should be seated and erect. The plane of nose and forehead should normally be nearly horizontal but guard against contributory thoracic and lumbar spine movements. The *total* range in the flexion and extension plane is normally 130°, of which about a fifth occurs in the atlanto-axial and atlanto-occipital joints.

(3) Lateral flexion (normal = 45°). Ask the patient to tilt his head on to his shoulder. Lateral flexion, with slight shoulder shrugging, will allow the ear to touch the shoulder. Repeat on the other side, noting any difference. If lateral flexion cannot he carried out without forward flexion, this is indicative of involvement of the atlanto-axial and atlanto-occipital joints.

(4) Rotation (normal = 80°). Ask the patient to look over the shoulder. The movement may be encouraged with one hand, and movement of the shoulder restrained with the other. Normally the chin just falls short of the plane of the shoulders. About a third of rotation occurs in the first two cervical joints. Rotation is usually restricted and painful in cervical spondylosis.

Note. Recording motion in the cervical spine with any accuracy is difficult, but may be attempted (e.g. for medico-legal work) by asking the patient to hold a spatula in the clenched teeth. The legs of a goniometer may then be lined up with the spatula and the neutral plane, and a reading taken.

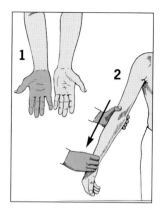

Thoracic outlet syndrome/cervical rib

(1) Begin by looking for evidence of ischaemia, such as coldness, discoloration or trophic changes. Bilateral changes are more in favour of Raynaud's disease.

(2) Palpate the radial pulse and apply traction to the arm. Obliteration of the pulse is not diagnostic but is suggestive when one-sided.

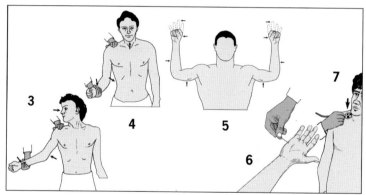

Adson's test. Abduct the shoulder to about 30° (3) and locate the radial pulse. Ask the patient to turn his head towards the affected side. He should then take a deep breath and hold it. Next, he should exhale, look forwards and lower the arm to the side (4). The radial pulse at the beginning of the manoeuvre should be compared with the pulse at the end. Obliteration or reduction, especially if accompanied by duplication of the patient's symptoms is usually significant, but compare the sides. The test may also be tried with the head rotated to the opposite side.

The Roos test. The arms should be held in the so-called 'surrender' position (5), and the hands clenched and unclenched slowly for up to 3 minutes. Neurological and/or vascular symptoms, and early disappearance of the radial pulse on the affected side are highly significant. Look for any evidence of neurological disturbance, including hypothenar wasting, sensory impairment (6) or disturbance of sweating. Auscultate over the subclavian artery (7). A murmur is suggestive of a mechanical obstruction, but repeat on the other side. Examine radiographs for the presence of a cervical rib. CAT and MRI scans are particularly helpful where clavicular problems are suspected.

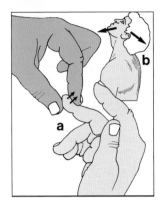

NEUROLOGICAL EXAMINATION

(A) Suspected nerve root involvement. Pay particular attention to myotomes and dermatomes.

(B) Suspected cord compression. In cervical myelopathy, flexor plantar responses are late in onset, and the sensory deficit is *not* dermatomal: there is often hypoalgesia or analgesia of the whole hand, wrist and forearm.

Other tests

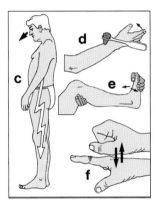

Hoffmann's test. (a) Rapidly extend the distal phalanx of the middle finger by flicking its anterior surface (pulp). In a positive test (indicating corticothalamic dysfunction), the IP joints of the thumb and index flex. Flexing and extending the neck (b) may facilitate this.

Lhermitte's test. (c) Flexion or extension of the neck produces electric shock like sensations, particularly in the legs.

Inverted radial reflex. (d) This highly specific test is positive if the fingers flex when the radial reflex is elicited.

Clonus. (e) This is a significant finding.

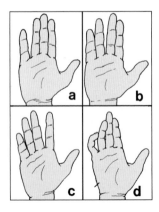

Note also if there is a *myelopathy hand*, indicative of pyramidal tract damage. This has two elements: (i) In the *kinetic myelopathy hand* (f) there is inability to rapidly flex and extend the fingers. The normal rate is in excess of 20 cycles in 10 seconds. (ii) In the *postural myelopathy hand* (a,b,c,d) there is deficient adduction, and often extension, of the ulnar 1–3 fingers. In the mildest cases when the fingers are extended, the little finger lies in a slightly abducted position (a). If it can adduct, this position cannot be held for long. The power of abduction is normal, distinguishing it from ulnar nerve palsy. In more severe cases, the little, ring (b) and sometimes the middle fingers (c) may abduct, and/or the same fingers may flex (d) and lose their power of extension.

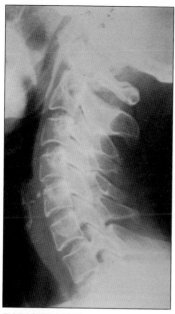 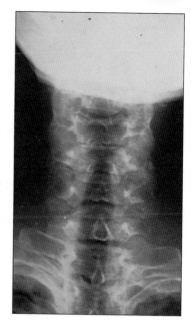

RADIOGRAPHS

The standard projections are a lateral and AP, with an additional through-the-mouth AP view of C1–3 (see later).

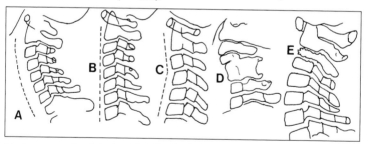

Begin your study of the lateral projection by noting the *cervical curvature*, which is normally slightly convex anteriorly (**A**); straightening of the curve (loss of cervical lordosis, **B**) may be due to posture, positioning or protective muscle spasm. It is a rather unreliable sign of the latter. An abrupt localised change in the curve (kinking, **C**) may be due to a local lesion (such as a subluxation) or from intense local muscle spasm.

Now look at the general *shape of the vertebral bodies*, comparing one with the others. Note, for example, a congenital vertebral fusion (**D**) (e.g. in the Klippel–Feil syndrome); or vertebral collapse (**E**) from TB, tumour or fracture.

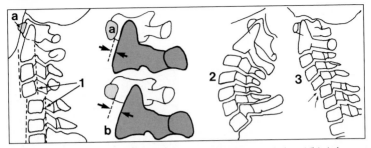

Note the *relationship of each vertebra* to the one above and below. This is best done by tracing the *posterior margins* of the bodies (1). Displacement occurs in dislocations, and may in fact be quite small when the facet joints on one side only are involved. In the case of the upper cervical vertebrae, note that the anterior arch of the atlas (a) lies in front of the lower cervical vertebrae. The distance between the arch and the axis is normally 1–4 mm. A greater distance (b) suggests rupture or laxity of the transverse ligament (e.g. from trauma, rheumatoid arthritis or infection).

Where instability is suspected at any level in the cervical spine, every lateral projection *must be supervised* to reduce the risks of neurological complications. If the first films are normal, repeat the examination with the neck first in unforced extension (2), and then in flexion (3) (flexion and extension views). These should reveal any latent instability.

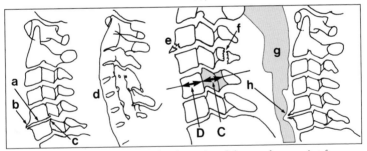

Examine the *disc spaces and the related margins of the vertebrae*, noting for example (a) disc space narrowing, (b) anterior lipping and (c) posterior lipping (all typical of cervical spondylosis). Note (d) the presence of any interbody fusion, typical of ankylosing spondylitis; (e) fracture of an osteophyte or the anterior margin of a vertebral body, suggestive of an extension injury of the neck; (f) fracture of a spinous process, suggestive of a flexion injury. Syringomyelia (which can produce pain in the head, neck and limbs) may cause vertebral body erosions and dilatation of the canal. The diameter of the canal at C5 (C) should not exceed the vertebral body diameter (D) by more than 6 mm (see also Pavlov ratio). Note the *pharyngeal shadow* (g) which normally lies fairly close to the bodies of the vertebrae. Displacement (sometimes with dysphagia) may occur with osteophytes (h), or a retro-pharyngeal haematoma, tumour or abscess.

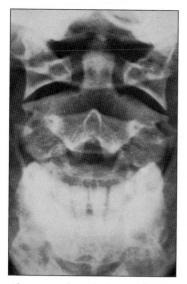
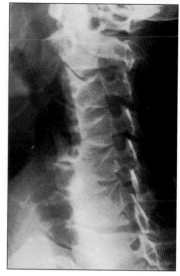

Above are a through-the-mouth AP projection of the upper cervical vertebrae, and one of normally two oblique projections of the cervical spine.

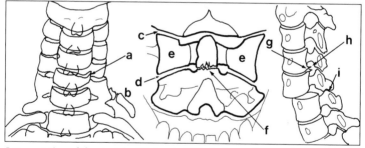

Interpretation of the *straight AP* view is difficult due to the complexity of the superimposed structures. Examine the shape of the vertebral bodies, noting for example any lateral wedging (a). Look for any abnormality in the *facet* or *uncovertebral joints* showing in this projection, and note any cervical rib (b). In the *through-the-mouth AP view of C1–3*, note (c) the atlanto-occipital joints, (d) the atlanto-axial joints and (e) the lateral mass of the atlas. Note any lack of symmetry in the alignment of the odontoid process with the atlas, and look for any evidence of fracture (f). Occasionally, congenital abnormalities of the odontoid process (such as hypoplasia or failure of fusion between its ossification centre and the main mass of the axis) may cause difficulties in interpretation. *Right* and *left oblique projections* are invaluable in demonstrating localised lipping in the uncovertebral joints (joints of Luschka) (g) which may be obstructing the neural foramina (h). They may also show locked facet joints (i) in cervical subluxations.

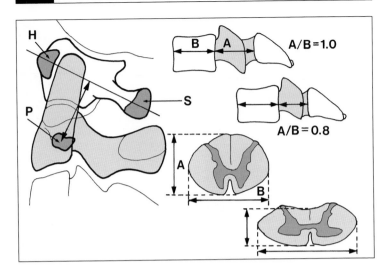

Specialised studies

Suspected advanced rheumatoid arthritis of the proximal cervical spine.

Having noted any atlanto-axial subluxation, look for any upward (cranial) migration of the odontoid process. In the adult this may be assessed by measuring the distance between the pedicle (**P**) of C2 and a line connecting the spinous process (**S**) with the arch (**H**) of Cl. If this is less than 11.5 mm, upward migration is considered to be present.

Suspected cervical myelopathy.

Normally, the depth (**A**) of the cervical canal, as seen in the lateral projection, is as great as that of its related vertebral body (**B**), giving a *Pavlov ratio* (**A/B**) of 1.0, and more than adequate room for the spinal cord. A Pavlov ratio of 0.8 or less indicates a developmentally narrow cervical canal, with risk of cord compression. If the ratio is reduced, check the lumbar spine, as there may well be an associated lumbar spinal stenosis.

If there are axial MRI scans (or post-myelographic CAT scans) which show the cord at the suspect levels, the presence and degree of cord compression may be assessed by working out the *cord compression ratio*. This is calculated by dividing the (sagittal) diameter (thickness) (**A**) of the cord by its width (**B**). (As this is a ratio, the reduction effects of the scans are immaterial.) Note also that the cord may be considerably distorted, so use its *minimal* sagittal diameter (as shown bottom right) for the calculation. A value of 0.4 is indicative of a serious degree of compression, and if decompression surgery is planned it is best done before a figure as low as this is reached. However, be aware that degenerative changes are common in the cervical spine and increase with age (occurring in over 85% of those over 60). These are most often symptom-free, even when there is evidence of disc protrusion and cord compression!

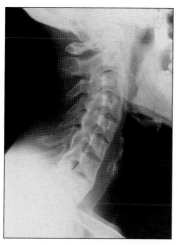
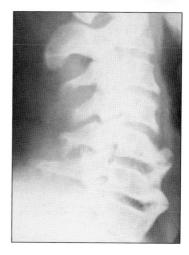

Examples of pathology

Left: ankylosing spondylitis. There is widespread fusion of the facet joints, and the anterior longitudinal ligament is calcified. **Right: cervical spondylosis.** There is gross anterior lipping of C5, 6 and 7, and the pharyngeal shadow is distorted. Similar appearances are found in Forestier's disease, typified by excessive osteophyte formation and abnormal ligamentous calcification.

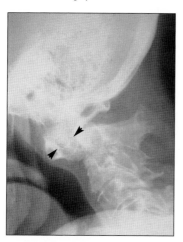
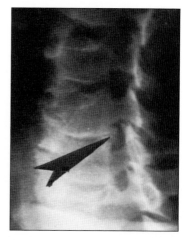

Left: rheumatoid arthritis. This flexion view shows extensive demineralisation and an excessive gap between the anterior arch of the atlas and the odontoid process due to an atlanto-axial subluxation. **Right: cervical spondylosis**, with osteophytes arising from the uncovertebral joint causing unilateral compression of the C6 nerve root.

Basic features 40
Common pathology round
   the shoulder 41
Assessment 44
Radiographs 51

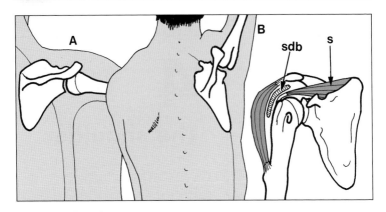

BASIC FEATURES

Glenohumeral movement (A) occurs at the beginning of abduction, and accounts for about half of the total range. It can be slightly increased by external rotation which delays the impingement of the greater tuberosity on the glenoid. **Scapulothoracic movement (B)** accounts for most abduction beyond 90°, and is only possible if there is freedom at the acromioclavicular and sternoclavicular joints, and between the scapula and the chest wall. When the arm is at the side, the deltoid acting alone is incapable of initiating abduction: its contraction tends to raise the head of the humerus relative to the glenoid. On the other hand, when the arm is at the side, the supraspinatus (**s**) is in its position of greatest mechanical advantage; with deltoid it forms a couple and initiates abduction (which is then taken over by deltoid). A tear of the supraspinatus (or relevant part of the shoulder cuff) will prevent the normal initiation of abduction which will then only be possible by trick movements. (**sdb**, subdeltoid bursa)

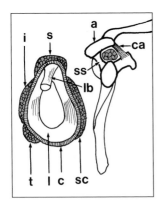

The shoulder cuff. The concavity of the glenoid is deepened by the labrum (**l**) which is attached to its peripheral margin along with the joint capsule (**c**). The capsule is reinforced with the musculotendinous insertions of supraspinatus (**s**), subscapularis (**sc**), infraspinatus (**i**) and teres minor (**t**). These muscles in fact fuse with the capsule, forming an annulus (the shoulder cuff). The supraspinatus is its most important part. It in effect runs through a tunnel formed by the spine of the scapula (**ss**), the acromion (**a**), and coracoacromial ligament (**ca**). It is partly separated from the acromion by the subdeltoid bursa. (**lb**, long head of biceps.)

COMMON PATHOLOGY ROUND THE SHOULDER

The commonest cause of shoulder pain is cervical spondylosis, with pain being referred from irritated nerve roots. On occasion both the neck and shoulder may be involved. The site of restriction of movements, and pain on movements are the most important differentiating factors.

Impingement syndromes

The rotator cuff may become compressed, resulting in pain and disturbance of scapulothoracic rhythm. The commonest site is subacromial, giving a painful arc of movement between 70° and 120° abduction. Compression may also occur beneath the acromioclavicular joint itself (when the painful arc is during the last 30° of abduction), or deep to the coracoacromial ligament. Symptoms may occur acutely (e.g. in young sportsmen) or be chronic, particularly in the older patient with degenerative changes in the acromioclavicular joint. It is common in those on haemodialysis due to subacromial amyloid deposits.

Rotator cuff tears

In the young athletic patient the shoulder cuff may be torn as the result of violent trauma. In the older patient, tears may occur spontaneously or follow more minor trauma, such as sudden arm traction. Most commonly the supraspinatus region is involved, and the patient has difficulty in initiating abduction of the arm. In other cases, the torn shoulder cuff impinges on the acromion during abduction, giving rise to a painful arc of movement. Limitation of rotation may supervene, so that many of these cases, particularly in the older patient, become ultimately indistinguishable from those suffering from frozen shoulder.

Rotator cuff arthropathy

If complete rotator cuff tears are neglected, the loss of soft tissue above the head of the humerus may lead to its proximal migration, with bony collapse and secondary osteoarthritis in the glenohumeral joint.

'Frozen shoulder'/idiopathic adhesive capsulitis

'Frozen shoulder' is a condition affecting the middle-aged, in whose shoulder cuffs degenerative changes are occurring. The outstanding feature is limitation of movements in the shoulder, accompanied in most cases by pain, which is often severe and may disturb sleep. There is often a history of a minor trauma which may produce some tearing of the degenerating shoulder cuff, thereby initiating the low-grade inflammatory changes with which the condition is associated. It is commoner on the left side, and may follow prolonged rest of the arm after a Colles' fracture. It may follow a silent or overt cardiac infarct, and is commoner in diabetics. Most cases resolve spontaneously over a prolonged period of up to two years, although exercise regimes are often helpful.

Calcifying supraspinatus tendinitis

Degenerative changes in the shoulder cuff may be accompanied by the local deposition of calcium salts. This process may continue without symptoms, although radiological changes are obvious. Sometimes, however, the calcified material may give rise to inflammatory changes in the subdeltoid bursa. Sudden, severe, incapacitating pain results; the shoulder becomes acutely tender, and is often swollen and warm to the touch. It is important to differentiate the condition from an acute infection or an acute attack of gout.

Osteoarthritis of the acromioclavicular joint

Arthritic changes in the acromioclavicular joint may give rise to prolonged pain associated with shoulder movements (with or without shoulder cuff involvement). There is usually an obvious prominence of the joint from arthritic lipping, with well-localised tenderness.

Osteoarthritis of the glenohumeral joint

Osteoarthritis of the glenohumeral joint is rare and occurs most frequently secondary to avascular necrosis of the humeral head. This may be of idiopathic origin or may follow a fracture of the proximal humerus. It can occur in caisson disease or result from radionecrosis following radiotherapy.

Rheumatoid arthritis of the shoulder

Rheumatoid arthritis is more common than osteoarthritis, and the features are similar to those of the condition in other joints.

Recurrent dislocation of the shoulder

There is a history of previous frank dislocations of the shoulder in which the causal trauma has usually become progressively less severe. It should be differentiated from habitual dislocation: in the latter the patient is often psychotic or suffering from a joint laxity syndrome.

Infections round the shoulder

Infections involving the shoulder joint are on the whole uncommon. *Staphylococcal osteitis* of the proximal humerus is probably the commonest. *Tuberculosis of the shoulder* is now rare. In the moist form, commonest in the first two decades of life, the shoulder is swollen, there is abundant pus production and sinuses may form. The progress is comparatively rapid and destructive. In the past a dry form, *caries sicca*, with little destruction or pus formation and affecting an older age group was recognised. It is now thought that these cases are likely in fact to have been suffering from frozen shoulder. *Gonococcal arthritis* of the shoulder is uncommon, but when it occurs there is moderate swelling of the joint and great pain which often seems out of keeping with the physical signs.

Miscellaneous conditions round the shoulder

Clavicle. Primary pathology in the clavicle is uncommon, but a common cause of confusion is a pathological fracture due to radionecrosis, years after treatment for breast carcinoma. The fracture may be preceded by pain for many months, and may be mistaken for metastatic spread.

Scapula: snapping scapula. A patient may complain of a grinding sensation arising from beneath the scapula. This is often due to a rib prominence, but in some cases it may be caused by an exostosis arising from the deep surface of the scapula. When symptoms are persistent, excision of such an exostosis may give relief.

High scapula. There are several related congenital malformations affecting the neck and shoulder girdle. In the most minor cases, one scapula may be a little smaller than the other and more highly placed; in more severe cases one or both shoulders are highly situated, the scapulae are small and there may be webs of skin running from the shoulder to the neck (Sprengel shoulder).

Klippel–Feil syndrome. In this condition the neck is short, there are multiple anomalies of the cervical vertebrae (which may include vertebral body fusions and spina bifida) and the scapulae are also highly placed. There may be other congenital lesions including diastomatomyelia, lumbosacral lipomata, and renal abnormalities.

Winged scapula. The patient complains of prominence of the scapula, which is raised along its vertebral border from the chest wall. This is due to weakness of the serratus anterior. The cause may be primarily muscular (as in progressive muscular dystrophy) or follow traumatic paralysis of the long thoracic nerve.

Ruptured biceps tendon. Rupture of the long head of biceps may occur spontaneously or as a result of a sudden muscular effort, usually in an elderly or middle-aged person in whom degenerative tendon changes are present. The biceps tendon may also give rise to symptoms if its anchorage is imperfect; this may allow it to displace causing local discomfort. Whether the result of this or not, the tendon may also undergo painful inflammatory changes.

Age incidence of the commonest problems around the shoulder

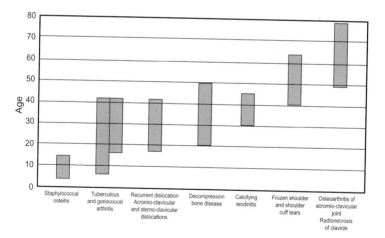

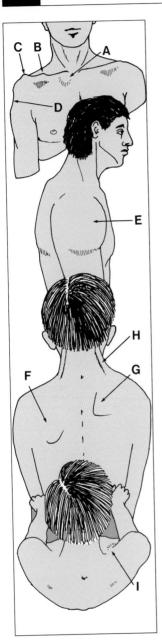

ASSESSMENT

Inspection

From the front. Note (**A**) any prominence of the sternoclavicular joint, suggestive of subluxation from old trauma.; (**B**) deformity of clavicle (e.g. from old fracture); (**C**) prominence of the acromioclavicular joint (e.g. from subluxation or osteoarthritis); (**D**) deltoid wasting (from disuse or axillary nerve palsy).

From the side. Note (**E**) if there is any swelling of the joint, suggesting infection, an inflammatory reaction (e.g. from calcifying supraspinatus tendinitis) or recent trauma.

From behind. Note (**F**) if the scapula(e) are normally shaped and situated, or (**G**) if the scapula(e) are small and highly placed as in Sprengel shoulder and the Klippel–Feil syndrome, or (**H**) if there is any webbing of the skin at the root of the neck, also typical of the Klippel–Feil syndrome. Note any winging of the scapula due to paralysis of serratus anterior.

From above. Note (**I**) any deformity of the clavicle, swelling of the shoulder or asymmetry of the supraclavicular fossae.

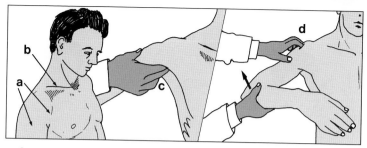

Palpation

(a) Look for tenderness over the anterior and lateral aspects of the glenohumeral joint. If *diffuse* and marked, this may be due to infection or calcifying supraspinatus tendinitis; *local* tenderness is commoner in shoulder cuff tears and frozen shoulder. (b) Look for tenderness over the clavicle: *medially* this may occur in sternoclavicular dislocations and infections (particularly tuberculosis); *centrally*, over tumours, and radionecrosis; and *laterally* over the acromioclavicular joint— e.g. after recent subluxations or where there are arthritic changes (often accompanied by lipping) and crepitus on movement. (c) Palpate the upper humeral shaft and head via the axilla. Exostoses of the proximal humeral shaft may often be detected via this route. (d) Press below the acromion and abduct the arm. Sudden tenderness during a portion of the arc of movement is found in tears and inflammatory lesions involving the shoulder cuff and/or the subdeltoid bursa.

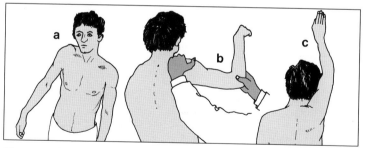

Movements

Begin by asking the patient to abduct both arms. A full, free and painless range is rare in the presence of any significant pathology in the shoulder region. *Difficulty in initiating abduction* (a) is suggestive of a major shoulder cuff tear. A history of violent injury may be obtained in the young adult. In the middle-aged or elderly patient, a tear may follow comparatively minor trauma or occur spontaneously in a shoulder cuff weakened by attrition from chronic impingement. If the patient cannot abduct the arm actively, attempt to do so passively (b), remembering to externally rotate it while doing so. A full range indicates an intact glenohumeral joint. Ask the patient to hold the arm himself in the vertical position (c). If he can do so, deltoid and the axillary nerve are likely to be intact. If the patient has passed the last test, ask him to lower the arm to the side. Again note the presence of any painful arc of movement.

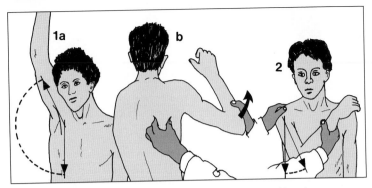

(1) Abduction (normal = 0–170°). In the normal shoulder, the arm can touch the ear with only slight tilting of the head (**a**). Compare the sides. If both active and passive movements are restricted, fix the angle of the scapula with one hand and try to abduct the arm with the other (**b**). Absence of movement indicates a fixed glenohumeral joint, with any previously noted movements being scapular.

(2) Adduction in extension (normal = 50°). Place one hand on the shoulder and swing the arm, flexed at the elbow, across the chest.

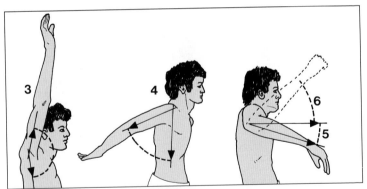

(3) Forward flexion (normal = 0–165°). Ask the patient to swing the arm forwards and lift it above his head. View the patient from the side.

(4) Backwards extension (normal = 0–60°). Ask the patient to swing the arm directly backwards, again viewing and measuring from the side.

(5) Internal rotation in abduction (normal = 70°). Abduct the shoulder to 90°, and flex the elbow to a right angle. Ask the patient to lower the forearm from the horizontal plane.

(6) External rotation in abduction (normal = 100°). From the same starting position with the forearm parallel to the ground, ask the patient to raise the hand, keeping the shoulder in 90° abduction.

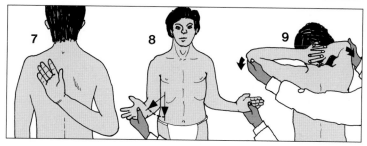

(7) Internal rotation in extension (normal = can touch the opposite scapula). Note where he reaches and compare the sides. Severe restrictions occur in frozen shoulder, and the patient may not be able to get his hand behind his back at all. This is an invaluable screening test.

(8) External rotation in extension (normal = 70°). Place the elbows into the sides and flex to 90°, with the hands facing forwards. Move them laterally, comparing one side with the other. An increase in external rotation in extension is a feature of tears of the subscapularis muscle.

(9) External rotation at 90° abduction (normal = the hand can be placed behind the head with the elbow pulled fully back). Ask the patient to place both hands behind the head. If the shoulders are in horizontal flexion, try to pull the elbows backwards gently so that they lie in the plane of the shoulders.

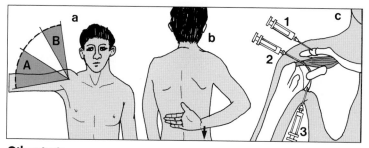

Other tests
The shoulder cuff. (a) Note pain during abduction (which may have to be assisted): **(A)** during the arc 70–120°, suggestive of shoulder cuff impingement in the region of the acromion; **(B)** during the latter phase of abduction, suggestive of shoulder cuff impingement in the region of the acromioclavicular joint or coracoacromial ligament, or from osteoarthritis of the acromioclavicular joint. **(b)** To test subscapularis (which may be torn by violent external rotation, hyperextension or anterior dislocation of the shoulder), ask the patient if he can draw the hand away from contact with the back, when in the position shown. **(c)** Where there is shoulder pain related to movement and the source is uncertain, serial injections with local anaesthetic may be tried. Start with the acromioclavicular joint **(1)**. If pain on movement is not relieved after 5–10 minutes, proceed to the upper part of the shoulder cuff **(2)**. If this also fails, infiltrate the glenohumeral joint **(3)**.

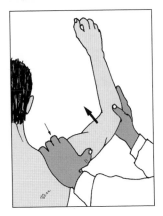

Osteoarthritis about the shoulder.

Place one hand over the shoulder, with the middle finger lying along the acromioclavicular joint. Abduct the arm with the other hand. Look for crepitus arising from the shoulder, and try to locate its source (glenohumeral or acromioclavicular). Repeat while the arm is actively abducted, and if in doubt, auscultate. Clicking may arise from a number of sources, including scapular exostoses and coracoid impingement. (The latter may cause shoulder pain and coracoid tenderness.)

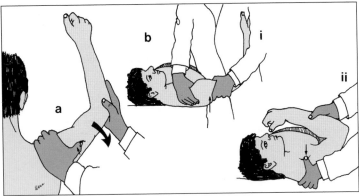

Glenohumeral stability

(a) The apprehension test. Stand behind the seated patient and abduct the shoulder to about 90°. Slowly externally rotate the shoulder, while pushing the head of the humerus forwards with your thumb. Apprehension, fear or refusal to continue is evidence of chronic anterior instability of the shoulder.

(b) Drawer tests of Gerber and Ganz. For *anterior* instability **(i)**: support the (supine) patient's relaxed arm against your side, with his shoulder in 90° abduction, slight flexion and external rotation. Steadying the scapula with the thumb on the coracoid and the fingers behind, try to move the humeral head anteriorly with your other hand. Note movement, clicks or patient apprehension. Compare the sides: axial radiographs may be taken during the procedure, which is sometimes performed under anaesthesia. Where recurrent *posterior* dislocation is suspected **(ii)**, place the thumb just lateral to the coracoid. Now internally rotate the shoulder and flex it to about 80°, pressing the humeral head backwards with the thumb; any backward displacement of the humeral head should be detected, but X-ray confirmation may also be made.

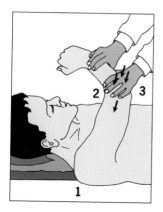

(c) The jerk test for posterior instability. With the patient's shoulder over the edge of the examination couch **(1)**, flex both the shoulder and elbow to 90°. With one hand on the elbow **(2)**, push downwards **(3)** and attempt to sublux the humeral head posteriorly. If this occurs, indicating instability, a jerk or jump will be felt. If negative, repeat with the shoulder adducted and internally rotated.

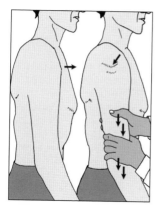

(d) The sulcus sign for inferior instability. With the patient standing, grasp the arm and pull it downwards. If there is inferior laxity then a depression will become obvious between the humeral head and the acromion. This is of greater significance if the sign is absent or less on the good side, or if accompanied by pain and apprehension on the affected side. A positive test is commoner when there is multidirectional instability in the shoulder.

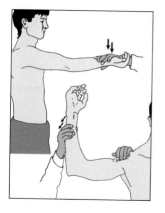

Biceps tendon instability test (see illustration lower right). The shoulder is abducted to 90° and the elbow flexed to a right angle. The tendon is then located in the region of the bicipital groove. Keeping the examining fingers in position, the patient's shoulder is internally rotated. If the tendon is unstable it may be felt to move out of position, and this may be accompanied by an audible click, often accompanied by discomfort.

Biceps tendinitis: the Speed test (see illustration upper left). With the patient's elbow fully extended and in supination, try to extend the shoulder. This manoeuvre causes pain if the tendon is inflamed.

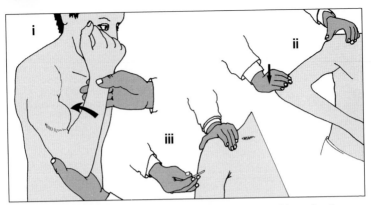

The long head of biceps. Support the patient's elbow with one hand. Grasp his wrist, and ask him to pull toward his shoulder, while you resist this movement (**i**). If the long tendon of biceps is ruptured, the belly of biceps will appear globular in shape. Compare the two sides.

Deltoid and the axillary nerve. Ask the patient to try to keep the arm elevated in abduction while you press down on his elbow (**ii**). Look and feel for deltoid contraction. If axillary nerve palsy is suspected, test for sensory loss in the 'regimental badge' area on the lateral aspect of the arm (**iii**).

The long thoracic nerve. Check this if there is winging of the scapula due to paralysis of serratus anterior (See Ch. 2).

The suprascapular nerve. Check as described in Chapter 2. Apart from brachial plexus injuries, paralysis of supraspinatus and infraspinatus may be caused by a ganglion in the greater scapular notch. Confirm with an MRI scan.

The cervical spine. Always screen the cervical spine in examining a case of shoulder pain. This is doubly important if shoulder movements are found to be normal.

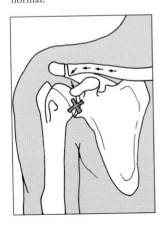

Aspiration. Consider if pus is suspected. **Method:** with the patient supine, follow the clavicle laterally and find the coracoid, which lies about 5 cm obliquely below the acromioclavicular joint. Now rotate the arm, when you should be able to feel the head of the humerus. After local infiltration, pass a large bore needle directly backwards into the joint just inferior to the coracoid.

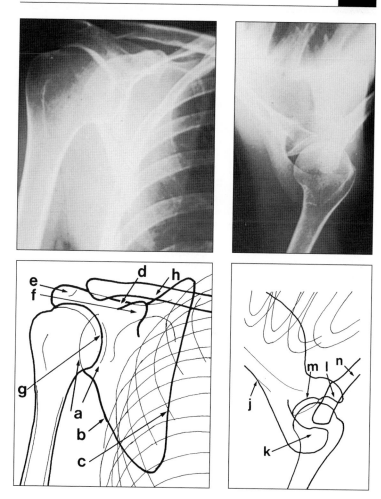

RADIOGRAPHS

The standard shoulder projection is the anteroposterior taken in recumbency (left). Examine the radiograph methodically by identifying **(a)** the glenoid, **(b)** the lateral border of the scapula, **(c)** the medial border, **(d)** its spine, **(e)** the acromion and **(f)** the coracoid. Note the relations of **(g)** the humeral head and **(h)** the clavicle to the glenoid and the acromion.

The normal *axial (per-axillary or axillary) lateral* gives the most useful additional information but is dependent on the patient being able to abduct the arm. It is very helpful in clarifying the relationships of the glenoid and humeral head: **(j)** lateral border, **(k)** acromion, **(l)** coracoid, **(m)** glenoid, **(n)** clavicle.

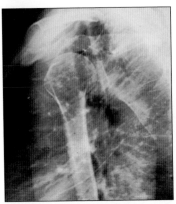
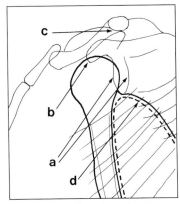

If the patient is not able to have the arm abducted, a *translateral* may be taken. In this projection, note (a) glenoid, (b) coracoid, (c) acromioclavicular joint and superimposed clavicular shadows. Note the parabolic curve (d) formed by the humeral shaft and the lateral border of the scapula. This is disturbed in most shoulder dislocations and subluxations. Unfortunately, detail is often poor, especially in the stout patient, and some prefer an *apical oblique projection*; this duplicates and foreshortens the features seen in the AP but helps clarify the glenohumeral relationship. Where subluxation of the acromioclavicular joint is suspected, a *standing AP projection*, showing both shoulders on the one film, should be taken with the patient holding weights in both hands.

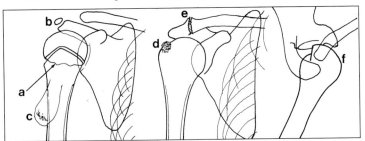

Features. In the child or adolescent, do not mistake (a) the margins of the epiphyseal plate for fracture, or (b) the acromial ossification centre for a loose body. Note (c) any simple exostosis (ossifying chondroma) of epiphyseal plate origin; (d) calcification in the supraspinatus tendon; (e) arthritic changes in the acromioclavicular joint; (f) a hatchet head (Hill–Sachs) deformity of the humeral head (best seen in an axial lateral) and typically found in cases of recurrent dislocation of the shoulder.

Special investigations. In suspected infections, perform white cell and differential blood counts, blood culture, ESR, chest X-ray and aspiration of the joint to exclude pyogenic, gonococcal and tubercular infections. In undiagnosed mechanical problems or painful arc syndromes, perform a CAT scan or MRI scan, arthroscopy, examination under anaesthesia or arthrography.

CHAPTER

5

The elbow

Common pathology round
the joint 54
Assessment 55
Radiographs 59

COMMON PATHOLOGY ROUND THE JOINT

Tennis elbow

This is by far the commonest cause of elbow pain in patients attending orthopaedic clinics, and is usually associated with a strain of the common extensor origin or fibrosis in extensor carpi radialis brevis. The patient is usually in the 35 to 50 age group and complains both of pain on the lateral side of the elbow and difficulty in holding any heavy object at arm's length. In *golfer's elbow*, pain and tenderness involve the common flexor origin on the medial side of the elbow.

Cubitus varus and cubitus valgus

Decrease or increase in the carrying angle of the elbow generally follows a supracondylar or other elbow fracture in childhood. If this fails to remodel, the deformity may be unsightly, and there is tendency to tardy ulnar nerve palsy.

Tardy ulnar nerve palsy

This form of ulnar nerve palsy is of slow onset and progression. It often declares itself between the ages of 30 and 50, and there is commonly a history of childhood injury such as a fracture about the elbow.

Ulnar neuritis and the ulnar tunnel syndrome

Ulnar neuritis, often with small muscle wasting and sensory loss in the hand, may occur as a complication of local trauma at the elbow or at the wrist, but in a number of cases there may be no obvious cause. It may be seen at the elbow if the nerve is abnormally mobile or subject to pressure as it passes between the two heads of flexor carpi ulnaris. In the hand it may be compressed in the ulnar tunnel, e.g. from a ganglion. Nerve conduction studies may help in localisation.

Olecranon bursitis

Swelling of the olecranon bursa is common in carpet-layers and others who repeatedly traumatise the posterior aspect of the elbow joint. In rheumatoid arthritis, there may be associated nodular masses in the proximal part of the forearm.

Pulled elbow (See page 311.)

Osteoarthritis and osteochondritis dissecans

Primary osteoarthritis of the elbow joint is not uncommon in heavy manual workers; secondary osteoarthritis may follow fractures involving the joint surfaces or complicate osteochondritis dissecans. In all cases loose bodies may form, and these may restrict movements or cause locking of the joint.

Rheumatoid arthritis

This may affect either one or both elbows. If both are involved, the functional disability may be great. When there is gross destruction, the ulnar nerve may be affected, and the joint may become flail.

Tuberculosis of the elbow

This is now very uncommon. If present, there is marked swelling of the elbow with profound local muscle wasting, which is usually so striking that there is unlikely to be delay in further investigation by aspiration and synovial biopsy.

Myositis ossificans

This occurs most commonly after fractures or dislocations about the elbow, with calcification appearing in the haematoma which forms at the front of the joint. It is particularly common in association with head injuries and may also follow over-vigorous physiotherapy. It leads to a mechanical block to flexion.

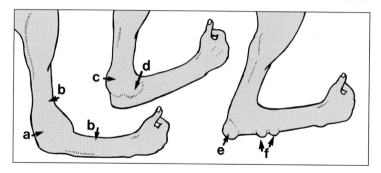

ASSESSMENT

Inspection

Look for **(a)** generalised swelling of the joint and **(b)** muscle wasting, both suggestive of infective arthritis (e.g. tuberculosis) or rheumatoid arthritis. The swollen elbow is always held in the semiflexed position. Note **(c)** the earliest sign of effusion is the filling out of the hollows seen in the flexed elbow above the olecranon; **(d)** the next sign is swelling of the radiohumeral joint. Fluid may be squeezed between these two areas. Observe any localised swellings round the joint, such as **(e)** olecranon bursitis or **(f)** rheumatoid nodules.

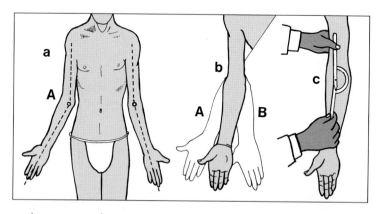

The carrying angle. Normal, males = 11° (range 2–26°); females = 13° (range 2–22°). Ask the patient to extend both elbows and compare the sides **(a)**. Any small difference between them will then be obvious. In cubitus valgus **(A)** there is an increase in the carrying angle, while in cubitus varus **(B)** there is a decrease **(b)**. The commonest cause of unilateral alteration is an old supracondylar fracture. Measure any departure from normal using a goniometer **(c)**.

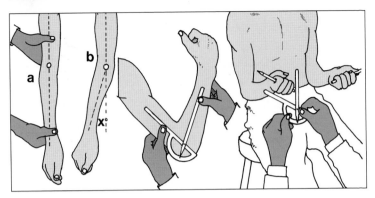

Movements

Extension (normal = 0°). Full extension (0°) is present if the arm and forearm can be made to lie in a straight line **(a)**. Loss of full extension is especially common in osteoarthritis, rheumatoid arthritis and after fractures. If the elbow can be extended beyond the neutral position, record as 'X° hyperextension' **(b)**. Up to 15° is accepted as normal, especially in women, but if more than this, look for hypermobility in other joints (e.g. Ehlers–Danlos syndrome). **Flexion (normal = 145°).** Restriction is common in arthritis and after fractures. **Pronation (normal = 75°); supination (normal = 80°).** An accurate assessment may be made by asking the patient to keep the elbows in at the sides, and lining up the legs of a goniometer with the vertical and the line of a pen grasped in the hand.

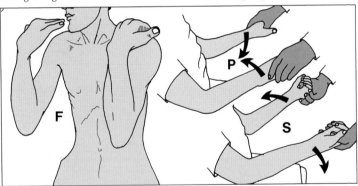

Screening tests of movement. Flexion (F): ask the patient to attempt to touch both shoulders. A slight difference in flexion between the sides is then usually obvious. **Pronation (P):** ask the patient to hold the elbows closely to the sides. Turn the palms downwards into pronation, comparing the sides. **Supination (S):** repeat, turning the palms upwards. Pronation/supination movements may be reduced after fractures at the elbow, forearm and wrist (e.g. most commonly after Colles' fracture). Loss may also occur after dislocation of the elbow, rheumatoid and osteoarthritis, and in pulled elbow in children (pure supination loss only).

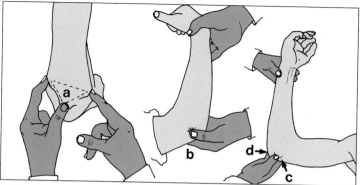

Palpation

Begin by locating the epicondyles and the olecranon. These form an equilateral triangle (a) which is disturbed in elbow subluxations. Now palpate the *lateral epicondyle* (b) with the thumb. Sharply localised tenderness here or just distally is almost diagnostic of tennis elbow. Tenderness over the *medial epicondyle* (c) occurs after local injury, in golfer's elbow, and in tears of the ulnar collateral ligament. Tenderness over the *olecranon* (d) is uncommon, apart from fracture and infected olecranon bursitis, both of which are usually obvious.

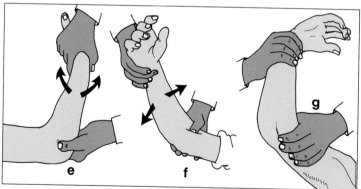

Palpate the *radiohumeral joint* (e) by pressing the thumb firmly into the space on the lateral side of the elbow between the radial head and humerus. Now pronate and supinate the arm. Tenderness here is common after injuries of the radial head, osteoarthritis and osteochondritis dissecans. Examine the *antecubital fossa* (f) by feeling on both sides of the biceps tendon while flexing and extending the elbow through 20°. Note the presence of any abnormal masses (e.g. myositis ossificans, loose bodies). Roll the *ulnar nerve* (g) under the fingers behind the medial epicondyle. If there is any thickening or increased sensitivity, check nerve function. Inspect the nerve while flexing and extending the elbow, looking for abnormal mobility. Note any cubitus valgus or varus deformity.

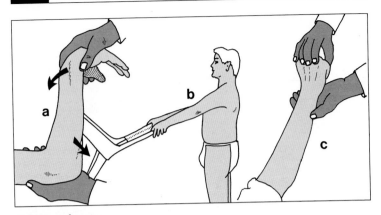

Additional tests

Tennis elbow. (a) Flex the elbow and fully pronate the hand. Now extend the elbow. Pain over the lateral epicondyle is almost diagnostic of tennis elbow. As an alternative, pain may be sought by pronating the arm with the elbow fully extended. (b) The chair test: ask the patient to attempt to lift a chair (of about 3.5 kilos in weight) with the elbows extended and the shoulders flexed to 60°. Difficulty in performing this manoeuvre, with complaint of pain on the lateral aspect of the affected elbow, is suggestive of tennis elbow. (c) Thomsen's test. Ask the patient to clench the fist, dorsiflex the wrist and extend the elbow. Try to force the hand into palmar flexion while the patient resists. Severe pain over the external epicondyle is again most suggestive of tennis elbow. Repeat, only this time attempting to flex the extended middle finger rather than the wrist.

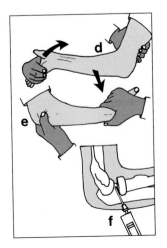

Golfer's elbow. Flex the elbow, supinate the hand and then extend the elbow (d). Pain over the medial epicondyle is very suggestive of golfer's elbow. A good response to local injections of hydrocortisone may sometimes help to confirm the diagnosis.

Aspiration of the elbow joint. The most direct and safest approach is from the lateral side. Flex the elbow to 90°; to locate the radial head, pronate and supinate the arm, and feel with the thumb for its rotation (e). After infiltration of the area with local anaesthetic, introduce the aspirating needle (f) in the area of the palpable depression between the proximal part of the radial head and the capitulum.

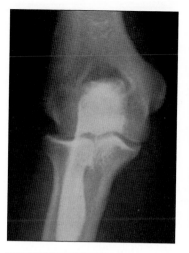
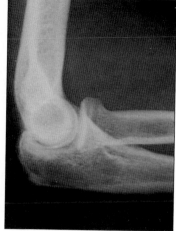

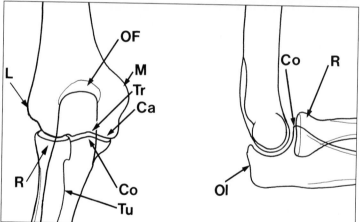

RADIOGRAPHS

The standard projections are the AP and lateral. In examining the AP, trace out the outline of medial epicondyle (**M**), olecranon and coronoid fossae (**OF**), lateral epicondyle (**L**), capitulum (**Ca**), radial head (**R**), tuberosity of the radius (**Tu**), coronoid process of ulna (**Co**) and trochlea (**Tr**). In the lateral, note the radial head (**R**), coronoid process of the ulna (**Co**) and olecranon (**Ol**). For the X-ray appearances of the elbow in the growing child, see Chapter 20.

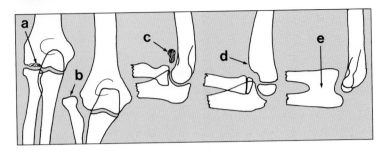

Examples of pathology

Look for **(a)** any defects in the capitulum—the commonest cause is an osteochondritis dissecans, which in some cases may be secondary to old trauma; **(b)** an old Monteggia fracture (fracture of the ulna and dislocation head of radius), where there may be persistent loss of alignment between the radial head and the capitulum, usually associated clinically with reduction of pronation and supination; **(c)** loose bodies, single or multiple—these are usually secondary to osteoarthritis or osteochondritis dissecans, and clinically may lead to a mechanical block to flexion (sometimes of an intermittent character when the loose bodies retain their mobility); **(d)** an incompletely remodelled supracondylar fracture (usually associated with loss of flexion); **(e)** a congenital synostosis (with inevitably complete absence of pronation and supination).

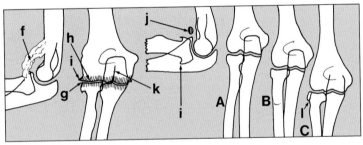

Note the presence of myositis ossificans **(f)**; the abnormal mass of bone may bridge the joint, with loss of all flexion and extension (although pronation and supination may sometimes be retained); any osteoarthritic changes with, for example, joint space narrowing **(g)**, sclerosis of the bone margins **(h)**, osteophytes **(i)**, loose body formation **(j)**, or evidence of a previous (and perhaps causal) fracture **(k)**. Where the radial head is suspect, radiographs should be taken in the anteroposterior plane **(A)** in mid-position, **(B)** in supination, **(C)** in pronation. The point is that these different projections can bring a suspect area (e.g. of osteochondritis of the radial head or an old fracture **(l)**) into profile.

Common syndromes 62
Assessment 64
Radiographs 68

COMMON SYNDROMES
Colles' fracture

For complications occurring after Colles' fractures, see under 'Fractures' (p. 337).

Ganglions

Ganglions are extremely common about the wrist and hand. In many cases they may have a tenuous communication with a carpal joint or tendon sheath. Fluctuations in the size of ganglions and their rupture from trauma are well known. The diagnosis is not usually difficult, except in the case of small ganglions on the back of the wrist. Here local swelling and tenderness may only be obvious when the wrist is palmar flexed. Ganglions in proximity to peripheral nerves may cause neurological complications.

de Quervain's disease

Tenosynovitis involving abductor pollicis longus and extensor pollicis brevis is known as de Quervain's disease. It occurs in the middle-aged, and the patient complains of pain on certain movements of the wrist, and weakness of grip.

Extensor tenosynovitis

Acute frictional tenosynovitis occurs most frequently in the 20 to 40 age group, generally following a period of excess activity. Any or all of the extensor tendons may be involved. The condition has a benign course and usually settles if the wrist is immobilised in a cast for three weeks.

Osteoarthritis of the wrist

Osteoarthritis of the wrist is surprisingly uncommon considering the frequency with which the joint is involved in fractures. It is seen most often after avascular necrosis of the scaphoid following fracture of that bone, non-union of the scaphoid, comminuted fractures involving the articular surface of the radius, and Kienbock's disease (spontaneous avascular necrosis of the lunate).

Rheumatoid arthritis

Rheumatoid arthritis of the wrist is common, and extensive synovial thickening of the joint and related tendon sheaths leads to gross swelling, increased local heat, pain and stiffness. Fluctuation can sometimes be transmitted from just above the wrist to the palm, the synovial fluid being displaced from one level to the other underneath the flexor retinaculum (compound palmar ganglion). With progressive joint involvement, the carpus tilts into ulnar deviation and subluxes in a palmar direction. The head of the ulna displaces dorsally, disrupting the inferior radioulnar joint, and causing painful and reduced pronation and supination.

Carpal tunnel syndrome

This condition occurs most commonly in women in the 30 to 60 age group. Basically there is compression of the median nerve which leads to symptoms and signs related to its distribution. In some cases, premenstrual fluid retention, early rheumatoid arthritis with synovial tendon sheath thickening and old Colles' or carpal fractures may be responsible by restricting the space left for the nerve in the carpal tunnel. It is sometimes seen in association with myxoedema, acromegaly and pregnancy. However, in many cases, no obvious cause can be found.

The patient complains of paraesthesia in the hand: often all the fingers are claimed to be involved, although theoretically at least the little finger should always be spared. Paraesthesia may also radiate proximally to the elbow. There may be pain in the same areas, and weakness in the hand. The symptoms may become most marked in the early hours of the morning, often waking the patient from sleep and causing her to shake the hand or hang it over the side of the bed. In some cases it may be difficult to differentiate the patient's symptoms from those produced by cervical spondylosis; a trial period of immobilisation of the wrist in a cast, the use of a cervical collar, or nerve conduction tests may be helpful. The latter is being employed with increasing frequency in the practice of defensive medicine.

Note that on rare occasions the median nerve may be compressed proximal to the carpal tunnel. Above the elbow this may be due to a supracondylar bony spur (obvious on radiographs); just distal to the elbow, by the origin of pronator teres; and in the proximal part of the forearm, by the sublimis. Proximal lesions of the median nerve give rise to the anterior interosseous nerve syndrome.

Ulnar tunnel syndrome

The ulnar nerve may be compressed as it passes through the ulnar carpal canal, between the pisiform and the hook of the hamate. Both the sensory and motor divisions of the nerve may be affected, but often one only is involved. The symptoms therefore may include small muscle wasting and weakness in the hand with sensory disturbance on the volar aspect of the little finger. In all cases every effort should be made to exclude a more proximal cause for the patient's symptoms (e.g. ulnar neuritis at the elbow, cervical spondylosis). Nerve conduction studies are often of particular value in this situation. The commonest causes of nerve involvement at the wrist are ganglionic compression, occupational trauma, ulnar artery disease and old carpal or metacarpal fractures.

The Ehlers–Danlos syndrome

This is the name given to a number of closely related connective tissue disorders which are due to a collagen abnormality. The condition is comparatively rare with a strong (autosomal dominant) hereditary tendency. It may be found in association with Marfan's syndrome and osteogenesis imperfecta. The skin has a velvety feel, and is fragile and hyperelastic; when grasped it can be raised and stretched by a remarkable amount. Wound healing is poor, leading to abnormal and somewhat keloid scarring, evidence of which may be widespread. Cases vary in severity, but in some healing may be so poor that surgery is contraindicated. The walls of blood vessels are affected, and bruising is a common problem. Ligaments lose their resistance to stretching, so that there is usually a striking increase in the range of movements in the affected joints; there may be instability, leading to sprains and dislocations.

Tuberculosis of the wrist

Tuberculosis of the wrist is now rare in Britain. Marked swelling of the joint is followed by muscle wasting in the forearm, bone erosion and destruction, and anterior subluxation of the carpus. The diagnosis is confirmed by synovial biopsy. Monarticular rheumatism is the only condition likely to cause difficulty in diagnosis.

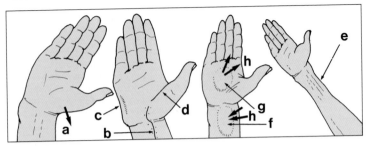

ASSESSMENT

Inspection

Anteriorly: note any *radial deviation deformity* of the hand (**a**), common after Colles' fracture and striking in congenital absence of the radius. *Ulnar deviation* is common in rheumatoid arthritis. Note any surgical or other *scarring* (**b**), *hypothenar* (**c**) or *thenar* (**d**) wasting. Muscle *wasting of the forearm* (**e**) occurs in rheumatoid arthritis and tuberculosis, and is bilateral in muscular dystrophy and many neurological disorders. Note any *generalised swelling* of the wrist and hand, or any *colour change*.

Note any *localised swellings* suggestive of ganglion (**f**), rheumatoid nodule or tumour. If there is swelling at the wrist and also in the palm (**g**), try to demonstrate cross-fluctuation (**h**). This is a feature of compound palmar ganglion, seen most often in rheumatoid arthritis and tuberculosis.

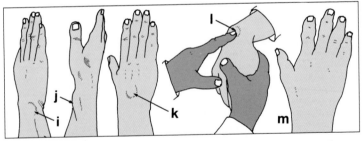

Medially: note any *undue prominence of the ulna* (**i**): this is common after Colles' fractures or in Madelung's deformity.

Laterally: note any distal radial swelling, e.g. in de Quervain's disease (**j**). Note also any *anterior tilting* of the plane of the wrist (common after Smith's fractures), or any *backward tilting* (e.g. after Colles' fractures); and note any *anterior subluxation* (e.g. in rheumatoid arthritis, old carpal injuries and infective arthritis).

Dorsally: most ganglions (**k**) in relation to the wrist, carpus and extensor tendons may be easily identified by inspection, but if inconspicuous they may be rendered obvious by palmar flexion of the wrist (**l**). Diffuse swelling and tenderness of the wrist (**m**) is typical of rheumatoid arthritis, infections and Sudeck's atrophy. The latter is seen most often after trauma (such as Colles' fractures).

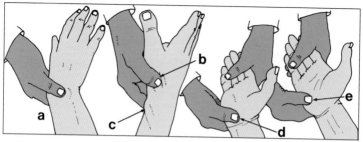

Palpation

Diffuse tenderness about the wrist is common in all inflammatory lesions (e.g. rheumatoid arthritis and tuberculosis of the wrist) and in Sudeck's atrophy. *Localised tenderness* is found (**a**) over the inferior radioulnar joint when it is disrupted, e.g. after Colles' fracture or rheumatoid arthritis; (**b**) in the anatomical snuff box, after scaphoid fractures and wrist sprains; (**c**) over the sheaths of abductor pollicis longus and extensor pollicis brevis, where there is often local thickening, in de Quervain's tenosynovitis; (**d**) over the median nerve, often with the production of paraesthesia in the fingers and hand, in the carpal tunnel syndrome; (**e**) over the ulnar nerve, often with paraesthesia, in the ulnar tunnel syndrome.

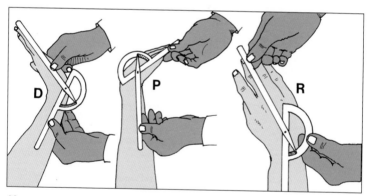

Movements

Dorsiflexion (D) (normal = 75°).
Palmar flexion (P) (normal = 75°). If the range exceeds this, look for other signs of joint hypermobility.
Radial deviation (R) (normal = 20°).
Ulnar deviation (normal = 35°). (Radial and ulnar deviation are the angles formed between the forearm and the middle metacarpal.)
Pronation (normal = 75°).
Supination (normal = 80°). (See page 56 for details of measurement.)

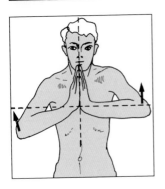

Screening tests for movement

Dorsiflexion: ask the patient to press the hands together in the vertical plane in a prayer-like fashion, and to raise the elbows to the horizontal. This should quickly reveal any loss of dorsiflexion.

Palmar flexion: ask the patient to put the backs of the hands in contact, and then to bring the forearms into the horizontal plane. Any loss of palmar flexion should be obvious.

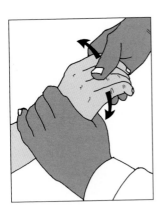

Other tests

Crepitus. While grasping the wrist, flex and extend the fingers. Ask the patient to repeat these movements on his own. Crepitus, fine in character, occurs in tenosynovitis of the extensor tendons. Auscultation over the tendons may reveal characteristic grating sounds. Feel also for crepitus in the radiocarpal and the inferior radioulnar joints on movement, indicative of arthritic change.

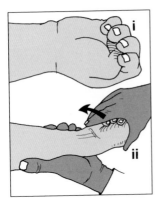

de Quervain's tenosynovitis. This condition involves the tendons of abductor pollicis longus and extensor pollicis brevis, and their sheath which runs obliquely across the radius in its distal third. If the history suggests this, look for local swelling and tenderness, and confirm the diagnosis with the following test: ask the patient to flex the thumb and close the fingers over it **(i)**. Now move the hand into ulnar deviation **(ii)**. The test is positive if this manoeuvre produces excruciating pain in the region of the tendon sheath.

Carpal and ulnar tunnel syndromes. See Chapter 2.

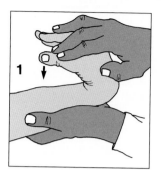

Tests for joint hypermobility

(1) Try to bring the thumb into contact with the forearm and measure any gap. The average separation is 4.5 cm at age 17½, and it increases with age (as the ligaments lose some of their elasticity). While the thumb contacting the forearm suggests hypermobility, this is nevertheless said to occur in 56% of normal subjects.

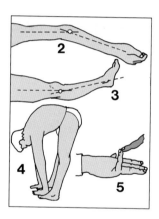

(2) Check the elbow and (3) the knee to see if they can hyperextend by 10° or more. (4) Check if the spine can be flexed so that the palms of the hands can be placed on the floor. (5) Test if the little finger can be passively dorsiflexed to 90° or more.

Joint laxity is diagnosed if any three of these tests (1–5) are present.

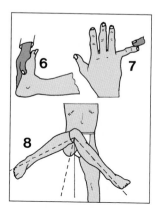

Other evidence of hypermobility includes: (6) hyperextension of the ankle beyond 45°; (7) an abnormal range of abduction of the little finger; (8) an increase in hip rotation in a child (from 90–93° to about 110°), with the centre of the range being displaced in favour of internal rotation.

Joint hypermobility is a feature of the Ehlers–Danlos syndrome, Marfan's disease, osteogenesis imperfecta and Morquio–Brailsford's disease.

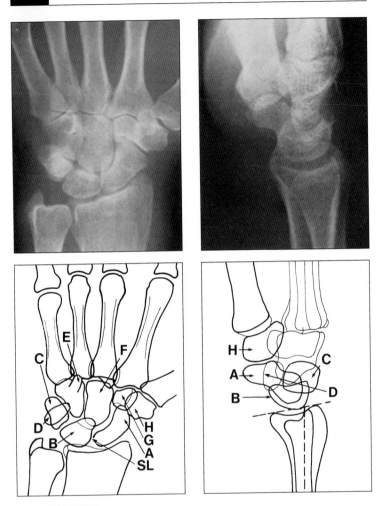

RADIOGRAPHS

AP and lateral are the standard projections, although at least one additional oblique projection is usually advised. In the AP, identify the carpal bones and note their shape, density and position: **(A)** scaphoid; **(B)** lunate; **(C)** triquetral; **(D)** pisiform; **(E)** hamate with its hook; **(F)** capitate; **(G)** trapezoid; **(H)** trapezium. Note the gaps between the various carpal bones, particularly between the scaphoid and lunate **(SL)**. In spite of bony superimposition, in the lateral it is usually possible to make out **(H)** the trapezium; **(A)** the tubercle and mass of scaphoid; **(D)** pisiform; **(B)** crescent of lunate; **(C)** triquetral. Note that the plane of the wrist joint has normally a 5° anterior tilt.

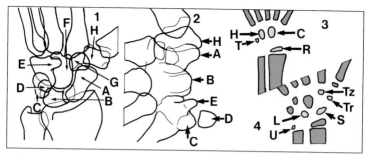

Oblique projections (1) are advised when the carpus is suspect. These are of particular value in detecting hairline crack fractures of the carpal bones. Note (A) scaphoid; (B) lunate; (C) triquetral; (D) pisiform; (E) hamate; (F) capitate; (G) trapezoid; (H) trapezium. A **tangential projection** (2) may be useful in the investigation of the carpal tunnel, and may show arthritic lipping or causal pathology. Note (A) scaphoid; (B) lunate; (C) triquetral; (D) pisiform; (E) hook of hamate; (H) trapezium. During growth the changing patterns of ossification may give difficulty in interpretation. In the **first year of life** (3), the capitate (F) and hamate (E) appear at 2 months, the radius (R) at 6 months, and the triquetral (C) at 10 months. **After the first year** (4), the lunate (L) appears at 2, the trapezium (Tr) at 2½, the trapezoid (Tz) and scaphoid (S) at 3, and the distal ulna (U) at 4½ years.

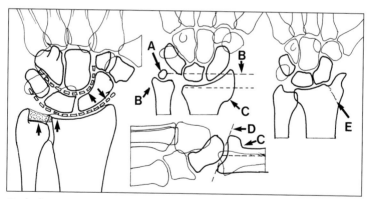

Pathology

In the AP, note the *smooth curves* formed by both the proximal and distal margins of scaphoid, lunate and triquetral. Note that the distal end of the ulna stops short of the radius to make room for the triangular fibrocartilage. Look for *evidence of previous injury*. In the malunited Colles' fracture, there may be (A) non-union of the ulnar styloid; (B) prominence of the distal ulna secondary to (C) distortion and resorption at the radial fracture. The joint line (D) may be tilted away from the normal. Osteoarthritic changes are uncommon after Colles' fracture, but are seen after radial styloid fractures (E).

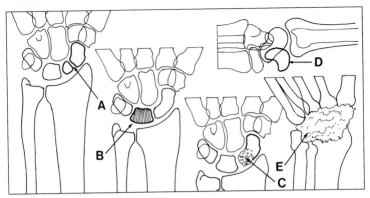

Look for *non-union of a scaphoid fracture* (**A**). (Osteoarthritis may not always follow such pathology.) Note increased bone density and deformity in *Kienbock's disease* (**B**) of the lunate or in *avascular necrosis of the scaphoid* (**C**), both of which are almost invariably accompanied by osteoarthritis. Note any carpal malposition, *dislocation of the lunate* (**D**) being the most common. Gross porotic changes are seen most often in *rheumatoid arthritis* and in *Sudeck's atrophy*, while gross destructive changes are seen in *tuberculosis* (**E**) and other infections.

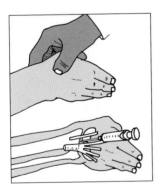

Aspiration of the wrist joint. This is indicated in suspected infections. Begin by feeling with the thumb for the depression at the back of the wrist lying between the distal end of the radius and scaphoid. Then locate the gap at right angles to this, between extensor digitorum communis and extensor carpi radialis brevis. Infiltrate with local anaesthetic and insert the aspiration needle at this spot. Incline the needle at 60°, with its tip directed in the direction of the elbow, to enter the radiocarpal joint.

CHAPTER

7

The hand

Common syndromes 72
Assessment 75

COMMON SYNDROMES

Dupuytren's contracture

In this condition there is nodular thickening and contracture of the palmar fascia. The palm of the hand is affected first, followed at a later stage by the fingers. In some cases there is corresponding thickening of the plantar fascia. It mainly affects men over the age of 40; there is a hereditary predisposition, and in some cases there may be an association with epilepsy, diabetes or alcoholic cirrhosis. Below the age of 40 in either sex, the onset may be precipitated by trauma and pursue a particularly rapid course.

Vibration syndromes

Prolonged exposure to high frequency vibration may affect bone, nerves and blood vessels. There may be (rarely) new bone formation and hair-line fractures. Involvement of the peripheral nerves may lead to pain and paraesthesia, numbness, tremor, loss of fine touch sensation, proprioception and discrimination. Disturbance of the autonomic control of the peripheral blood vessels makes the arterioles of the hand hypersensitive to cold and vibration, and in typical cases there are attacks in which one or more fingers turn white on exposure to cold ('episodic blanching'), with reactive hyperaemia on warming. The hand becomes weak and clumsy, and with impaired sensation and proprioception the patient has difficulty in dressing and handling small objects.

Tendon and tendon sheath lesions

Mallet finger. In a mallet finger the distal interphalangeal joint is held in a permanent position of flexion, and the patient is unable to extend the distal joint actively: either not at all or incompletely. The problem is due to rupture of the distal slip of the extensor tendon or avulsion of its bony attachment.

Mallet thumb. Delayed rupture of the extensor pollicis longus tendon may follow Colles' fracture or rheumatoid arthritis.

Boutonnière deformity. Flexion of the proximal interphalangeal joint of a finger with extension of the distal interphalangeal joint characterises this deformity which is due to detachment of the central slip of the extensor tendon (which is attached to the base of the middle phalanx). It is most commonly seen in rheumatoid arthritis.

Extensor tendon division in the back of the hand. With appropriate treatment, extensor tendons divided on the back of the hand carry an excellent prognosis.

Profundus tendon injuries. (i) Isolated avulsion injuries are uncommon and are treated surgically. (ii) In open wounds in the palm, repair by direct suture is usually feasible and the prognosis good. In the flexor tendon sheaths, there is risk of adhesions spoiling function, and a number of techniques have been developed to try to overcome this. Accompanying digital nerve divisions may have to be treated.

Trigger finger and thumb. This results from thickening of a fibrous tendon sheath or a nodular thickening in a flexor tendon. In adults, the middle or ring finger is most frequently involved. When all the fingers are extended, the affected one lags behind and then quite suddenly straightens. A nodular thickening, always at the level of the MP joint, may be palpable.

Rheumatoid arthritis

As it progresses, this condition may involve joints, tendons, muscles, nerves and arteries, producing severe deformities and crippling effects on hand function. In the earliest phases, the hands are warm and moist; later the joints become obviously swollen and tender. Synovial tendon sheath and joint thickenings with effusion, muscle wasting and deformity then become apparent. Tendon ruptures and joint subluxations are the main factors leading to the more severe deformities.

Osteoarthritis of the interphalangeal joints

Nodular swellings situated dorsally over the bases of the distal phalanges (Heberden's nodes), or less commonly over the bases of the middle phalanges (Bouchard's nodes) are a sign of osteoarthritis of the finger joints. They occur most frequently in women after the menopause, and are often familial. They are not related to osteoarthritis elsewhere. In many cases they are symptom free, but they may be associated with progressive joint damage which does cause pain.

Carpometacarpal joint of the thumb

Osteoarthritic changes are common between the thumb metacarpal and the trapezium, and may give rise to disabling pain and impaired function in the hand.

Tumours in the hand

The commonest tumours in the hand include:

Ganglions occur in the fingers, most commonly along their volar aspects. They are small, spherical and tender to the touch.

Implantation dermoid cysts are also most commonly sited along the volar surfaces of the fingers and palms.

Glomus tumours are small, vascular and exquisitely tender swellings which occur most often in the region of the nail beds.

Mucous cysts are always found on the dorsal surfaces of the distal interphalangeal joints.

Osteoid osteoma may involve a distal phalanx (or a carpal bone), and has a typical X-ray appearance. If there is doubt about the diagnosis, an isotope bone scan will show it up as a 'hot spot'.

Chondroma, a common benign tumour, occurs in the metacarpals and phalanges, and is generally confined to bone (enchondroma). It may give rise to a pathological fracture, or to gross swelling and deformity. It is often solitary, but multiple tumours of a similar nature are found in Ollier's disease, which has a hereditary diathesis.

Metastatic tumours are uncommon but have a tendency to involve the distal phalanges. Lung and breast are the commonest primary sites.

Infections in the hand

Paronychia. This is the commonest of all infections in the hand and occurs between the base of the nail and the cuticle.

Apical infections occur between the tip of the nail and the underlying nail bed.

Pulp infections occur in the fibro-fatty tissue of the finger tips and are extremely painful. If unchecked, infection frequently leads to involvement of the terminal phalanx.

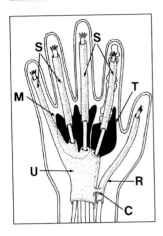

Tendon sheath infections. Infection within a tendon sheath (**S**) leads to rapid swelling of the finger and build up of pressure within the tendon sheath; there is always a serious risk of tendon sloughing or disabling adhesion formation. In the case of the little finger there may be retrograde spread of infection to involve the ulnar bursa (**U**) in the hand. In the case of the thumb, infection may also spread proximally to involve the radial bursa (**R**). In either case, swelling appears in the palm and in the wrist proximal to the flexor retinaculum. It should also be noted that in 70% of cases there is a connection (**C**) between these two bursae, allowing spread from one to the other.

Web space infections. Web space infections are usually accompanied by great pain and systemic upset. There is redness and swelling in the affected web space. Infection may spread along the volar aspects of the related fingers or to adjacent web spaces across the anterior aspect of the palm. If seen early, most web space infections respond to antibiotics, splintage and elevation, but drainage is sometimes necessary.

*Midpalmar (**M**) and thenar (**T**) space infections.* These two compartments of the hand lie between the flexor tendons and the metacarpals. Infection may spread to them from web space or tendon sheath infections: dissemination through the hand is then rapid and potentially crippling. In either case, there is usually gross swelling of the hand and a severe systemic upset. Unless there is a rapid response to antibiotics, elevation and splintage, early drainage is essential for the preservation of function in the hand.

Tuberculosis and syphilis. On rare occasions either of these two infections may produce spindle-shaped deformity of a finger. Spindling of a finger is much more common, however, in rheumatoid arthritis, gout or collateral ligament trauma.

Occupational infections. Superficial infections are common in certain trades and the following may be noted:

- pilonidal sinus in barbers
- erysipeloid in fishmongers and butchers
- 'butcher's wart' (tuberculous skin lesions) in butchers and pathologists
- malignant pustule (anthrax) in hide sorters and tanners.

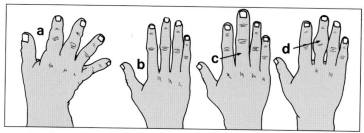

ASSESSMENT
Inspection

Look at the general shape of the hand and its proportions: the fingers are short and stumpy in *achondroplasia* (**a**); the hand is large and coarse in *acromegaly*; and in myxoedema, the hand is often podgy and the skin dry. In *Marfan's syndrome*, the proximal phalanges in particular are long and thin (**b**); in *Turner's syndrome* the ring metacarpal is often very short. In *hyperparathyroidism* the finger tips may be short and bulbous, while in *Down's* and *Hurler's* syndromes the little fingers are incurved. Note the presence of any *hypertrophy of a finger* (**c**): this may occur in *Paget's* disease, neurofibromatosis and local arteriovenous fistula. Note any *fusiform swelling* (**d**). The commonest causes are *collateral ligament tears* and *rheumatoid arthritis*. Less commonly this is seen in *syphilis*, *TB*, *sarcoidosis* and *gout*. In *psoriatic arthritis*, the distal joints are usually involved.

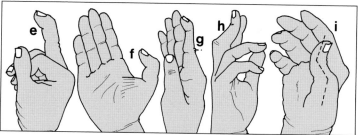

Look for other deformities of the fingers: In *mallet finger* (**e**), the distal interphalangeal joint is flexed. It cannot be actively extended fully, although passive extension is usually possible. In *mallet thumb* (**f**) there is loss of active extension in the interphalangeal joint of the thumb, due to rupture of extensor pollicis longus. This is seen as a late complication of Colles' fracture, from rheumatoid arthritis or wounds of the wrist or the thumb with tendon division. In *swan-neck deformity* (**g**), common on rheumatoid arthritis, the distal interphalangeal joint is flexed and the proximal interphalangeal joint is hyperextended. In *boutonnière deformity* (**h**), the proximal interphalangeal joint is flexed and the distal joint extended. It occurs when the central extensor tendon slip to the middle phalanx is affected, by a wound on the dorsum of the finger, by traumatic avulsion or rupture in rheumatoid arthritis. Again, commonly in rheumatoid arthritis, in the *Z-deformity* (**i**), the thumb is flexed at the metacarpophalangeal joint and hyperextended at the interphalangeal joint.

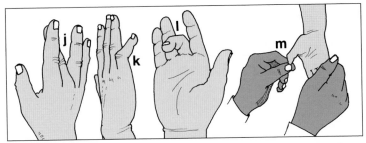

Flexion of a finger at the metacarpophalangeal joint, with inability to extend, follows *rupture or division of an extensor tendon* (**j**). Flexion of the little finger at the proximal IP joint, is seen in *congenital contracture of the little finger* (**k**). Flexion of the middle or ring fingers at the proximal IP joint, with sudden extension on effort or with assistance, is seen in *trigger finger* (**l**). There is usually a palpable nodular thickening over the corresponding MP joint. In infants and young children, flexion of the IP joint of the thumb is usually due to a *stenosing tenovaginitis* (**m**) involving flexor pollicis longus. A nodular thickening is usually palpable over the MP joint. The condition is acquired and triggering is not a feature.

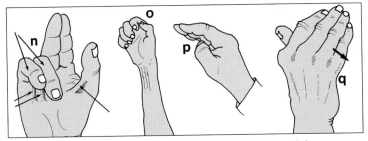

Flexion of the fingers at the MP and IP joints, associated with nodular thickening in the palm and fingers, is characteristic of *Dupuytren's contracture* (**n**); thickening in the palm often precedes finger involvement. The thumb is occasionally affected. *Volkmann's ischaemic contracture* (**o**) occurs as a late sequel (i.e. after several months) to brachial artery damage, often after a supracondylar fracture. There is clawing of the thumb and fingers, and forearm wasting. The fingers can be extended if the wrist is flexed. Ischaemia in the forearm (e.g. in a compartment syndrome secondary to an over-tight cast) may lead to fingers which become flexed at the MP joints and extended at the IP joints. The thumb is adducted into the palm (**p**). Ulnar deviation of the fingers at the MP joints occurs in rheumatoid arthritis, and in the later stages these joints may dislocate (**q**).

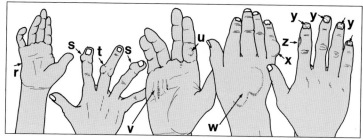

Unilateral intrinsic muscle wasting (**r**) suggests a root, plexus or nerve lesion. Exclude a generalised peripheral neuropathy, syringomyelia, multiple sclerosis or muscular dystrophy. *Heberden's nodes* (**s**) on the dorsal surface of the distal IP joints occur in osteoarthritis of the fingers, and there may be deviation of the distal phalanges. The proximal IP joints may be similarly affected (*Bouchard's nodes* (**t**)). Note any swellings: firm, pea-like *ganglions* (**u**) occur along the line of the tendon sheaths; nodular swellings of the palm and fingers (**v**) occur in Dupuytren's contracture. Isolated nodules or synovial swellings are common in rheumatoid arthritis (**w**). *Enchondroma* (**x**), is one of the commonest bone tumours in the hand. Note any disturbance of nail growth or sign of fungal infection or psoriasis (**y**); finger burns or trophic ulceration, suggestive of neurological disturbance (**z**); any alteration of skin colour, suggesting circulatory involvement from local arterial or sympathetic nerve supply disturbance.

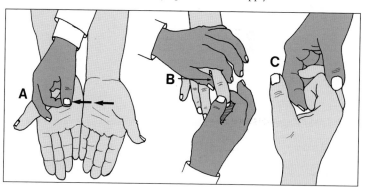

Palpation

Note any generalised or local disturbance of temperature or sweating in the palm or volar surfaces of the fingers (**A**). The other hand may be used for comparison. Palpate the individual finger joints (**B**) between the finger and thumb, looking for thickening, tenderness, oedema and increased local beat. Note that in gouty arthritis a single joint only may he affected. Try to tuck each finger into the palm (**C**), and ask the patient to repeat this unaided. Loss of active (but not passive movements) is usually due to nerve or tendon discontinuity, while passive loss may be due to joint or tendon adhesions or arthritis.

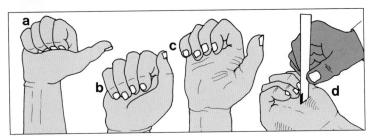

Movements

Composite movements. As all the joints of all the fingers are involved in grasping and holding, begin by asking the patient to make a fist. This usefully screens movements in all three joints of all the fingers. **Normal = (a).** The distal phalanges should 'tuck-in', touching the palm at right angles to it. Only a slight loss at any level is sufficient to prevent 'tuck-in'. All the fingers may be involved **(b)**, but if a single finger is affected its prominence will be obvious. Greater reduction in movements **(c)** will prevent the fingers from reaching the palm and indicates more serious impairment of the patient's ability to grasp and hold. This important restriction of functional ability may be measured by noting the distance that the fingers stand proud of the palm **(d)** on maximum flexion.

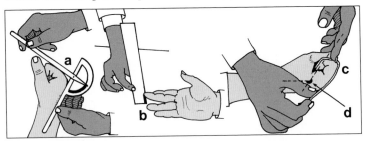

Individual finger joint movements. Measurement and recording of both active and passive movements in the individual joints of the fingers may be required for medicolegal purposes and for the assessment of progress.

- **Metacarpophalangeal joint (normal = 0–90°).** Passive hyperextension up to 45°.
- **Proximal interphalangeal joint (normal = 0–100°).**
- **Distal interphalangeal joint (normal = 0–80°).**

Flexion in the joints may be measured with a goniometer **(a).** Extension loss may also be measured with a ruler **(b).** When passive extension is possible, loss of active extension suggests division, rupture or displacement of the extensor tendons, or a posterior interosseous palsy if all the fingers are affected. If a length of malleable wire is moulded round the flexed finger **(c)**, the wire may then be placed on the case record and a tracing made round it. Later measurements may be superimposed. The total flexion capability of a finger **(d)** is also a useful measurement and is a little less than the sum of movements in the individual joints: **TAM (Total active range of movements). Normal = 250°.**

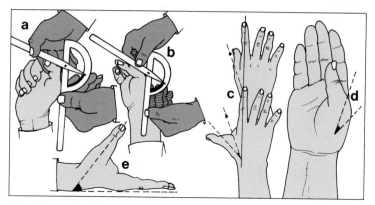

Thumb movements

- **(a) Interphalangeal joint (normal range = –20° to 80°)**, i.e. the normal interphalangeal joint can be flexed 80° and extended 20° (both actively and passively) from the neutral.
- **(b) Metacarpophalangeal joint (normal range = 0–55°)**. Passively, 5° of hyperextension is usually possible.
- **Carpometacarpal joint. (c) Extension (normal = 20°)**. The starting point is with the thumb contacting the side of the index finger. Flexion **(d)** is difficult to measure, but is in the order of 15°. **(e) Abduction (normal = 60°)**. The hand is placed on a table, palm up, and the patient asked to point the thumb at the ceiling.

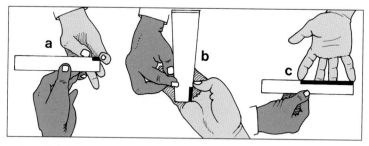

Other movements. **Opposition** involves abduction at right angles to the palm, flexion and rotation. Normally the thumb should be able to touch the tips of the fingers in succession, ending with the little finger. Loss of opposition may be assessed by measuring the distance between the tip of the thumb and little finger **(a)**, or between the tip of the thumb and the MP joint of the little finger **(b)**. **Finger abduction** may he assessed by measuring the spread between index and little fingers **(c)**, or the spread between individual fingers. Excessive abduction of the little finger is found in the Ehlers–Danlos syndrome.

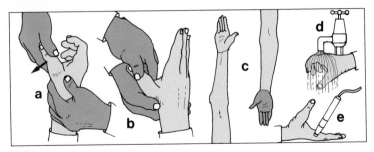

Other tests

Ulnar collateral ligament of the thumb: extend the joint and stress the medial collateral ligament (**a**). Compare the sides. Excess mobility can be very disabling and may follow ligament tears ('gamekeeper's thumb'), or as a complication of rheumatoid arthritis. **Carpometacarpal joint:** while lightly grasping the joint, flex and extend the joint, feeling for crepitus (**b**). This occurs in carpometacarpal joint osteoarthritis. **Vibration syndromes:** in vibration white finger, although little clinical abnormality may be found, note (**c**) if the hand becomes pale on elevation (for 30 seconds) and the speed with which it pinks up on depression; (**d**) see if an attack is precipitated by holding the hand under cold water for two minutes; (**e**) check the flow in the digital vessels with a Doppler flowmeter. Remember that the peripheral circulation may be disturbed by oral antihypertensives.

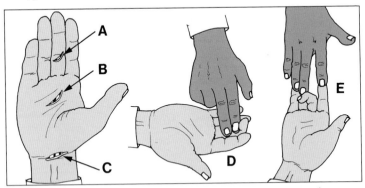

Flexor tendon injuries in the fingers. Note first the position of any wound and try to work out the structures at risk, e.g. (**A**) flexor profundus, (**B**) sublimis, and if deeper, profundus, (**C**) median nerve, flexor carpi radialis longus, sublimis, and more deeply the profundus tendons. If a *profundus tendon* is suspect, support the middle phalanx, either by grasping it or by pressing it against a flat surface. Now ask the patient to bend the tip (**D**). Loss occurs when the flexor digitorum profundus tendon is divided. If the *sublimis tendon* is suspect, hold all the fingers except the suspect one in a fully extended position (to neutralise the effect of flexor profundus). If the patient is able to flex the finger at the proximal interphalangeal joint, then sublimis is intact (**E**).

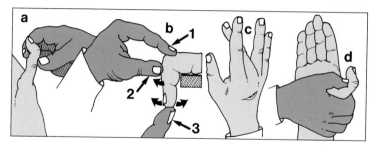

Extensor tendon injuries of the fingers. *Terminal slips:* there will be a mallet finger deformity. Confirmation: support the middle phalanx and ask the patient to attempt to straighten the finger (**a**). *Middle slip:* Elson's test (**b**)—flex the PIP joint of the finger over the edge of a table and steady the proximal phalanx (**1**). Ask the patient to try to extend the PIP joint and feel for any activity (**2**): this occurs if the middle slip is intact, and the DIP joint will be flail (**3**). If the middle slip is ruptured, extension at the PIP joint does not occur and the DIP joint stiffens and extends. *Proximal whole tendon lesions:* there will be a characteristic deformity (**c**), with the finger flexed at the MP joint, and extended at the IP joints (due to lumbrical action). Active extension will not be possible. *Tendon injuries of the thumb:* to test flexor and extensor pollicis longus, support the proximal phalanx and ask the patient to bend and straighten the tip (**d**).

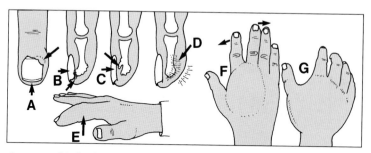

Suspected infections. *Paronychia* is the commonest infection. Pain is aggravated by pressure on the end of the nail (**A**). *Apical infections* give pain which is aggravated by downward pressure on the nail (**B**). A *subungual exostosis* (**C**) (which can be confirmed by radiographs) may sometimes cause confusion. *Pulp infections* (**D**) are exquisitely tender and may lead to destruction of the distal phalanx. *Tendon sheath infections* lead to a fusiform flexed finger (**E**). Tenderness is marked and localised (usually at the base of the sheath), and any attempt to straighten the finger causes pain. In *web space infections* (**F**), there is usually marked swelling of the back of the hand and the web, with spreading of the fingers. In thenar and midpalmar space infections (**G**) there is gross swelling of the hand involving both the dorsal and palmar surfaces. In the case of the thenar space, the swelling may be more pronounced on the radial side of the palm.

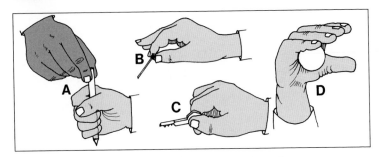

Assessment of the principal functions of the hand:

(A) Grasp. Ask the patient to grasp a pen firmly in the hand, using the thumb and fingers. Attempt to withdraw the pen and note the resistance offered. Where finger flexion is restricted, repeat using an object of greater diameter.

(B) Pinch grip. Ask the patient to pick up a small object between the tips of the thumb and index. Intact sensation is necessary for a satisfactory performance. The patient should be asked to repeat the test with his eyes closed.

(C) Thumb to side of index grip. The patient should be asked to grip a key between the thumb and side of the index in the normal fashion. Test the firmness of the grip by attempting to withdraw the key, using your own pinch grip.

(D) Palmar grasp. Test the cupping action of the hand by asking the patient to grasp a small ball in the palm of the hand and note his ability to resist its removal.

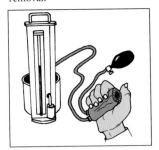

Grip strength. The power of grip (which is in effect the strength of the grasp) is ideally assessed quantitatively with a dynamometer. If one is not available, inflate a rolled sphygmomanometer cuff to 20 mmHg and ask the patient to squeeze it as hard as he can. When the hand is normal it should be possible to achieve a reading of 200 mmHg or over.

Bilateral function. While the function in one hand may be assessed as described, it is important to note that impairment of function in one hand may clearly affect many activities which normally involve both. The degree of overall functional impairment may be investigated by enquiring about, or testing, the patient's ability to perform certain tasks. The following list (adapted from tests devised by Lamb et al) may be found to be helpful, either selected or as a whole. Each of these may be scored on a scale (0–5 or 0–10) and summed: (1) unscrew top from bottle; (2) fill cup and drink; (3) open tin with tin-opener; (4) remove match from box and light it; (5) use knife and fork for eating; (6) apply paste to toothbrush and clean teeth; (7) put on jacket; (8) do up buttons; (9) fasten belt round waist; (10) tie shoe laces; (11) sharpen pencil; (12) write messages; (13) use telephone; (14) staple papers together; (15) wrap string round parcel; (16) use playing cards.

8

The thoracic and lumbar spine

Common syndromes 84
Commoner causes of back
    complaints in the various
    age groups 92
Assessment 93
Radiographs 102

COMMON SYNDROMES

Back pain

Back pain is one of the commonest and most troublesome of complaints; its causes are legion and an exact diagnosis is often difficult. It may be helpful to assess any case of back pain under three headings:

1. Back pain, where there is clear cut spinal pathology, such as vertebral infections, tumours, ankylosing spondylitis, polyarthritis, Paget's disease and primary neurological disease.
2. Back pain with associated nerve root symptoms, with the commonest cause being an intervertebral disc prolapse.
3. Back pain caused by disturbance of the mechanics of the spine (mechanical back pain). In some cases the cause may be well defined (e.g. osteoporotic spinal fractures, spondylolisthesis, Scheuermann's disease and osteoarthritis. In others, although the symptoms may be identical in character, the cause cannot be determined with any accuracy. This is the default diagnosis of a very high proportion of cases and is settled on only after appropriate investigation.

History taking

1. Note the patient's age and occupation: both may be relevant.

2. Ask about the onset of the pain:
   (a) When did the symptoms commence?
   (b) Was the onset slow and insidious, rapid, or sudden?
   (c) Was there a history of an injury, such as, for example, a sudden twist or strain, or a sneeze occurring when the patient was in a flexed position? (This is a common history in cases of intervertebral disc prolapse.)

3. Ask about any directly relevant previous history:
   (a) Is there a history of a previous similar attack?
   (b) Is there a history of any previous trouble with the spine?

4. Ask about the site and nature of the pain:
   (a) Where is the pain situated? Is it well localised or diffuse?
   (b) Is the pain always present or does it disappear at times?
   (c) Are there any factors which aggravate or alleviate the pain?

5. Ask about radiation of the pain:
   (a) Does the pain radiate in to the legs?
   (b) If so, exactly how far down does the pain go, and what area is involved? (Note that the commonly affected roots of the sciatic nerve (L4, L5, S1) supply the skin *below* the knee.)
   (c) What is the pain like?
   (d) Is there paraesthesia?

   Note that pain radiating in to the legs is not necessarily due to nerve root involvement. Pain arising from nerve roots is usually sharp and knife-like, and in addition, in the case of the commonly affected L5 and S1 roots, it often extends below the knee to the ankle or foot. In the common situation where there is involvement of one or, at the most, two nerve roots, the whole limb cannot be affected.

6. Ask about motor involvement.
   (a) Has the patient noted any weakness in the lower limbs, or any muscle wasting or fibrillation?
   (b) Has there been any disturbance of gait or balance, any tendency to giving-way of the legs or any sign of drop foot?

7. Make enquiries in the following areas:
   (a) Has there been any malaise, fever or involvement of other joints?
   (b) Has there been any weight loss?
   (c) Has the patient had any bowel or other gastrointestinal problem?
   (d) Have there been any genitourinary symptoms?
   (e) Has the patient had any respiratory difficulty?

A positive answer to any of these questions will generally necessitate appropriate further investigation. The possibility of an invasive primary tumour or metastatic lesion must always be kept in mind, and examination of the abdomen, rectum and common sites of primary tumour is wise if there is any likelihood of malignancy.

The spine should then be examined clinically; if the symptoms have remained unchanged over a two week period, radiological examination and estimation of the sedimentation rate should be carried out. Plain films of the spine will generally allow the detection of any disturbance in vertebral alignment or of the architecture of the vertebrae. At this stage, any well-defined spinal pathology should be detected (such as spondylolisthesis, ankylosing spondylitis, osteitis of the spine, etc). If conditions such as these have been eliminated, the question whether the symptoms are due to a prolapsed intervertebral disc should be considered. The history, clinical findings and plain radiographs of the spine should be in harmony before it is reasonable to make this diagnosis. By the process of elimination, if a diagnosis has not yet been made, the patient is likely to be suffering from mechanical back pain: but note that both the history and findings should be in accord with this. If not, caution must be exercised, close surveillance should be maintained, and further investigation may be indicated.

Other imaging techniques

CAT scans. Because the images can be presented in the sagittal and coronal planes, CAT scans can further clarify bony anatomy. It can be helpful in fracture cases, in spondylolisthesis and where internal fixation devices are present.

MRI scans. These afford the most sensitive means of examining for the presence of spinal pathology, especially in cases where intervertebral disc and nerve root involvement is suspected; it is generally the investigation of choice.

Myelography. This invasive procedure, with its (slight) risks of infection or of chronic arachnoiditis has been largely superseded by MRI scanning. Nevertheless, it may sometimes be used to allow dynamic assessment of nerve compression (e.g. when standing in extension and flexion), and is especially valuable when followed by a CAT scan.

Bone scanning with SPECT (single-photon-emission computed tomography). This allows the identification of increased osteoblastic activity and is therefore a good screening test for the presence of degenerative disease or tumour, or determining the principal source of the problem in the presence of multiple pathology.

Discography. This painful procedure, with screening and CAT scanning, is of limited use. While it may reveal disc fissuring and other local pathology, perhaps its greatest value is when it duplicates the patient's pain.

Scoliosis

Scoliosis is a lateral curvature of the spine. If the vertebrae are normal (non-structural scoliosis) the deformity may be: *compensatory*, due to tilting of the pelvis from real or apparent shortening of one leg; *sciatic*, from protective muscle spasm (e.g. in a disc prolapse); or *postural*, which occurs most commonly in adolescent girls.

In structural scoliosis, there is alteration in vertebral shape and mobility, and the deformity cannot be corrected by alteration of posture. This may be: (i) *congenital*, e.g. from a hemivertebra; (ii) *paralytic*, secondary to loss of the supportive action of the trunk and spinal muscles, nearly always as a sequel to anterior poliomyelitis; (iii) *neuropathic*, which is seen as a complication of neurofibromatosis, cerebral palsy, spina bifida, syringomyelia and Freidrich's ataxia; (iv) *myopathic* (e.g. in muscular dystrophy, arthrogryposis); (v) *metabolic*, in cystine storage disease, Marfan's syndrome and rickets; (vi) *idiopathic*, whose cause remains obscure. *This is the commonest and by far the most important of the structural scolioses.*

Several vertebrae at one or less commonly two distinct levels are affected (*primary curve*). In the area of the primary curve there is loss of mobility (the fixed curve) and rotational deformity of the vertebrae (the spinous processes rotate into the concavity, and the bodies, which carry the ribs in the thoracic region, rotate into the convexity).

Above and below the fixed primary curves, *secondary* curves (which are mobile) develop in an effort to maintain the normal position of the head and pelvis. Once scoliosis has appeared in the growing child the natural tendency is to deterioration, and the prognosis of a given case is dependent on the age of onset, the level of the spine affected, the size and number of the primary curves, and the type of structural scoliosis (e.g. idiopathic or congenital). Generally speaking, the higher the level of the spine involved in the primary curve and the younger the patient, the worse the prognosis. However, in some cases occurring in infancy there is spontaneous recovery, favourable factors being left-sided curves in the first year of life in males and where there is a rib–vertebral angle of less than 20°.

In all cases of structural scoliosis, appropriate investigation, radiographic measurement of the curves and careful observation is essential. Note in particular:

1. Syringomyelia is present in 25% of cases of juvenile idiopathic scoliosis. As decompression may lead to improvement, an MRI scan is mandatory in all cases occurring within this group.
2. At its onset, scoliosis is not normally a painful condition. When there is pain (especially night pain relieved by aspirin), the commonest cause in the adolescent is an osteoid osteoma of a pedicle.

Kyphosis

Kyphosis is the term used to describe an increased convexity of the thoracic spine, usually obvious when the patient is viewed from the side. Several vertebrae are usually affected, and the increased curvature is then said to be *regular*. In *angular* kyphosis, where one or two vertebrae only are affected, there is an abrupt alteration in the thoracic curvature which is usually accompanied by undue prominence of a spinous process (gibbus).

Where mobility is normal, the deformity is most frequently postural. In some cases it is secondary to an increased lumbar lordosis. Less commonly, kyphosis may result from muscle weakness (e.g. after polio and in muscular dystrophy).

When the thoracic curvature is fixed, the most frequent causes are Scheuermann's disease, ankylosing spondylitis, senile kyphosis and Paget's disease. When there is an angular kyphosis, the most common causes are TB or other infections of the spine, fracture (traumatic or pathological) or tumours. In adults the commonest tumour is the metastatic deposit, and in children it is the eosinophilic granuloma.

Scheuermann's disease (spinal osteochondrosis)

This condition results in a growth disturbance of the thoracic vertebral bodies, which in lateral radiographs of the spine are seen to be narrower anteriorly than posteriorly (anterior wedging). The diagnostic protocol for the condition specifies that not less than three adjacent vertebrae should be involved. The epiphyses of the vertebral bodies are often irregular and may be disturbed by herniation of the nucleus pulposus. Nuclear herniation may occur into the centre of the bodies (Schmorl's nodes). Mobility is impaired, thoracic kyphosis is regular, and secondary osteoarthritic changes may supervene.

Calvé's disease

Back pain in children may be accompanied by gross flattening of a single vertebral body. Symptoms resolve spontaneously. In many cases the pathology is that of an eosinophilic granuloma.

Ankylosing spondylitis

In this disease there is progressive ossification of the joints of the spine; its aetiology is unknown, but there is a hereditary tendency. The incidence is greatest in males during the third and fourth decades. Unlike rheumatoid arthritis it is comparatively rare in women.

The sacroiliac joints are almost invariably involved at an early stage, and there may be fusion of the manubriosternal joint. The costovertebral joints are usually affected, leading to a reduction in chest expansion and vital capacity. Stiffness of the back and pain are the presenting symptoms in the majority of cases, and this usually progresses to complete ankylosis of the spine. There may be a history of iritis or its sequelae, and on occasion involvement of the knees or hips may be the first thing to attract attention.

The sedimentation rate is high (40 to 120 mm), rheumatoid factor is not present and estimations of HLA-B27 are usually positive. There is often associated anaemia, muscle wasting and weight loss.

Diffuse idiopathic skeletal hyperostosis (DASH)

This comparatively benign condition, also known as Forestier's disease, is sometimes mistaken for ankylosing spondylitis. It is characterised and diagnosed by the presence of flowing calcification and ossification along the anterolateral borders of at least four contiguous vertebral bodies. However, the disc spaces are preserved (unlike in ankylosing spondylitis), without loss of height or other degenerative changes, and the sacroiliac and the facet joints do not ankylose.

Senile kyphosis

In true senile kyphosis, the ageing patient becomes progressively stooped and shorter in stature through degenerative thinning of the intervertebral discs. Pain may occur if there is associated osteoarthritis. In elderly women, the kyphosis may be aggravated by senile osteoporosis or osteomalacia which lead to anterior vertebral wedging and often pathological fracture. There is usually radiographic evidence of decalcification, the serum chemistry may be disturbed, and pain is a feature if fractures are present.

Paget's disease

Paget's disease of the spine is comparatively uncommon, and although the diagnosis is made on the radiological findings, it may be suggested clinically by other stigmata of the disease. Paget's disease may lead to disturbance of cord function, which may often be successfully treated with biphosphonates.

Tuberculosis of the spine

Bone and joint tuberculosis is uncommon in Britain, but the incidence is increasing. The factors responsible include an increase in numbers of immunosuppressed individuals, the development of drug-resistant strains of the organism and an ageing population. HIV is the leading risk factor for the reactivation of latent tuberculous infections. About a fifth of newly diagnosed cases of tuberculosis are extrapulmonary, and the spine is involved in 50 per cent of cases.

The onset is often slow, with aching pain in the back and stiffness of the spine. There may be fever and weight loss.

Radiographs taken in the earliest stages show narrowing of a single disc space; later, as the anterior portions of the vertebral bodies become progressively involved, they collapse, leading to angulation of the spine. The local abscess may expand and track distally. The spinal cord may be compromised, with weakness of the limbs or paraplegia.

Initial investigation should include radiographs of the chest, culture of urine and any sputum, Mantoux testing, brucellosis complement-fixation testing, and in the case of the lumbar spine at least, an IVP (renal spread being not uncommon). CAT and MRI scans of the spine are also invaluable in demonstrating the extent of bone and soft tissue involvement. As the clinical and radiological features of localised tuberculosis of the spine are mimicked in the early stages by other infections (especially staphylococcal), the only certain method of establishing the diagnosis in the majority of cases seen at this stage is by obtaining specimens for histological and bacteriological examination. Computed tomography-guided needle aspiration biopsy may be employed if this facility is available.

Pyogenic osteitis of the spine

Pyogenic osteitis of the spine is relatively uncommon. In the early stages of the disease, differentiation from tuberculosis of the spine is often extremely difficult, so that the diagnosis may not be clearly established unless material is provided for bacteriological examination (e.g. by needle biopsy). In the late stages, exuberant new bone formation may appear, favouring the diagnosis of pyogenic osteitis.

Metastatic lesions of the spine

Metastatic disease of the spine is seen particularly in the elderly and may be complicated by paraplegia. The diagnosis is usually by means of X-rays.

Spondylolysis, spondylolisthesis

In the erect position, there is a tendency for the body of the fifth lumbar vertebra (carrying the weight of the trunk) to slide forwards on the corresponding surface of the sacrum, as the plane of the L5–S1 disc is not horizontal but slopes downwards anteriorly. This is usually prevented by the articular processes. This supportive mechanism may fail if there is a fracture or defect in the part of the fifth lumbar vertebra lying immediately anterior to its inferior articular process (the pars interarticularis). Before any slip has occurred the condition is known as *spondylolysis*, and after, as *spondylolisthesis*. Less commonly, the fourth lumbar vertebra may be involved. Both congenital and developmental factors have been recognised in the causation, with local fractures due to trauma or fatigue being important factors. They give rise to low back pain which radiates into the buttocks.

A number of patients may suffer from concurrent neurological disturbances in the lower limbs (cauda equina syndrome), with low back pain radiating into the buttocks, spinal stiffness, hamstring spasm, gait abnormalities, and disturbance of bladder and bowel control. This may be due to an associated disc protrusion, or by the cauda equina and roots of the lumbosacral plexus being stretched over the prominent upper edge of the fifth lumbar vertebra or the sacrum. These complications necessitate an immediate decompression procedure.

Osteoarthritis (osteoarthrosis)

Primary osteoarthritis of the spine is extremely common, especially in the elderly, and is often asymptomatic. In the majority of cases there are no obvious causes. In secondary osteoarthritis, previous pathology in the spine accelerates normal wear and tear processes. Osteoarthritis may be localised to one spinal level (e.g. at the site of a previous fracture or prolapsed intervertebral disc), but more often involves many. It may be accompanied by disc degeneration, anterior and posterior lipping of the vertebral bodies, narrowing and lipping of the facet joints, and sometimes abutment of the vertebral spines (kissing spines).

When osteoarthritis gives rise to symptoms, these are usually of pain and stiffness in the back; once other conditions have been eliminated, the radiological appearances are diagnostic.

Rheumatoid arthritis

Rheumatoid arthritis may affect the spine: other peripheral sites are normally involved so that the diagnosis is not normally difficult. The radiographs generally show widespread osteoporosis, disc space narrowing, narrowing of the facet joints and often reduction in the height of vertebral bodies.

Spina bifida

Spina bifida is a condition in which there is a congenital failure of fusion of the posterior elements of the spine, through which the contents of the spinal canal may herniate. The grosser forms in the newly born child present no difficulty in diagnosis. There may be associated hydrocephalus, neurological problems and the risk of ascending meningitis. The older child or adult may present with spina bifida occulta, the diagnosis being confirmed by X-ray examination. Many cases are symptom-free. In some the only manifestation may be the presence of pes cavus. In others there may be progressive bladder dysfunction, weakness and incoordination of the legs, or trophic changes in the feet.

Spinal stenosis

A decrease in the sagittal diameter of the spinal canal, perhaps associated with narrowing of the nerve root tunnels, may give rise to symptoms of vague backache and morning stiffness. There may be temporary motor paralysis or neurogenic claudication where there are lower limb pains, cramps and paraesthesia related to walking or exercise. The claudication distance is variable, and pain may be rapidly relieved by forward flexion of the spine or by sitting. The sensory loss is segmental, and impulse symptoms are usually present, while in claudication due to vascular insufficiency, the claudication distance is constant, the peripheral pulses are usually absent and the sensory loss is generally of stocking type. Clinically, the straight leg raising test is hardly ever affected, but motor disturbances and absence of the knee jerks are frequent. It is commonest in osteoarthritis of the lumbar spine, spondylolisthesis, Paget's disease, previous fracture or spinal surgery, and achondroplasia. The diagnosis may be confirmed by CAT and MRI scans, which reliably demonstrate the space available within the spinal canal for the neurological structures.

The prolapsed intervertebral disc (PID)

In the commonest pattern of intervertebral disc prolapse, a tear in the annulus allows protrusion of the semi-liquid nucleus pulposus. This may be limited by intact fibres at the periphery of the annulus (contained prolapse). In other cases, extrusion of the nucleus is usually more extensive, and the prolapsed material may be cut off from its source (sequestered disc prolapse). Confirmation is usually obtained by an MRI scan. The investigative findings must be interpreted in conjunction with the history and clinical findings. The disc at L5/S1 is most commonly involved, followed in order by L4/L5 and L3/L4.

In a typical case there is a pain in the lumbar region, with tenderness between the spines at the affected level and sometimes at the sides over muscles in spasm. There may be loss of lumbar lordosis, restriction of movements in the lumbar spine and a protective scoliosis. The extruding nucleus frequently presses on a lumbar nerve root, giving rise to pain and paraesthesia in the leg, and sometimes muscle weakness, sensory impairment and diminution or abolition of the ankle jerk. At higher levels, the knee jerk may be lost. The neurological disturbance is *segmental in pattern, and is dependent on the level of the prolapse*. Impulse symptoms are common. When the prolapse is large and central, the cauda equina may be affected, producing bladder disturbance, diminished perineal sensation and even paraplegia. Such an occurrence is a surgical emergency, and immediate exploration imperative.

In the adolescent, there is striking restriction of movements in the lumbar spine, which becomes almost completely rigid. Occasionally, also in the young, the nucleus pulposus may herniate into the substance of the vertebral bodies (Schmorl's nodes), giving rise to mild backache without root symptoms.

In the thoracic spine, prolapses are rare and have a variety of presentations, often with a confusing clinical picture. A number are misdiagnosed as multiple sclerosis or amyotrophic lateral sclerosis. The diagnosis is established by MRI scan.

In the long term, the extrusion of disc material from between the vertebral bodies leads to narrowing of the disc space. The facet joints are disturbed and tend to develop secondary arthritic changes which decrease the mobility of the spine at that level, and themselves become a source of pain and sometimes nerve root irritation.

Mechanical back pain

The diagnosis is made largely by a process of elimination: it is back pain which is not due to a prolapsed intervertebral disc or any other clearly defined pathology. The patient is usually in the 20–45 age group and complains of dull backache aggravated by activity. There is often a history of morning stiffness which is gradually relieved as the patient moves about. Extensive radiation of pain is not a feature. Physical signs are often slight, and there are no positive neurological signs. Acute cases may be precipitated by a traumatic incident, and there may be a period where there is intense protective muscles spasm. In chronic cases there is often a long history of intermittent low back pain over a number of years.

Coccydynia

There is often a history of a fall in the seated position on to a hard surface; consequently in a number of cases radiographs may reveal a fracture of the end piece of the sacrum, or show the coccyx to be subluxed into the anteverted position. Symptoms of pain on sitting and defecation are often protracted for 6–12 months, but tend to resolve spontaneously.

COMMONER CAUSES OF BACK COMPLAINTS IN THE VARIOUS AGE GROUPS

Children
- Scoliosis
- Spondylolisthesis
- Pyogenic or tuberculous infections
- Calvé's disease

Adolescents
- Scheuermann's disease
- Scoliosis (idiopathic and postural)
- Mechanical back pain
- Adolescent intervertebral disc syndrome
- Pyogenic or tuberculous infections

Young adults
- Mechanical back pain
- Prolapsed intervertebral disc
- Spondylolisthesis
- Spinal fracture
- Ankylosing spondylitis
- Coccydynia
- Pyogenic or tuberculous infections
- Spinal stenosis

Middle-aged
- Mechanical back pain including primary osteoarthritis
- Prolapsed intervertebral disc
- Scheuermann's disease and old fracture
- Spondylolisthesis
- Rheumatoid arthritis
- Spinal stenosis
- Paget's disease
- Coccydynia
- Spinal metastases
- Pyogenic osteitis of the spine

Elderly
- Osteoarthritis, primary and secondary
- Spinal stenosis
- True senile kyphosis
- Osteoporosis, with or without fracture
- Osteomalacia, with or without fracture
- Spinal metastases

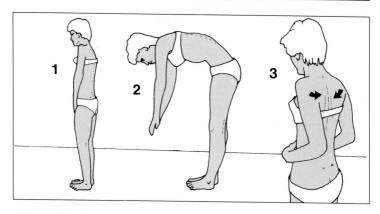

ASSESSMENT

Inspection from the side

Assessing thoracic posture. With the patient standing, look at the spine from the side. Although normal posture is difficult to define, try to make an assessment of the thoracic curvature. Note if there is any excess curvature (kyphosis) (1), and if there is, whether the resulting curve is regular.

Assessing mobility in a curve. Ask the patient to bend forwards (2), carefully examining the flow of movement in the spine and whether any curvature that has been detected increases. Any increase in flexion is indicative of a *mobile kyphosis.* (As the range of flexion in the thoracic spine is small, it may also help to check rotation: see later.) Now ask the patient to brace back the shoulders (3) to produce extension in the thoracic spine. If the curve corrects, this also suggests that it is a mobile one. *Postural kyphosis* is one of the commonest causes of a non-fixed increased regular curvature of the thoracic spine. It may be associated with a degree of *postural scoliosis.*

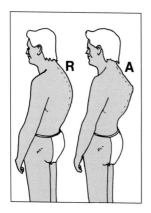

If your examination fails to detect any alteration in a thoracic curve on movement, then the curve is likely to be a fixed or relatively immobile one. The commonest causes of a *regular fixed kyphosis* (R) are senile kyphosis (sometimes associated with osteoporosis, osteomalacia or pathological fracture), Scheuermann's disease and ankylosing spondylitis.

If the spine is found to be angled at one level, then the deformity is one of *angular kyphosis* (A). The prominent vertebral spine forms a gibbus. The commonest causes are fracture (traumatic or pathological), tuberculosis of the spine or a congenital vertebral abnormality.

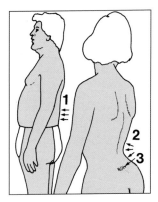

Assessing lumbar posture. Note the lumbar curvature. The normal modest concavity (lumbar lordosis) may be *flattened* (**1**) or *reversed*, particularly in PID, osteoarthritis of the spine, infections of the vertebral bodies and ankylosing spondylitis. Flexion of the spine, hips and knees (Simian stance) is suggestive of spinal stenosis. *An increase in the lumbar curvature* (**2**) is often normal in women, but if found with prominence of the distal vertebral spines (**3**), suspect spondylolisthesis. It may also occur where there is a flexion deformity of the hip(s), which should always be screened.

Inspection from behind

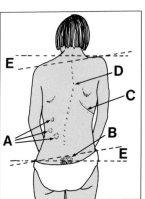

Note (**A**) cafe-au-lait spots which may suggest neurofibromatosis where there is often an associated scoliosis; (**B**) a fat pad or hairy patch, suggestive of spina bifida; (**C**) scarring suggestive of previous spinal surgery or a thoracotomy (and a possible thoracogenic scoliosis). Note (**D**) the presence of any lateral curvature (scoliosis), often with some associated diminution in height. The commonest scoliosis is a protective scoliosis (or list) in the lumbar region secondary to a PID. Note whether the shoulders and hips are level or not (**E**).

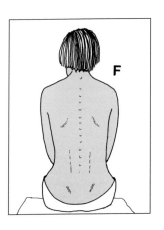

In considering other causes of scoliosis, examine the spine with the patient sitting. Obliteration (**F**) of an abnormal curve suggests that the scoliosis is *mobile* and secondary to shortening of a leg. (Check the relative leg lengths.) If on sitting the scoliosis persists, ask the patient to bend forwards. If the curve disappears, this also indicates that it is mobile and most likely to be postural in origin. If the curvature remains, this suggests that the scoliosis is fixed (structural scoliosis). If a *rib hump* is present, this confirms the diagnosis. Note that syringomyelia is present in about a quarter of cases of juvenile idiopathic scoliosis, and an MRI scan is mandatory.

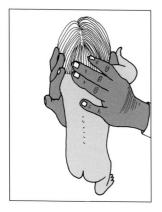

In the case of infantile scoliosis, assess the rigidity of a curvature by noting any alteration as the child is lifted by the armpits. Radiographs of the spine should be examined, and at the apex of the curve the angle between the vertebral columns and the line of the ribs should be measured on both sides. A difference of 20° or more suggests that the curve is likely to be progressive. An improvement over a three-month period carries a good prognosis. The best prognosis is in males where the onset occurs in the first year of life and the RVAD (rib–vertebral angle difference) is less than 20°.

Palpation

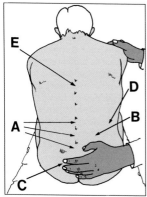

Ask the patient to lean forwards. Look for tenderness: (A) between the lumbar vertebral spines, especially at the lumbosacral junction, while at the same time noting if there is any vertebral prominence suggestive of spondylolisthesis; (B) over the lumbar muscles (common in PID and in cases of mechanical back pain); (C) over the sacroiliac joints (common in cases of mechanical back pain and in sacroiliac joint infections); (D) in the renal area, requiring further investigation; (E) high in the spine, e.g. from vertebral body infections.

Movements

Flexion: normal thoracic 45°; normal lumbar 60°. Ask the patient to try to touch his toes, while watching the flow of movement and any areas of restriction. Note that hip flexion (H) can account for apparent motion in a rigid spine. Flexion may be recorded by noting where the fingers reach relative to the ground (G) or the legs (L), e.g. 'the patient flexes to within 10 cm from the floor'. (**Normal = 7 cm or less.**) *This is an indication of the summation of thoracic, lumbar and hip movements; it does not distinguish between them and is under voluntary control.*

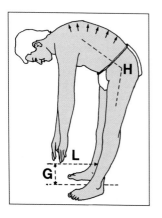

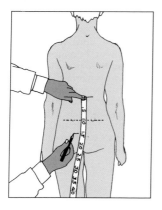

Modified Schober's method of assessing flexion (normal = 5 cm or more). When the spine flexes, the distances between successive vertebral spines increase. By measuring the spine when the patient is erect, and then when bent forwards, any gain gives unequivocal evidence of spinal flexion. The commonest practice in the UK is to employ a 15 cm length of spine: this has been shown to give the most reliable results. Begin by positioning a tape measure with the 10 cm mark level with the dimples of Venus (which mark the posterior superior iliac spines). Mark the skin at the end of the tape—i.e. at zero and also at 15 cm.

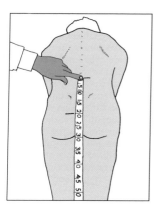

Anchor the top of the tape with a finger and ask the patient to flex as far forward as he can. Note where the 15 cm mark strikes the tape and work out the increment, which is entirely due to lumbar spine flexion. This is normally about 6–7 cm. Less than 5 cm is indicative of organic spinal pathology. Do not eliminate the skin marks and repeat the test later with the patient sitting up on the examination couch. This may help distinguish a genuine loss of movement from one due to overlay. Flexion in the thoracic spine (between the vertebra prominens and L1) may be similarly assessed. This is usually in the order of 3 cm only.

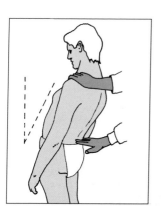

Extension (normal = 60° maximum). Ask the patient to arch his back. Assist him by steadying the pelvis and pulling back on the shoulders. Accurate measurement with a goniometer is difficult, but the maximum range is in the order of lumbar 35° and thoracic 25°; in practice, extension is usually appreciably less. Assessment of lumbar spine flexion may also be made by noting the decrease in the previously marked 15 cm length of spine. Pain on extension is common in intervertebral disc prolapses.

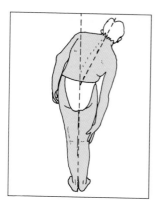

Lateral flexion (normal = 30° to both sides). Ask the patient to slide the hands down the side of each leg in turn and record the point reached, either in centimetres from the floor or the position that the fingers reach in the legs. Alternatively, measure the angle formed between a line drawn through T1 and S1, and the vertical. The contributions of the thoracic and lumbar spine are usually roughly equal.

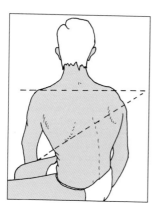

Rotation (normal = 40° maximum to both sides). The patient should be seated and asked to twist round to each side. (Some claim a more accurate assessment can be made if the test is carried out with the patient's arms folded across the chest.) Rotation is measured between the plane of the shoulders and the pelvis. *Nearly all movement in this plane is thoracic* with a maximum lumbar contribution of 5° or less.

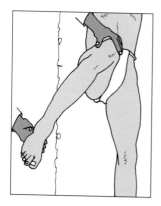

Special tests
Suspected prolapsed intervertebral disc. Always start by screening the hips. Osteoarthritis of the hip and prolapsed intervertebral disc are frequently confused. A full range of rotation in the hips, with absence of pain at the extremes, is generally all that is required to eliminate osteoarthritis of the hip as the source of the symptoms.

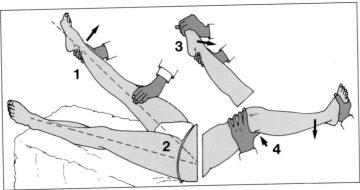

Straight leg raising test. Raise the leg from the couch (1) while watching the patient's face. Stop when he appears to have pain and ask if this is in the back or legs. (Distinguish this from hamstring tightness which can be ignored.) The production of paraesthesia or radiating root pain is highly significant, indicating nerve root irritation. Make a note of the result (2) (e.g. SLR (R) +ve at 60° or straight leg raising (R) full (no pain)). *Note the site of pain*—back pain suggests a central disc prolapse, leg pain a lateral protrusion. *Repeat on the good side.* If well-leg raising produces pain and paraesthesia on the affected side, this is highly suggestive of root irritation. Note that pain *must be below the knee* if the roots of the sciatic nerve are involved. Passive dorsiflexion of the foot (3) increases tension on the nerve roots, generally aggravating any pain or paraesthesia; try this and record the response. Alternatively, once the level of pain has been reached, slightly flex the knee and apply firm pressure with the thumb in the popliteal fossa over the stretched tibial nerve (4): radiating pain and paraesthesia in the leg suggest nerve root irritation (bowstring test).

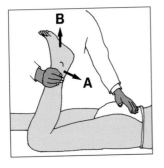

Reverse Lasegue test. The patient should be prone. Flex each knee in turn (A). This puts tension on the roots of the femoral nerve, giving rise to pain in its distribution. The test is positive in *high lumbar disc lesions.* If pain is produced, this is normally aggravated by extension of the hip (B), and this should be noted. High disc lesions are rare compared with those affecting the L5–S1 and L4–L5 spaces. Note also that pain in the *ipsilateral buttock or thigh* on full knee flexion may occur in more distally situated disc prolapses.

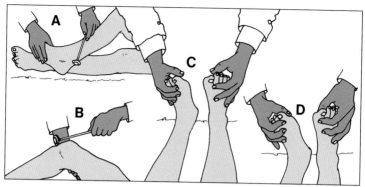

Look for further evidence of neurological involvement. **(A)** A reduced or absent ankle jerk (S1, 2) or **(B)** knee jerk (L3, 4) is a highly significant finding, especially if this accompanies a positive straight leg raising or positive reverse Lasegue test. Root pressure from a disc prolapse usually affects myotomes and dermatomes in a selective fashion; begin by noting the presence of any muscle wasting. Ask the patient to dorsiflex both feet **(C)**, and then attempt to force them into plantar-flexion against his resistance (L4, 5). Shift the grip to the great toes **(D)**, and test the power of dorsiflexion. Repeat with the lesser toes. (L4, 5). Now test the power of plantar-flexion of the great and lesser toes (S1, 2).

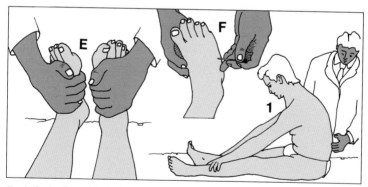

Encircle the feet with the hands **(E)**, and test the power of the peronei against the patient's resistance (L5, S1). Test the power of the quadriceps (L3, 4) when a high disc lesion is suspected. Test sensation to pin-prick **(F)** in the dermatomes of the lower limb. Diminution of sensation at the side of the foot (S1) is one of the commonest findings in lumbosacral disc prolapse.

Suspected functional overlay. **(1)** If there is some doubt regarding the severity or genuineness of the patient's complaints, ask him to sit up under the pretext of examining the back from behind. (*Flexion of the spine may also be re-measured in this position.*) The malingerer will have no difficulty, but the genuine patient will either flex the knees or fall back on the couch with pain (*flip test*).

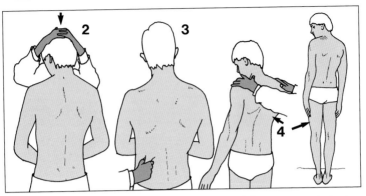

Apply pressure to the head (2). Overlay is suggested if this aggravates the back pain. (3) Pinch the skin at the sides. Such superficial stimulation should not produce deep-seated back pain, but if this occurs it is hard to explain on an organic basis. (4) Note the amount of rotation required to produce pain in the back. Now ask the patient to keep his hands firmly at his sides and repeat: the major part of the movement will now take place in the legs ('simulated rotation'). Pain occurring with the same amount of apparent rotation again suggests overlay. (5) Note the distribution of any motor or sensory loss. Any claimed loss should be segmental and localised. Widespread weakness and/or stocking anaesthesia also suggest overlay (but do carry out a thorough neurological and circulatory examination). In many centres, if three or more of the preceding tests are positive, surgery is considered to be contraindicated.

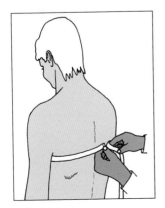

Suspected ankylosing spondylitis.

Check the patient's chest expansion at the level of the fourth interspace. The normal range in an adult of average build is at least 6 cm. Less than 2.5 cm is regarded as highly suggestive of ankylosing spondylitis. In addition, look for evidence of iritis which is often associated with this condition.

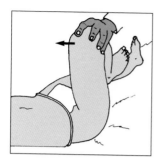

Suspected sacroiliac joint involvement. Flex the hip and knee, and forcibly adduct the hip. Pain may accompany this manoeuvre in early ankylosing spondylitis, tuberculosis and other infections, and Reiter's syndrome, but false positives are common. Alternatively, with the patient in the prone position, place the side of one hand over the sacrum and upper natal cleft; press down hard, using the other hand to assist. True sacroiliac pain may occur in women shortly before and after childbirth.

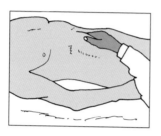

Additional tests
Abdominal examination. This is an essential part of the investigation of all cases of back pain. Rectal or vaginal examination may be required if indicated by the history or any other elements of the case.

The *sacrococcygeal joint* may be examined by first grasping the coccyx between the index (in the rectum) and the thumb outside, and then gently moving the joint. In coccydynia, marked pain normally accompanies this manoeuvre.

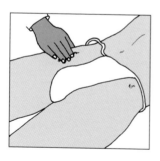

Circulation. The peripheral pulses and circulation should also be checked in all cases. Back and leg pain caused by arterial insufficiency are usually aggravated by activity, and absence of femoral pulsation is of particular significance.

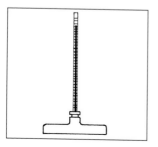

Sedimentation rate. Estimation of the sedimentation rate is a valuable screening test in the investigation of all spinal complaints. It is normal in prolapsed intervertebral disc, mechanical back pain and Scheuermann's disease, but elevated in ankylosing spondylitis, many infections and neoplasms. It is best if 25 mm is taken as the upper limit of normal. False positives are not uncommon, but false negatives are rare.

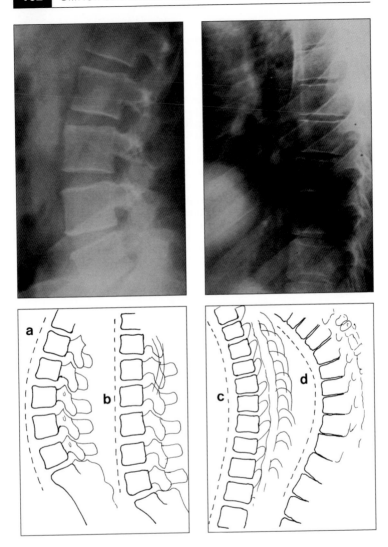

RADIOGRAPHS
Normal lateral projections. (1) Curves. *Lumbar:* note a normal curve (**a**); loss of lordosis (**b**) (often due to muscle spasm). *Thoracic:* note typical normal curve (**c**); an increased but regular curve (**d**), typical of senile kyphosis and Scheuermann's disease. The upper limit of normal is taken as 45° (measured by the Cobb method).

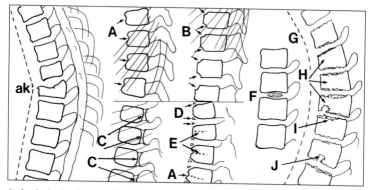

In both the lumbar and thoracic spine, note any sharp alteration in the curvature (angular kyphosis, **ak**), found typically where there is pathology restricted to one or two vertebral bodies, e.g. from fractures, TB or other infections, tumour and osteomalacia with local collapse.

(2) Bodies and discs. Be aware of the following normal appearances in children: **(A)** anterior clefts; **(B)** anterior notches; **(C)** incomplete fusion of elements; **(D)** epiphyses; **(E)** vascular tracks (which may persist). Note **(F)** disc calcification; typical Scheuermann's disease, with **(G)** kyphosis, **(H)** anterior wedging of not less than 5° in at least three sequential vertebrae, **(I)** ragged appearance of the epiphyses, and **(J)** a central disc herniation (Schmorl's node).

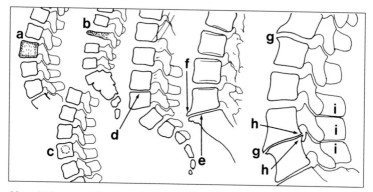

Note: **(a)** increased density and 'picture-frame' appearance of vertebrae seen in *Paget's disease*; **(b)** marked narrowing and density seen in *Calvé's disease*; **(c)** a space occupying lesion in a vertebral body, usually due to *tumour*, *infection* or *Schmorl's nodes*; **(d)** disc narrowing at any level in the spine, amongst other things the earliest evidence of *tuberculosis* and other infections; **(e)** narrowing at L5–S1, or less frequently the two spaces above, commonly seen in *long-standing PID*; **(f)** lipping seen in chronic disc lesions at the same level. Note **(g)** anterior and **(h)** posterior lipping, both common at all levels of the spine in *osteoarthritis*, along with **(i)** impingement of spinous processes ('kissing spines').

Normal AP views of the lumbar and thoracic spine

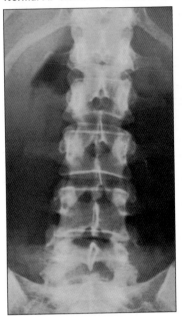
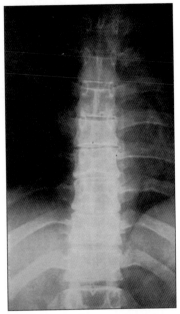

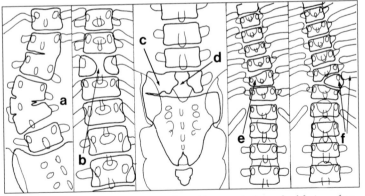

Note any congenital abnormalities such as: **(a)** *congenital vertebral fusion*, often associated with a congenital scoliosis; **(b)** *anterior spina bifida* in which there is failure of fusion of the vertebral body elements; **(c)** anomalies of the lumbosacral articulation, such as *partial sacralisation of the fifth lumbar vertebra*, a possible cause of low back pain; **(d)** *(posterior) spina bifida*; any localised *lateral angulation* of the spine **(e)** due to lateral vertebral collapse, e.g. from fracture, infection, tumour, osteoporosis or other causes; **(f)** *hemivertebra*, with extra rib.

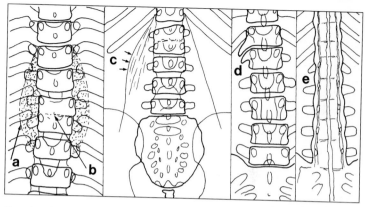

Examine the soft tissue shadows at the sides of the vertebrae, observing, for example, (**a**) a fusiform area of increased density, typical of a *tuberculous abscess*. Note also obliteration of disc spaces (**b**) and any early lateral wedging. Examine the psoas shadows for symmetry. Lateral displacement of the edge of the shadow (**c**), and increased density within the main area occupied by the psoas suggests a *psoas abscess*, typically found in tuberculosis of the lumbar or lowermost thoracic spine. Look for lateral lipping: at D12–L1 (**d**), it may be an early sign of *ankylosing spondylitis*, but there and elsewhere it usually indicates osteoarthritis. 'Bamboo spine' (**e**) is however diagnostic of ankylosing spondylitis. Note the body and facet joint fusions and ligament calcification.

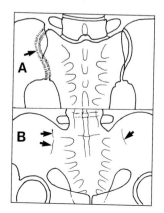

Look at the sacroiliac joints. (**A**) Unilateral involvement, with for example, blurring of the joint margins, sclerosis or destruction may occur in *tuberculosis* and *pyogenic infections*. Any asymmetry should be investigated by oblique projections and, if necessary, CAT scans (or tomography). Bilateral involvement may occur in rheumatoid arthritis, but obliteration and fusion of the joints (**B**) is almost diagnostic of *ankylosing spondylitis*: so much so that some are unwilling to accept the diagnosis of ankylosing spondylitis if this is not present.

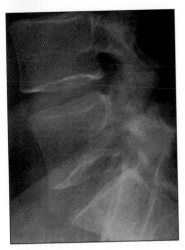
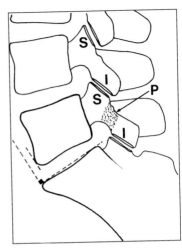

Normal localised view of the lumbosacral junction. Note that the pars interarticularis (**P**), lying between (**S**) the superior and (**I**) the inferior articular facets, is normally intact, and a line from the anterior margin of the sacrum lies in front of L5. If spondylolisthesis is suspected, the lateral should be taken erect.

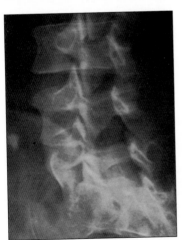
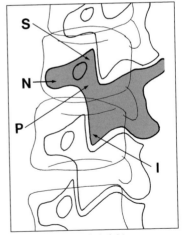

Normal oblique view of the lumbar spine. This is helpful in diagnosing spondylolysis and spondylolisthesis. Identify the 'Scotty dog' shadows. The nose (**N**) is formed by a transverse process, the ear (**S**) by a superior articular process, the front legs (**I**) by an inferior articular process and the neck (**P**) by the pars interarticularis.

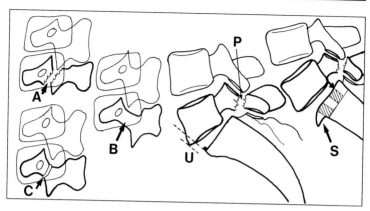

In *spondylolisthesis* (**A**) the 'dog' becomes decapitated due to forward slip, and the inferior articular process of the vertebra above encroaches on the neck. In *spondylolysis*, where no slip has occurred, the neck (**B**) is elongated or (**C**) develops a collar. (These views are only likely to be successful when the radiographs are taken with the beam in the plane of any defect. CT scans with a reverse gantry angle may be helpful.) Looking again at the straight lateral, note any defect (**P**) and forward slip (**U**). Note that new bone formation (**S**) (buttressing) may make use of the anterior edge of the sacrum as a reference point unreliable. Instead, note the relation of the *posterior* edge of the slipping vertebra to the one below. The example shows a forward slip of 25%. The deformity may occur between L5 and S1 and much less frequently between L4/L5 or L3/L4. Backward vertebral slip (retrospondylolisthesis) is uncommon, always of a minor degree and is usually associated with disc degeneration.

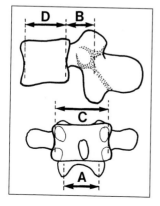

Spinal stenosis. Where spinal stenosis is suspected, calculate the canal to body ratio, AB:CD, where **A** = the interpedicular distance, **B** = the depth of the spinal canal from front-to-back (measure to the root of the spinous process), **C** = the width of vertebral body, **D** = the front-to-back measurement of the vertebral body. The normal range is from approximately 1:2 to 1:4.5. Values greater than 1:4.5 suggest spinal stenosis, but other investigations (particularly CAT scanning) may be indicated to give a clearer visualisation of the canal and its contents.

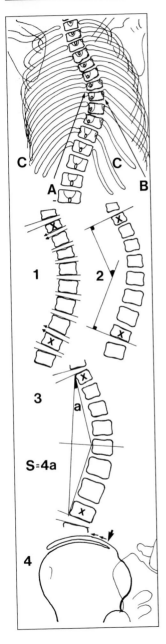

Scoliosis. Note any structural scoliosis with (**A**) on the concavity, displacement of spines and narrowing of pedicles; (**B**) on the convexity, widening of disc spaces; (**C**) in the thorax, rib cage distortion. Identify primary curves clinically or by lateral flexion radiographs (to identify absence or presence of mobility).

To assess the severity of a scoliotic curve and to monitor its progress, it is necessary to measure the deformity. The *Cobb method* is most popular. Find the upper and lower limits of the primary curve by drawing tangents to the bodies and noting where the disc spaces begin to become widened on the concavity of the curve (**1**). Now erect perpendiculars from the vertebrae which form the limits of the curve (marked 'X'). Note the angle between them (**2**). This is a measure of the primary curve. Kyphotic curves may be measured in a similar way.

Capasso's method of measuring scoliotic curves is said to be more sensitive and accurate (**3**). The magnitude of the scoliotic curve (**S**) in degrees is determined by multiplying by four the angle (**a**) subtended by a line joining the ends of the curves, with one running from the centre of the curve to one end of the curve.

Risser's sign. In late adolescence the appearance and progressive fusion of the iliac apophysis from behind forwards (**4**) heralds skeletal maturity. It would appear, however, that very slight growth may continue in the spine for up to ten years after cessation of limb growth. This, along with disc degeneration and other factors can lead to late deterioration in scoliotic curves, particularly those greater than 60°, so that this sign is of somewhat limited value.

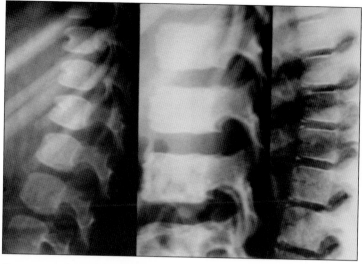

Representative radiographs

These three radiographs show anterior clefts, anterior notches, epiphyses, and vascular tracks—normal features of the growing spine.

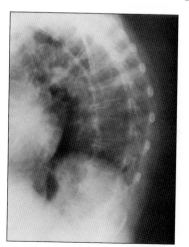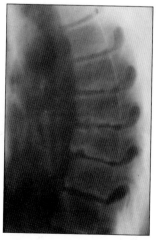

Left: there is a regular dorsal kyphosis with anterior vertebral lipping and a degree of osteoporosis typical of *senile kyphosis*. *Right:* there is a regular kyphosis, with slight anterior wedging of the vertebral bodies, irregularity of the disc margins and central disc herniation (Schmorl's nodes) typical of *Scheuermann's disease*.

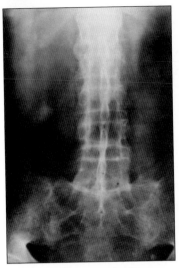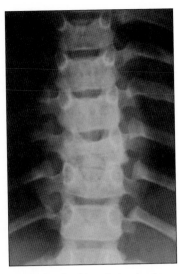

Left: the thoracic and lumbar vertebral bodies are fused, with early bambooing of the spine. The facet joints and the sacroiliac joints have been obliterated and there is ossification of the interspinous ligaments due to *ankylosing spondylitis*. *Right:* there is loss of a disc space, slight vertebral wedging and a fusiform abscess shadow on both sides of the spine due to *tuberculosis*.

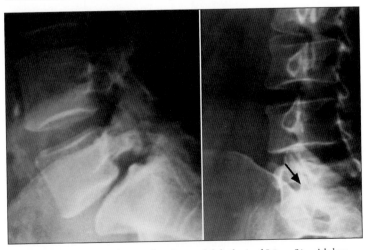

The lateral radiographs show a *chronic spondylolisthesis* of L5 on S1, with less than 25% forward slip. There is an obvious defect in the pars interarticularis, and the 'Scotty dog' in the oblique projection has been decapitated.

Common conditions around
   the hip 112
Other conditions affecting
   the hip 115
Conditions associated with
   total hip joint
   replacements 115
Hip assessment 116
Radiographs 127
Perthes' disease 130
DDH 132
Representative radiographs
   134

COMMON CONDITIONS AROUND THE HIP
Developmental dislocation of the hip (DDH)

Terminology. 'Developmental dislocation of the hip' is used to describe a condition which occurs in the perinatal period and involves displacement of the femoral head relative to the acetabulum. If untreated it disrupts the normal development of the hip joint. The term 'congenital dislocation of the hip' (CDH) is now less frequently used, but is for the main part virtually synonymous. (Note however that the abbreviation 'DDH' may be somewhat confusingly used for 'developmental dysplasia of the hip'.)

The term 'neonatal instability of the hip' (NIH) is of particular value as it is clearly defined: it describes a condition in which the hip is dislocated, able to be dislocated or is unstable at examination during the first five days after delivery. Similarly, 'late diagnosed DDH' is used to describe a dislocated or dislocatable hip diagnosed after the age of one week.

Aetiology. The condition is much commoner in girls than boys; there is a familial tendency and a well-established geographical distribution of the disorder. It is commoner after breech presentations, and it may occur in conjunction with other congenital defects.

Diagnosis. A simple test devised by Ortolani in the 1960s was found to show instability in the hips of some newborn children, and it was thought that in every case this was directly related to a dislocation of the hip, whether this was already present or going to happen. As a result it was considered that if all newborns could be screened with this test and treated promptly if instability were found, the condition would no longer pose a problem. Unfortunately, later experience showed that a number of children who had passed the screening test went on to develop hip dislocations. It also became clear that some unstable hips could resolve without treatment; and that treatment itself (in an abduction splint) was not free from complications (about 10% developing avascular necrosis).

When ultrasound screening is added to the clinical examination, there is a dramatic increase in the number of positive results, most of which resolve without treatment.

To accommodate these confusing facts, a number of regimes have been developed. One typical example recommends the following:

1. All children should be examined during the first 3 months of life on at least two occasions, by those expert in the performance of the screening tests.
2. Ultrasound screening should be added if the child is in a high-risk group. This group includes the following:
   i.   those with a family history of DDH
   ii.   breech presentations
   iii. those with a clicking hip
   iv.   where the birth has been by Caesarean section
   v.   where there are other deformities
   vi.   where there has been oligohydramnios
   vii. where there has been foetal growth retardation.
   (Note that in some centres ultrasound examination is offered routinely in all cases.)
3. If some doubt remains, the hips should be X-rayed at 3–4 months. Note that X-ray examination of the hips is not of much diagnostic value at birth (due to skeletal immaturity) but can be helpful by about 3–4 months.

4. If still negative, the hips should be re-examined clinically at 6 months and when weight bearing commences.

If the hip is clearly dislocated, then treatment should be commenced immediately (by appropriate splintage). If the hip is not dislocated but *can* be dislocated (Barlow's test), it should be re-examined at weekly intervals for 3 weeks. If instability remains, then some recommend that splintage (in abduction) should then be commenced, although others prefer to have both X-ray and ultrasound confirmation.

DDH in the older child

This must be suspected in any child where there is disturbance of gait or posture, shortening of a limb or indeed any complaint in which the hip might be implicated.

DDH in the adult

Where treatment in childhood has been unsuccessful or even where the condition has not been diagnosed, a patient may seek help during the third and fourth decades of life. Symptoms may arise from the hips or the spine. In the hips, secondary arthritic changes occur in the false joint which may form between the dislocated femoral head and the ilium with which it comes in contact. In the spine, osteoarthritic changes are a result of long-standing scoliosis (in the unilateral case), increased lumbar lordosis (in both unilateral and bilateral cases), or excessive spinal movements which occur in walking.

The dysplastic hip

Hip dysplasia is a condition in which the principal feature is that the femoral head is imperfectly contained by the acetabulum. The acetabular slope is frequently greater than normal, and the acetabulum may be relatively small in comparison with the femoral head. In early life this may be a major factor in developmental dislocation of the hip, but even if the hip does not dislocate it may nevertheless give trouble later in life from osteoarthritis or instability.

The irritable hip

In childhood there are a number of conditions affecting the hip which may be indistinguishable in their initial stages. They all give rise to a limp, restriction of movements and sometimes pain in the joint (irritable hip). The commonest conditions responsible for irritable hip are transient synovitis, Perthes' disease and tuberculosis of the hip.

Transient synovitis. This is the commonest cause of the irritable hip syndrome. The child presents with a limp, and there is sometimes a history of preceding minor trauma which in some cases at least is probably coincidental. There is no systemic upset and the sedimentation rate is generally normal. Radiographs of the hip sometimes give confirmatory evidence of synovitis as does ultrasound examination. Raised blood interferon levels have been described, suggesting the presence of a viral infection, but no other pathology is usually demonstrable.

Perthes' disease. In this condition there is a disturbance of the blood supply to the epiphysis of the femoral head so that a variably sized portion undergoes a form of avascular necrosis. The cause is unknown, and it is commoner in boys than girls. As a rule, radiological changes are well established by the time the child presents with symptoms, and these will confirm the diagnosis. The severity of the condition is dependent on the position and extent of the area of the femoral head involved.

Tuberculosis. Tuberculosis of the hip is now rare in Britain. The affected child walks with a limp and often complains of pain in the groin or knee. Night pain is a feature. Rotation in the hip becomes limited, a fixed flexion deformity develops and muscle wasting occurs. Radiographs of the hip in the early stages show rarefaction of bone in the region of the hip and widening of the joint space. As the disease advances, there is progressive joint destruction with abscess formation and sometimes dislocation. The diagnosis is usually confirmed by histological and bacteriological examination of synovial biopsy specimens, or by bacteriological examination of the aspirate.

Acute pyogenic arthritis of the hip

The *Staphylococcus* is the organism most frequently responsible and the infection is blood-borne. The onset is rapid, with high fever and toxaemia. All movements of the hip are severely impaired and accompanied by great pain and protective muscle spasm. The organism responsible may be isolated by blood culture or joint aspiration.

Osteitis of the symphysis pubis

In some cases of osteitis of the pubic symphysis (particularly those secondary to open wounds), organisms can be grown, but in the majority of cases attempts at culture fail. The condition may follow urological or gynaecological procedures, pregnancy, rheumatoid arthritis, trauma or sometimes intense athletic activity. Although most cases resolve spontaneously, there may be local pain and tenderness, clicking on walking and disturbance of gait.

Slipped femoral epiphysis

This is a disease of adolescence and is commoner in boys than girls. The attachment of the femoral epiphysis loosens, giving rise eventually to a coxa vara deformity. The cause is unknown, but there is often a history of preceding trauma or the suggestion of hormonal disturbance. Some cases have been noted to occur in those suffering from hypothyroidism.

Pain may occur in the groin or knee, and if the onset is very acute, weight-bearing may become impossible. There is usually restriction of internal rotation and abduction in the affected hip. The diagnosis is confirmed by X-rays.

The other hip should be kept under surveillance as there is bilateral involvement in 60% of cases.

Primary osteoarthritis of the hip

Primary osteoarthritis of the hip occurs in the middle-aged and elderly, and although often associated with overweight and overwork, its cause is usually uncertain. Pain is often poorly localised in the hip, groin, buttock or trochanter, and may be referred to the knee. There is increasing difficulty in walking and standing. Sleep is often disturbed and the general health of the patient becomes undermined as a result. Stiffness may declare itself in difficulty in putting on stockings and cutting the toenails. Fixed flexion and adduction contractures are common, with apparent shortening of the affected limb.

Secondary osteoarthritis of the hip
This occurs most often as a sequel to developmental dislocation of the hip, congenital coxa vara, hip dysplasia, Perthes' disease, tuberculous or pyogenic infections, slipped femoral epiphysis, and avascular necrosis secondary to femoral neck fracture or traumatic dislocation of the hip. A younger age group is generally involved than in the case of primary osteoarthritis.

Rheumatoid arthritis
The hip joints are frequently involved in rheumatoid arthritis. When both hips and knees are affected, the disability may be profound.

OTHER CONDITIONS AFFECTING THE HIP
Of the rarer conditions affecting the hip joint, the following are not infrequently overlooked.

- **Ankylosing spondylitis** may present as pain and stiffness in the hip in a young man. There may be no complaint of back pain, although there is almost invariably radiographic evidence of sacroiliac joint involvement.
- **Reiter's syndrome** may first present in the hip.
- **Primary bone tumours** are uncommon: of these, osteoid osteoma involving the femoral neck may be a cause of persistent hip pain.
- **The snapping hip**: 'clunking' sounds emanating from the region of the hip on certain movements may be a source of annoyance to a patient. In most cases this is due to the iliopsoas tendon snapping over a bony prominence, but if pain is a feature attempts should be made to localise the source of the problem.

The following important points should always be remembered in dealing with the hip joint:

- *The commonest cause of hip pain in the adult is pain referred from the spine, e.g. from a prolapsed intervertebral disc.* Hip movements are not impaired, and there are almost invariably signs of the primary pathology.
- *In the elderly, pain in the hip with inability to weight bear is frequently due to a fracture of the femoral neck or of the pubic rami.* In an appreciable number of cases there is no history of injury, and radiographic examination is essential.
- *Flexion contracture of the hip may result from psoas spasm secondary to inflammation or pus in the region of its sheath in the pelvis.* This is seen for example in appendicitis, appendix abscess or other pelvic inflammatory disease. Examination of the abdomen is essential.

CONDITIONS ASSOCIATED WITH TOTAL HIP JOINT REPLACEMENTS
Because of the success of hip joint replacement procedures, many of these operations have been performed, and complications (which occur in about 5% of cases) are being seen with increasing frequency. Excluding those which may arise in the immediate postoperative period, the following should be kept in mind:

Dislocation. The stability of the replacement is dependent on the precision with which the components have been aligned during their insertion, the time that has elapsed since surgery and the degree of violence to which the components have been subjected. After any hip replacement, the fibrous capsule which forms round the artificial joint thickens and strengthens as time progresses, leading to a progressive resistance to dislocation.

Component failure. Socket failure is relatively uncommon, and fracture of the stem of the femoral prosthesis is seen more often. Generally, there is immediate loss of the ability to weight-bear. If the greater trochanter has been reattached with wires, these may fracture and fragment, giving rise to local discomfort and sometimes episodes of sharp, jagging pain. The trochanter itself may fail to unite and may displace. This may cause local discomfort and a Trendelenberg gait.

Component loosening and infection. When this occurs, it is usually at the interface between the cement and bone. It is commonest in the area of the femoral stem, although both components may be affected. The complaint is of pain and impairment of function, and the diagnosis is usually made on the basis of the radiological appearances. Loosening may be the result of infection; in some cases this may be frank, and in others, organisms of low pathogenicity may be found in the affected area. In many cases, although an element of infection may be strongly suspected, no organism can be found and an alternative cause may be sought. In many, loosening may be associated with particulate wear debris.

HIP ASSESSMENT

A number of rating systems have been established to help gauge hip performance prior to or after hip surgery; many have elaborate scoring systems. There is general agreement over the factors that are of importance, and these may be profitably employed in the assessment of any hip problem.

Pain (which is subjective and hard to assess with accuracy) should be considered in terms of severity, how often it occurs and when it occurs (e.g. after a specific activity, at rest or at night).

Function includes gait and the need for walking aids; the distance that can be walked and the time taken; the ability to ascend and descend stairs and the method employed (e.g. one foot after the other or not, and the need to use a banister); the ability to rise from a chair; the capacity for standing; dressing capabilities, especially with regard to putting on socks and tying shoe laces; and the patient's ability to cut his own toenails.

Movements (on which dressing and the cutting of toenails depend), if lacking, may cause additional problems on their own, such as difficulty in using inside seats in public transport.

Deformity also affects gait and may in itself cause concern.

The radiographic findings are often of great importance in making a meaningful assessment, and many now advocate their inclusion in any system of hip assessment.

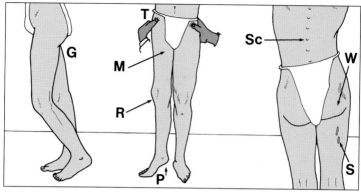

Gait

Observe the gait from the front, side (**G**) and behind. Analysis is often difficult, but grows from experience. In particular try to assess the stride and dwell time on each side, and the possible factors of pain, stiffness, shortening and gluteal insufficiency.

Inspection from the front. Examine the standing patient, noting (**T**) any pelvic tilting (e.g. from an adduction or abduction deformity of the hip, short leg or scoliosis); (**M**) muscle wasting (e.g. secondary to infection, disuse, polio); (**R**) rotational deformity (common in osteoarthritis); (**P**) plantar flexion of the foot.

Inspection from behind. Note (**Sc**) any scoliosis (possibly secondary to pelvic tilting, e.g. from an adduction deformity of the hip); (**W**) gluteal muscle wasting (e.g. from disuse or infection); (**S**) sinus scars (e.g. secondary to tuberculosis).

Inspection from the side. Note any increased lumbar lordosis suggestive of fixed flexion deformity of the hip(s).

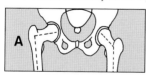

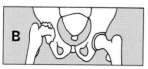

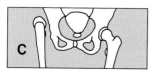

Shortening

It is important in the examination of the hip and the lower limb to determine the presence or absence of shortening. Shortening may be *true* or *apparent*.

True shortening. In this case the affected limb is physically shorter than the other, and the cause may be above or below the trochanters. *Causes above the trochanters* include (**A**) coxa vara (e.g. from femoral neck fractures, slipped upper femoral epiphysis, Perthes' disease, congenital coxa vara); (**B**) loss of articular cartilage (from infection or arthritis); (**C**) dislocation of the hip. Very rarely, *lengthening of the other limb* (e.g. from coxa valga or bone overgrowth from fracture or tumour) gives relative true shortening.

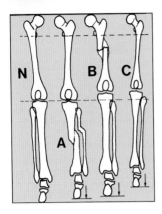

True shortening *distal to the trochanters* is most commonly due to the effects of a long bone fracture—e.g. of the tibia and, therefore, below the knee (**A**); or involving the femur and above the knee (**B**). Other causes include growth disturbance, e.g. from polio (**C**) where the whole limb above and below the knee may be affected, or from bone or joint infection or epiphyseal trauma. (**N**) = Normal side for comparison. True shortening may be compensated for by plantar flexion of the foot, or flexion of the knee on the contralateral side, or pelvic tilting (compensated in turn by a scoliosis).

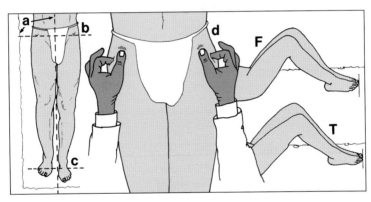

Examination in true shortening. The position of the patient should be adjusted to lie squarely on the couch, with the trunk and legs parallel to its edge (**a**). Check that the pelvis is not tilted (**b**) and note shortening betrayed by the position of the heels (**c**). If there is pelvic tilting due to an adduction contracture of the hip (as is the case in apparent shortening), it will not be possible to correct it. If there is pelvic tilting due to a postural scoliosis which is compensating some true shortening, it should be able to be overcome by adjusting the position of the patient and you may then proceed. Now hook the thumbs under the anterior spines and place the fingers on the greater trochanters (**d**). A lesser distance between thumb and fingers on the affected side suggests the cause of any true shortening lies *above* the trochanters. If none is discovered at this level (i.e. if no difference is found between the sides), then slightly flex both knees and hips, and bring the feet squarely together. Note the appearance of the legs at knee level: (**F**) indicates femoral shortening, and (**T**) tibial shortening.

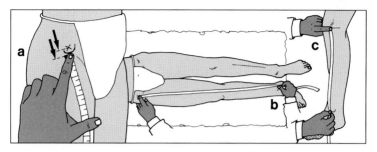

Measuring true shortening. To do this, it is important that clear landmarks are established. To obtain a fixed upper mark, place the metal end of a cloth measuring tape over the *centre* of the anterior spine and press it backwards until it slides distally, hooking under its inferior edge (**a**). For the lower mark, choose the middle or inferior border of the medial malleolus (**b**); the heel pad is less reliable. Compare the sides and always repeat the measurements until consistency is obtained. This measures *total true shortening*. Deformity of the pelvis (which is rare) may sometimes lead to errors in assessment. Pure *tibial shortening* may be assessed by measuring the distance between the knee joint and the medial malleolus (**c**). Assessment of pure *femoral shortening* may be attempted by measuring between the knee and greater trochanter, but this is somewhat unreliable unless the patient is very thin and the trochanters easily felt.

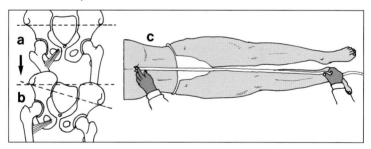

Apparent shortening. Here the limb is not altered in length, but appears short as a result of an adduction contracture of the hip (**a**) which has to be compensated by tilting of the pelvis (**b**). The presence and degree of apparent shortening may be indicated by the patient's position on the couch (with evidence of pelvic tilting and a difference in heel position). Apparent shortening may be roughly assessed by measuring the distance between the xiphisternum and the medial malleoli (**c**). There may be some additional true shortening. (If assessing this, adduct the sound leg while measuring between the anterior spines and the malleoli.) (Note that true shortening may also be measured: (1) in the standing patient by blocking up the short leg until both anterior superior iliac spines and the iliac crests lie horizontally, and the natal cleft is vertical; or (2) by radiographs of the hips, knees and ankles taken without altering the patient's position on the table.)

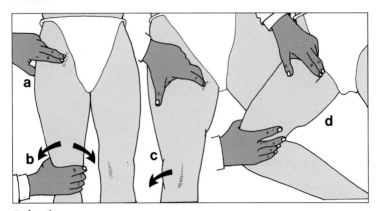

Palpation

Place the fingers over the head of the femur, just below the inguinal ligament and lateral to the femoral artery (**a**). Note any tenderness. Now rotate the leg medially and laterally (**b**), and feel for any crepitus arising from the hip joint (indicative of advanced osteoarthritis). Next, externally rotate the leg and palpate the lesser trochanter (**c**). Tenderness occurs here in strains of the iliopsoas which are often the result of athletic injuries. Now slightly flex and abduct the leg while palpating the origin of adductor longus (**d**). Tenderness is a feature of sports injuries (strain of adductor longus) and in patients developing adductor contractures in osteoarthritis of the hip. With the patient on his good side also palpate the region of the ischial tuberosity, looking for tenderness. Strains of the hamstring origin occur as a result of athletic activities, especially in children. Less commonly, athletic injuries may affect the anterior superior and anterior inferior iliac spines at the attachments of sartorius and rectus femoris.

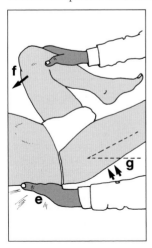

Movements

In making any assessment of hip movements it is necessary to take into account the possibility of *pelvic* movements (which occur in fact in the lumbar spine) giving a false impression. This is of importance in the case of flexion/extension and abduction/adduction. In assessing hip *extension*, it is necessary to see first of all whether the hip is not in fact permanently flexed. Place a hand (**e**) behind the lumbar spine so that you may assess its position. Now flex the *good* hip fully (**f**), observing with the hand that the lumbar curvature is *fully* obliterated. If the hip being examined rises from the couch (**g**), then it has lost full extension. (This is also described as a *fixed flexion deformity of the hip*). Any loss should he measured and recorded. This test is usually referred to as Thomas's test.

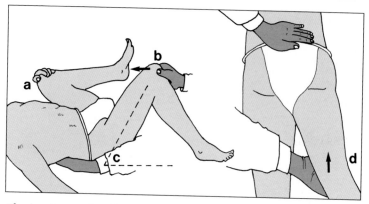

Flexion (normal = 120°). The *good* hip is first flexed (to obliterate the lumbar curve and to steady the pelvis), and the patient is asked to hold it in this position (**a**) while the one being examined (**b**) is fully flexed. The angle between the thigh and couch (**c**) is then measured.

Extension (normal = 5–20°). Turn the patient over on to his face and steady the pelvis with one hand. Lift each leg in turn and compare the range (**d**). A loss of extension is often the first detectable sign of effusion in the hip joint.

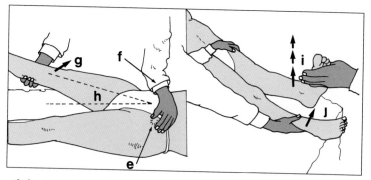

Abduction (normal 40°). The pelvis must be prevented from moving, and this may be done by holding one anterior superior iliac spine (**e**) and steadying the other with the forearm (**f**). (Alternatively, the good leg may be flexed at the knee, over the edge and against the side of the examination couch.) The leg is then abducted (**g**), measuring the angle between it and the midline (**h**).

Adduction (normal = 25°). Ideally an assistant should lift the good leg out of the way (**i**) to allow the affected leg to be adducted and the angle measured (**j**).

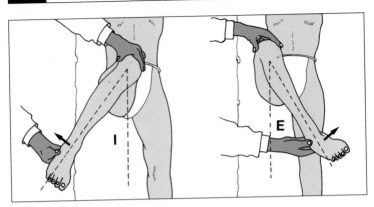

Internal rotation at 90° flexion (normal = 45°). Flex the hip and knee to 90° and move the foot laterally (**I**). *Do not be confused*: although the *foot moves laterally* (or externally), the *hip rotates internally* (or medially). The test may be carried out simultaneously on both sides to allow comparison. Loss of internal rotation is often the first sign of hip pathology.

External rotation at 90° flexion (normal = 45°). The position of the hip is the same as for testing internal rotation, but in this case the foot is moved medially (**E**). External rotation becomes limited in most arthritic conditions of the hip.

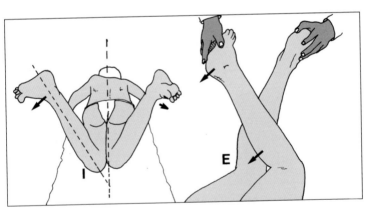

Internal rotation in extension (normal = 35°). The patient should be prone, with the knees flexed (**I**). The two sides can easily be compared and measurements taken.

External rotation in extension (normal = 45°). One leg requires to be flexed at the knee (**E**) more than the other (for clearance) if a direct comparison between the sides is being made—or each may be tested separately.

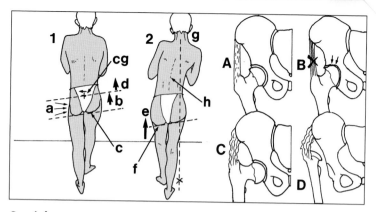

Special tests

Trendelenberg's test. Normally, when about to stand on one leg (**1**), contraction of the hip abductors (**a**) moves the centre of gravity (**cg**) at S2 over to the side, over the stance foot. This also tends to tilt the pelvis (**b**) and elevate the buttock on the non-stance side (**c**). The patient should be able to produce a _greater_ pelvic tilt (**d**) by being asked to lift the side higher, and _hold the position_ for 30 seconds.

To perform the test, ask the patient to stand on the affected side (**2**). (Any support (stick or hand) must be on the same side.) Now ask him to raise the non-stance leg further (**e**). Prevent excessive trunk movements. If the pelvis drops below the horizontal (**f**), or cannot be held steady for 30 seconds, the test is positive. Shoulder sway (**g**) and a scoliosis (**h**) may develop to maintain balance. The test is not valid below age 4: pain, poor cooperation or bad balance may give a false positive. The test is positive as a result of (**A**) gluteal paralysis or weakness (e.g. from polio, muscle-wasting disease); (**B**) gluteal inhibition (e.g. from pain arising in the hip joint); (**C**) from gluteal inefficiency from coxa vara or (**D**) DDH. False positives have been recorded in about 10% of patients.

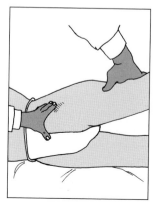

Duchenne sign. Note if the patient when walking lurches to one side. This may be an attempt to reduce pain by shifting the body weight over the affected hip. It is often also somewhat confusingly referred to as an abductor or Trendelenberg lurch. It is not invariably associated with a positive Trendelenberg sign.

Gluteal muscle function. Test the power of the abductors of the hip with the patient lying on the side, attempting to abduct the leg against resistance (left). Gluteus maximus may also be tested with the patient prone: ask him to extend the hip against resistance, at the same time feeling the tone in the contracting muscle.

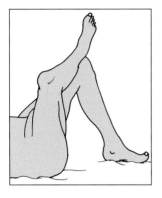

Patrick's test for early osteoarthritis. Basically, this is a variation of abducting the hip from a position of 90° flexion. Pain during the manoeuvre is regarded as being the very first sign of osteoarthritis in a hip. To perform (on the right), flex both hips and knees, place the right foot on the left knee, and gently press down on the right knee. This is also known as the fabere sign (**F**lexion, **AB**duction, **E**xternal **R**otation, **E**xtension).

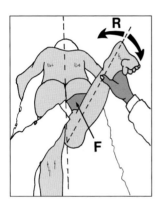

Assessing anteversion of the femoral neck. With the patient prone, flex the knee on the side being examined to 90°. Holding the leg with one hand, rock it from side to side (**R**) while simultaneously feeling the prominence of the greater trochanter with the other (**F**). When the trochanter is facing truly laterally, anteversion is equal to the angle between the leg and the vertical. This is the most accurate method of assessing anteversion.

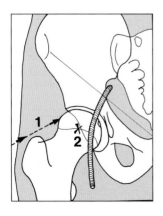

Aspiration. The hip may be aspirated by inserting a needle above the trochanter (**1**), allowing for femoral neck anteversion. Alternatively, a needle may be passed into the joint from in front, a little below the inguinal ligament and lateral to the femoral artery (**2**).

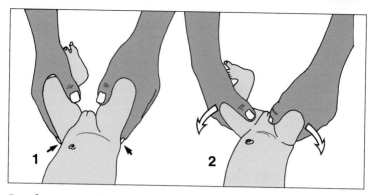

Developmental dislocation of the hip (DDH)

Ortolani's test. The examination must be carried out on a relaxed child, preferably after feeding. Flex the knees and encircle them with the hands so that the thumbs lie along the medial sides of the thighs and the fingers over the trochanters (1). Now flex the hips to a right angle, and starting from a position where the thumbs are touching, smoothly and gently abduct the hips (2).

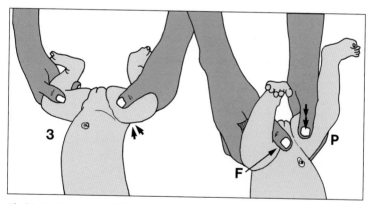

If a hip is dislocated, as full abduction is approached, the femoral head will be felt slipping in to the acetabulum (3). An audible click may accompany the displacement, but in no way must this be considered an essential element of the test. Note that restriction of abduction may be pathological and may represent an *irreducible* dislocation.

Barlow's provocative test. If the Ortolani test is negative the hip may nevertheless be unstable. Fix the pelvis between symphysis and sacrum with one hand (**F**). With the thumb of the other, attempt to dislocate the hip by gentle but firm backward pressure (**P**). Check both sides. If the head of the femur is felt to sublux backwards, its reduction should be achieved, either by reversing the direction of finger pressure or by wider abduction of the hip.

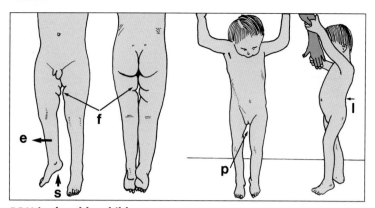

DDH in the older child

Posture and gait. The affected leg in a case of unilateral congenital dislocation of the hip may appear slightly shorter (s) and lie in external rotation (e); there may be asymmetry of the skin folds in the thigh (f), a sign of limited reliability. If both hips are involved, there is usually widening of the perineum (p). If the child has been walking, there will be a compensatory increase in lumbar lordosis (l). Trendelenberg's test will be positive, and in walking there will be excessive shoulder sway, with a gait dipping to the affected side in unilateral cases and waddling in bilateral cases.

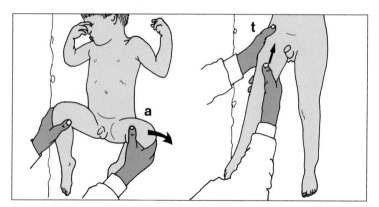

Hip abduction. Test the range of abduction (a) from a position of 90° flexion of the hip. Abduction is restricted in DDH in this position, and of course is most obvious in the unilateral case. Less than 60° of abduction is regarded as being of particular significance.

Telescoping. Attempt to elicit telescoping in the affected limb (t). Steady the pelvis with one hand, and push and pull along the axis of the femur with the other. Abnormal excursion of the limb is suggestive of DDH, but always compare the sides.

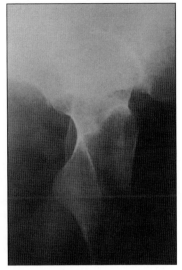

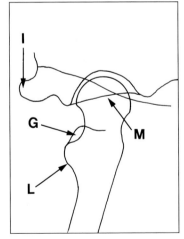

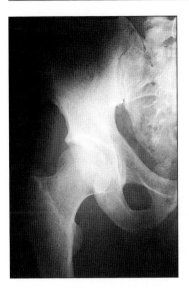

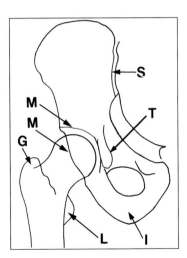

RADIOGRAPHS

The standard projections are the AP and lateral, but for simple screening, an AP projection of the pelvis allows direct comparison of the hips and is the most useful single investigation. Many prefer these three views to be taken routinely. Note the greater trochanter (**G**), lesser trochanter (**L**), sacroiliac joint (**S**), 'tear-drop' (**T**), acetabular margin (**M**) and ischium (**I**).

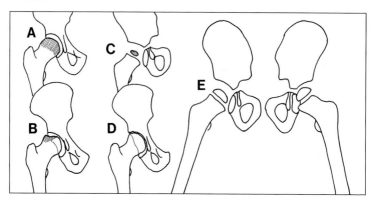

In the films, note in the first place any disturbance of bone texture (e.g. Paget's disease, osteoporosis or tumour), and note the relative *density* of the femoral head which may be *increased* in avascular necrosis (**A**), segmental avascular necrosis (**B**) and Perthes' disease (**C**). It may be *decreased* in rheumatoid arthritis, infection, and osteoporosis. Now note the joint space (which indicates the depth of articular cartilage and interposing fluid): this may be *decreased* in the later stages of infection and arthritis (**D**), and *increased* in Perthes' disease, synovitis and the early stages of infection (**E**).

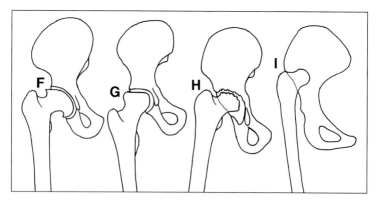

Examine the *shape of the femoral head* which may be, for example: (**F**) *buffer-shaped* after Perthes' disease, (**G**) *flattened* after avascular necrosis (total or segmental), (**H**) *irregular* or *destroyed* after infection, or (**I**) *atrophic* in persistent developmental dislocation of the hip.

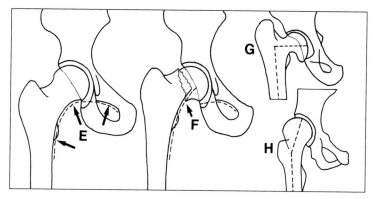

Note *Shenton's line* (**E**) which normally forms a smooth curve flowing from the superior pubic ramus to the femoral neck. Compare the sides if possible. Distortion occurs in many conditions involving the femoral neck and head, particularly fractures (**F**) and subluxations. Note the neck/shaft angle (normal: males = 128°, females = 127°). It is *decreased* in congenital coxa vara (**G**), and coxa vara secondary to rickets, Paget's disease, osteomalacia, fracture, etc. It is *increased* in coxa valga secondary to polio (**H**) and other neurological disturbances.

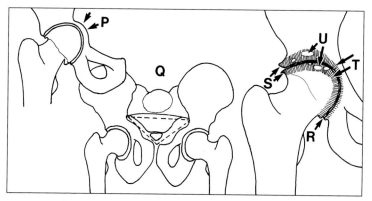

Note any *pelvic distortion*, such as in protrusio acetabuli (**P**) (which is often hereditary and accompanied by osteoarthritis) and in osteomalacia (**Q**) (and other diseases accompanied by bone softening, e.g. rickets and Paget's disease) which may lead to a so-called tri-radiate pelvis.

Note any evidence of *osteoarthritis*, such as joint space narrowing (**R**), marginal osteophytes (lipping) (**S**), marginal sclerosis (**T**) or cystic changes in the femoral head and acetabulum (**U**). Complete obliteration of the hip joint is a feature of ankylosing spondylitis and advanced joint infections.

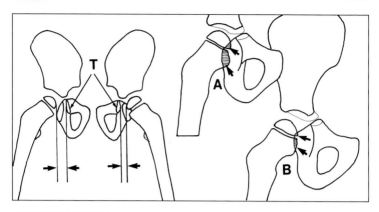

PERTHES' DISEASE

Earliest signs. The earliest radiographic sign is an *increase* in joint space: this is also a feature of synovitis of the hip and infective arthritis. Minor degrees of joint widening may be detected by comparing the distances between the 'tear drops' (**T**) and tangents to the femoral heads. If the 'tear drop' (which is formed by the anterior acetabular floor) is not clear, note (**A**) the overlap shadows of the head and neck on the acetabulum, comparing one hip with the other. Their relative decrease (**B**) is suggestive of joint distension.

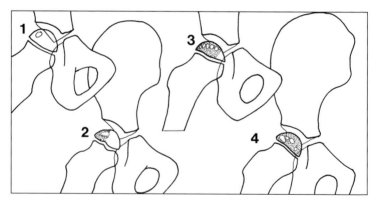

Catterall grading of Perthes' disease. This is the commonest method of assessing the severity of bone changes when they appear. **Grade 1:** cyst formation occurs in the anterolateral aspect of the capital epiphysis. Revascularisation may be completed without bone collapse, and the prognosis without treatment is good. **Grade 2:** a little more of the head is involved, and bony collapse is inevitable. **Grade 3:** most of the head is involved. **Grade 4:** the whole head is affected. Bony collapse is inevitable in grades 3 and 4, and the prognosis in these groups is poorer.

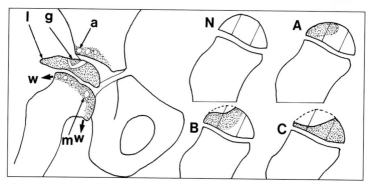

Other radiographic changes in Perthes' disease. Cysts may also appear in the acetabulum (**a**) and the metaphysis (**m**) which may widen (**w**). The femoral head often flattens and extrudes laterally (**l**). A sequestrum (**g**) which is surrounded by a 'V' of viable epiphysis may form (positive Gage sign). Lateral extrusions may be expressed as a percentage of the diameter of the metaphysis on the normal side.

Herring lateral pillar classification. During the fragmentation stage, divide the head in the AP radiograph into three columns (**N**); then if the lateral one is of normal height (Herring **A**) the prognosis is excellent. If it is depressed by up to 50% (even with the central column involved), Herring **B**, the results are generally good under age 9. In Herring **C**, the lateral pillar is less than 50%, and all develop permanent deformity.

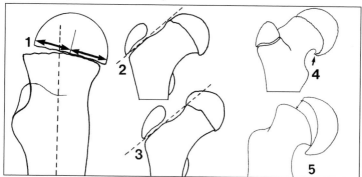

Slipped femoral epiphysis

The earliest signs are in the lateral projection. A line drawn up through the centre of the neck fails to meet the midpoint of the base of the epiphysis (**1**). Later, in the anteroposterior view, the first sign is that a tangent to the proximal femoral neck fails to strike the epiphysis (**2**) (while in a normal well-centred view, such a tangent (**3**) includes part of the epiphysis). Some weeks after the initial slip (so-called 'chronic slip' stage), there is distortion of the inferior part of the femoral neck with new bone formation ('buttressing') (**4**). So-called physeal separation (**5**), present in a minority, is associated with a high incidence of avascular necrosis.

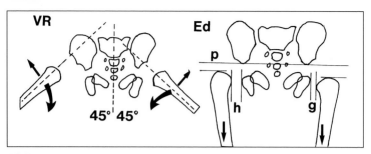

DDH
Radiographic examination of the neonate. Because of a degree of
unreliability and the risks of unnecessary radiation, reserve this for the
suspicious but uncertain case only. *Van Rosen method* (**VR**). An anteroposterior
view should be taken with the hips in at least 45° abduction and full internal
rotation. On the films, a line projected along the line of the femur in the normal
hip should strike the acetabulum, and in a case of dislocation, the region of the
anterior superior spine. *Edinburgh method* (**Ed**). An AP film is taken with the
child's legs held parallel, with slight traction and no external rotation. Centre the
beam at a standard distance of 100 cm. Measure the gap between the most
medial part of the femur and the lateral edge of the ischium (**g**): this is normally
about 4 mm. Over 5 mm (**h**) is suspicious; 6 mm is regarded as diagnostic of
DDH. Proximal migration (**p**) can also be measured in the same film.

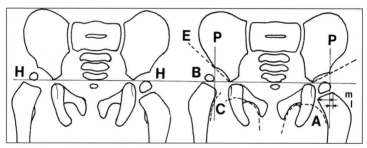

The older child. Draw a horizontal (**H**, Hilgenreimer) line across the pelvis.
On each side this should touch the downward pointing apex of the acetabular
element of the ilium. Draw vertical (**P**, Perkins) lines from the lateral limits of
each acetabulum. These divide each hip region into four. The epiphysis of the
femoral head should normally lie within the lower and inner quadrant (**A**), but in
DDH the head moves upwards and outwards (as at **B**). Note that the ossification
centre for the femoral head normally appears between 2 and 8 months, but is
often delayed in DDH. Shenton's line (**C**) may be disturbed. Dysplasia of the
acetabulum *increases* its slope (**E**). (In the normal hip the slope *decreases* with
growth from a normal of about 30°.) Assessment of MeP, the percentage lateral
displacement of the metaphysis (l/m × 100), is a reliable and valuable measure of
hip development. Additional information regarding the head, acetabulum and
limbus may be obtained by MRI scans or contrast arthrography.

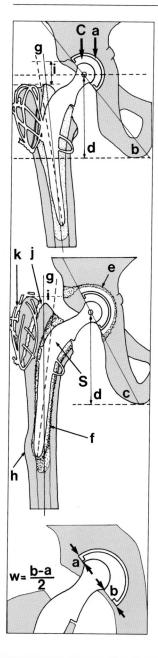

Total hip replacements

Component loosening and other problems (Charnley low friction arthroplasty illustrated):

The cup (C). The wire marker (**a**) sunk within the radiolucent cup aids the analysis of any radiographic series. The plane of the socket lies at an angle (**b**) to the plane of the pelvis, shown by a line drawn between the ischial tuberosities. This angle may be altered (**c**) by rotation of the cup if it loosens. The cup may also migrate proximally: look for any disturbance in the relationship between the wire marker and the fixed landmarks of the pelvis. An increase in the distance (**d**) between the centre of the cup and the ischium may be suggestive of migration, although errors of positioning and tube/film distances make this a little unreliable. Development of a radiolucent zone (**e**) (between cement and bone) exceeding 1 mm and extending right round the cup is a strong indicator of loosening. (Note that the appearance of a radiolucent line between the cement and a component is *diagnostic* of loosening.)

The stem (S). In detecting loosening, look for a radiolucent zone of more than 1 mm between cement and bone (**f**) or between the stem and the cement. Note any change in the angle between the axes of the femur and prosthetic stem (**g**), or any local bone disturbance (**h**). Check for sinking of the prosthesis by noting the distance between the greater trochanter (**i**) and the upper edge of the acetabulum. Non-union of the greater trochanter (**j**), and fracture and fragmentation (**k**) of any wires used to re-attach the trochanter should also be recorded.

Component wear (w). To assess, measure the gaps between the prosthetic head and the wire marker at their upper (**a**) and lower (**b**) limits. Half the difference between these is a measure of wear in the wall of the cup: 3 mm is indicative of an appreciable amount of wear.

REPRESENTATIVE RADIOGRAPHS

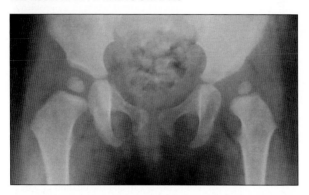

Developmental dislocation of the left hip (right side of illustration) with lateral and proximal displacement of the proximal femoral epiphysis.

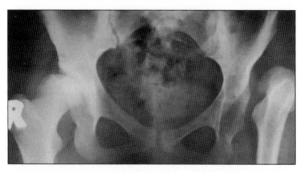

Untreated developmental dislocation of the left hip; dysplasia right hip, with a shallow, sloping acetabulum and early osteoarthritis.

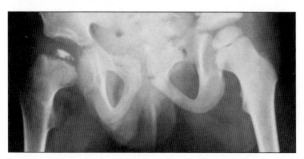

Perthes' disease, with a small, dense capital epiphysis and metaphyseal broadening.

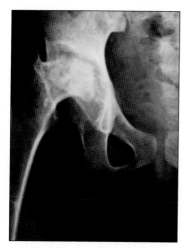 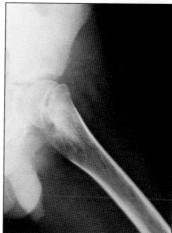

Left: Infective arthritis (tuberculosis) of the hip with gross destruction.
Right: Slipped femoral epiphysis (lateral X-ray projection of the hip).

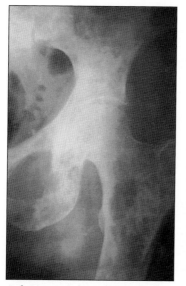 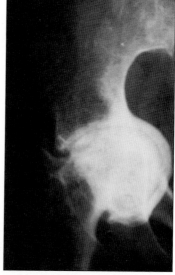

Left: Metastatic bone disease. *Right:* Protrusio acetabuli and osteoarthritis.

CHAPTER

10
The knee

Common pathology around
the knee 138
How to diagnose a knee
complaint 144
Assessment 147
Radiographs 165

COMMON PATHOLOGY ABOUT THE KNEE

Swelling of the knee

The knee may become swollen as a result of the accumulation within the joint cavity of excess synovial fluid, blood or pus (synovitis, haemarthrosis, pyarthrosis). Much less commonly the knee swells beyond the limits of the synovial membrane. This is seen in soft tissue injuries of the knee when haematoma formation and oedema may be extensive. It is also a feature of fractures, infections and tumours of the distal femur, where confusion may result either from the proximity of the lesion to the joint or because it involves the joint cavity directly.

Synovitis, effusion

The synovial membrane secretes the synovial fluid of the joint; excess synovial fluid indicates some affection of the membrane. Joint injuries cause synovitis by tearing or stretching the synovial membrane. Infections act directly by eliciting an inflammatory response. The membrane itself becomes thickened and its function disturbed in rheumatoid arthritis and villo-nodular synovitis; both are usually accompanied by large effusions. In long-standing meniscus lesions and in osteoarthritis of the knee, the synovial membrane may not be directly affected, and no effusion may be present. The recognition of fluid in the joint is of great importance. Effusion indicates damage to the joint, and the presence of a major lesion must always be eliminated. A tense synovitis may be aspirated to relieve discomfort.

Haemarthrosis

Blood in the knee is seen most commonly where there is tearing of vascular structures. The menisci are avascular, and there may be no haemarthrosis when a meniscus is torn. Bleeding into the joint will take place, however, if the meniscus has been detached at its periphery or if there is accompanying damage to other structures within the knee (e.g. the cruciate ligaments).

Pyarthrosis

Infections of the knee joint are rather uncommon, and usually blood-borne. Sometimes the joint is involved by direct spread from an osteitis of the femur or tibia; rarely the joint becomes infected following surgery or penetrating wounds.

In acute pyogenic infections, the onset is usually rapid and the knee very painful; swelling is tense, tenderness is widespread, and movement resisted. There is pyrexia and general malaise. Pyogenic infections in patients suffering from rheumatoid arthritis have often a much slower onset, often with suppressed inflammatory changes if the patient is receiving steroids.

Tuberculous infections of the knee (now relatively uncommon in the UK), have a slow onset, spread over weeks. The knee appears small and globular, with the associated profound quadriceps wasting contributing to this appearance. In gonococcal arthritis, great pain and tenderness (often apparently out of proportion to the local swelling and other signs), are the striking features of this condition.

When it is thought that there is pus in a joint, aspiration should be carried out to empty it and obtain specimens for bacteriological examination. If tuberculosis is suspected, synovial biopsy to obtain specimens for culture and histology is required.

The extensor mechanism of the knee

Extension of the knee is produced by the quadriceps muscle acting through the quadriceps ligament, patella, patellar ligament and tibial tubercle. *Weakness of extension* leads to instability, repeated joint trauma and effusion. There is often a vicious circle of pain → quadriceps inhibition → quadriceps wasting → knee instability → ligament stretching and further injury → pain. *Loss of full extension* also leads to instability, as there is failure of the screw-home mechanism.

Rapid wasting of the quadriceps is seen in all painful and inflammatory conditions of the knee. Weakness of the quadriceps is also sometimes found in lesions of the upper lumbar intervertebral discs, as a sequel to poliomyelitis, in multiple sclerosis and other neurological disorders, and in the myopathies. Quadriceps wasting may be the presenting feature of a diabetic neuropathy or secondary to femoral nerve palsy from an iliacus haematoma.

The term 'jumper's knee' is used to describe a number of conditions where there is pain in the patellar ligament or its insertion: it includes the *Sinding–Larsen–Johansson* syndrome, seen in children in the 10–14 age group, where there are X-ray changes in the distal pole of the patella. Note also *Osgood Schlatter's disease* (often thought to be due to a partial avulsion of the tibial tuberosity) which occurs in the 10–16 age group. In it there is recurrent pain over the tibial tuberosity, which becomes tender and prominent. Radiographs may show partial detachment or fragmentation. Pain generally ceases with closure of the epiphysis. In an older age group (16–30) the patellar ligament itself may become painful and tender. This almost invariably occurs in athletes, and there may be a history of giving-way of the knee. CT scans may show changes in the patellar ligament, the centre of which becomes expanded. (Disruption of the extensor mechanism is described later in Chapter 25.)

The ligaments of the knee

The cruciate, collateral, posterior and capsular ligaments, and the menisci form an integrated stabilising system which prevents the tibia from shifting or tilting under the femur in an abnormal fashion. It is important to detect ligament injuries as they may account for appreciable disability in the form of incidents of giving way of the joint, recurrent effusion, lack of confidence in the knee, difficulty in undertaking strenuous or athletic activities and sometimes trouble in using stairs or walking on uneven ground. The diagnosis and interpretation of instability in the knee is difficult as the main structures round the knee have primary and secondary supportive functions, and several may be damaged. Acute injuries are described in Chapter 25.

The medial ligament and capsule. The medial ligament has superficial and deep layers. Considerable violence is required to damage it. If only a few fibres are torn, no instability will be demonstrated, but stretching the ligament will cause pain. With greater violence, the whole of the deep part of the ligament ruptures, followed in order by the superficial part, the medial capsule, the posterior ligament, the posterior cruciate ligament and sometimes finally the anterior cruciate ligament. Minor tears of the medial ligament in the older patient may be followed eventually by calcification in the accompanying haematoma, and this may give rise to sharply localised pain at the upper attachment (Pellegrini–Stieda disease).

The lateral ligament and capsule. This ligament may be damaged by blows on the medial side of the knee which throw it into varus. As in the case of the medial ligament, increasing violence will lead to tearing of the posterior capsular ligament and the cruciates. In addition, the common peroneal nerve may be stretched and sometimes irreversibly damaged.

The anterior cruciate ligament. Impaired anterior cruciate ligament function is seen most frequently in association with tears of the medial meniscus. In some cases this is due to progressive stretching and attrition rupture. In others, the anterior cruciate ligament tears at the same time as the meniscus, and in the most severe injuries the medial ligament may also be affected (O'Donoghue's triad). Isolated ruptures of the anterior cruciate ligament are uncommon, but do occur.

Chronic laxity generally results from old injuries, and may cause problems from acute, chronic or recurrent tibial subluxations. There may be a history of giving way of the knee, episodic pain, and functional impairment. There is often quadriceps wasting and effusion, and secondary osteoarthritis may develop.

The posterior cruciate ligament. Posterior cruciate ligament tears are produced when in a flexed knee the tibia is forcibly pushed backwards (as for example in a car accident when the upper part of the shin strikes the dashboard). Instability is not uncommon, often leading if untreated to osteoarthritis of rapid onset.

Rotatory instability in the knee: tibial condylar subluxations. In this group of conditions, when the knee is stressed, the tibia may sublux forwards or backwards on either the medial or lateral side, giving rise to pain and a feeling of instability in the joint. The main forms are as follows:

1. *The medial tibial condyle subluxes anteriorly* (anteromedial rotatory instability). In the most severe cases, this follows tears of both the anterior cruciate ligament and the medial ligament and capsule. The medial meniscus may also be damaged and contribute to the instability.
2. *The lateral tibial condyle subluxes anteriorly* (anterolateral rotatory instability). In the more severe cases, the anterior cruciate ligament and the lateral structures are torn, and there may be an associated lesion of the anterior horn of the lateral meniscus.
3. *The lateral tibial condyle subluxes posteriorly* (posterolateral rotatory instability). This may follow rupture of the lateral and posterior cruciate ligaments.
4. *Combinations of these lesions* (particularly 1 and 2, and 2 and 3) may be found, especially where there is major ligamentous disruption of the knee.

Lesions of the menisci
Congenital discoid meniscus. This abnormality, most frequently involving the lateral meniscus, commonly presents in childhood. It may produce a very pronounced clicking from the lateral compartment, a block to extension of the joint and other derangement signs.

Meniscus tears in the young adult. The commonest cause is a sporting injury, when a twisting strain is applied to the flexed, weight-bearing leg. The trapped meniscus commonly splits longitudinally, and its free edge may displace inwards towards the centre of the joint (bucket-handle tear). This prevents full extension (with physiological locking of the joint), and if an attempt is made to straighten the knee, a painful elastic resistance is felt ('springy block to full extension'). In the case of the medial meniscus, prolonged loss of full extension may lead to stretching and eventual rupture of the anterior cruciate ligament.

Degenerative meniscus lesions in the middle-aged. Loss of elasticity in the menisci through degenerative changes associated with the ageing process may give rise to horizontal cleavage tears within the substance of the meniscus; these tears may not be associated with any remembered traumatic incident, and sharply localised tenderness in the joint line is a common feature.

Cysts of the menisci. Ganglion-like cysts occur in both menisci, but are much more common in the lateral. Medial meniscus cysts must be carefully distinguished from ganglions arising from the pes anserinus (the insertion of sartorius, gracilis and semitendinosus). In true cysts there is often a history of a blow on the side of the knee over the meniscus. They are tender, and as they restrict the mobility of the menisci, they render them more susceptible to tears.

Patellofemoral instability. The patella has always a tendency to lateral dislocation as the tibial tuberosity lies lateral to the dynamic axis of the quadriceps. Normally, at the beginning of knee flexion, the patella engages in the groove separating the two femoral condyles (the trochlea), which helps to keep it in place as flexion continues. This system may be disturbed in a number of ways: there may be an abnormal lateral insertion of the quadriceps, tight lateral structures, or an increase in the angle between the axis of the quadriceps and the line of the patellar ligament (e.g. as a result of knock-knee deformity or by a broad pelvis); the lateral condyle may be deficient, or the patella itself may be small and poorly formed (hypoplasia) or highly placed (patella alta). This is often associated with genu recurvatum. (Note that a low set patella—known as patella baja or infera—is uncommon and may follow certain surgical corrective procedures. It is not associated with any patellar instability.)

There are a number of conditions characterised by loss of normal patellar alignment:

- *Acute traumatic dislocation of the patella.* This injury most frequently occurs in adolescent females during athletic activities.
- *Recurrent lateral dislocation.* Further painful dislocations of the patella occur, often with increasing frequency and ease.
- *Congenital dislocation of the patella.* The patella may be dislocated at birth in association with other congenital abnormalities. The dislocation is irreducible.
- *Habitual dislocation of the patella.* The patella dislocates every time the knee flexes, and this is pain free. It often arises in childhood and may be due to an abnormal attachment of the iliotibial tract, from fibrosis in a quadriceps muscle, or as a feature of one of the joint laxity syndromes.
- *Permanent dislocation of the patella.* This is uncommon and may result from an untreated childhood or adolescent dislocation.

Retropatellar pain syndromes/chondromalacia patellae

These are characterised by chronic ill-localised pain at the front of the knee, often made worse by prolonged sitting, or walking on slopes or stairs. It is commonest in females in the 15–35 age group, and the pathology is often uncertain. In a number of cases there is softening or fibrillation of the articular cartilage lining the patella (chondromalacia patellae), and this may lead to patellofemoral osteoarthritis. There may be no obvious precipitating cause, but in some there is evidence of patellofemoral malalignment or other of the factors responsible for recurrent dislocation (even although there may be no history of frank dislocation).

Osteochondritis dissecans

This occurs most frequently in males in the second decade of life, and most commonly involves the medial femoral condyle. A segment of bone undergoes avascular necrosis, and a line of demarcation becomes established between it and the underlying healthy bone. Complete separation may occur so that a loose body is formed. The symptoms are initially of aching pain and recurring effusion, with perhaps locking of the joint if a loose body is present.

Fat pad injuries

The infrapatellar fat pads may become tender and swollen, and may give rise to pain on extension of the knee, especially if they are nipped between the articulating surfaces of femur and tibia. This may occur as a complication of osteoarthritis, but is seen more frequently in young women when the fat pads swell in association with premenstrual fluid retention.

Loose bodies

Loose bodies are seen most often as a sequel to osteoarthritis or osteochondritis dissecans. Much less commonly, numerous loose bodies are formed by an abnormal synovial membrane in the condition of synovial chondromatosis.

Osteoarthritis

The stresses of weight-bearing mainly involve the medial compartment of the knee, and it is in this area that *primary* osteoarthritis usually first occurs. Being overweight, the degenerative changes accompanying old age, and overwork are common factors. *Secondary* osteoarthritis may follow ligament and meniscus injuries, recurrent dislocation of the patella, osteochondritis dissecans, joint infections and other previous pathology. It is seen in association with knock-knee and bow-leg deformities, which throw additional mechanical stresses on the joint.

In osteoarthritis, the articular cartilage becomes progressively thinner, leading to joint space narrowing. The subarticular bone may become eburnated, and often small marginal osteophytes and cysts are formed. Exposure of bone and free nerve endings gives rise to pain and crepitus on movement. Distortion of the joint surfaces may lead to loss of movement and fixed flexion deformities.

Rheumatoid arthritis

Characteristically, the knee is warm to touch, there is effusion, limitation of movements, muscle wasting, synovial thickening, tenderness and pain. Fixed flexion, valgus and (less commonly) varus deformities are quite common.

Generally other joints are also involved, although the monoarticular form is occasionally seen.

Reiter's syndrome
This usually presents as a chronic effusion accompanied by discomfort in the joint. It is often bilateral, with an associated conjunctivitis, and there may be a history of urethritis or colitis.

Ankylosing spondylitis
The first symptoms of ankylosing spondylitis are generally in the spine, but occasionally the condition presents at the periphery, with swelling and discomfort in the knee joint. Stiffness of the spine and radiographic changes in the sacroiliac joints are nevertheless almost invariably present.

Disturbances of alignment
Genu varum (bow leg). This commonly occurs as a growth abnormality of early childhood, and usually resolves spontaneously. Rarely genu varum is caused by a growth disturbance involving both the tibial epiphysis and proximal tibial shaft (tibia vara). In adults genu varum most frequently results from osteoarthritis, where there is narrowing of the medial joint compartment. It also occurs in Paget's disease and rickets. It is less common in rheumatoid arthritis.

Genu valgum (knock knee). This occurs most frequently in young children where it is usually associated with flat foot. Nearly all cases resolve spontaneously by the age of 6. It is also seen in plump adolescent females and may be a contributory factor in recurrent dislocation of the patella. In adults, it most frequently occurs in rheumatoid arthritis, after uncorrected depressed fractures of the lateral tibial table, and as a sequel to a number of paralytic neurological disorders where there is ligament stretching and altered epiphyseal growth.

Genu recurvatum. Hyperextension at the knee is seen after ruptures of the anterior cruciate ligament and in girls where the growth of the upper tibial epiphysis may be retarded from much point work in ballet classes or from the wearing of high heeled shoes in early adolescence. In the latter cases there is corresponding elevation of the patella (patella alta), contributing to a tendency to recurrent dislocation or chondromalacia patellae. More rarely, the deformity is seen in congenital joint laxity, poliomyelitis and Charcot's disease.

Bursitis
Cystic swelling occurring in the popliteal region is usually referred to as enlargement of the semimembranosus bursa. This may communicate with the knee joint, and fluctuate in size. Rupture may lead to the appearance of bruising on the dorsum of the foot, and this may help to distinguish it from deep venous thrombosis or cellulitis. Fluctuant bursal swellings may also occur over the patella (prepatellar bursitis or housemaid's knee) or the patellar ligament (infrapatellar bursitis or clergyman's knee). Chronic prepatellar bursitis, with or without local infection, is common in miners where it is referred to as 'beat knee'; it is also associated with other occupations where prolonged kneeling is unavoidable (e.g. it is common in plumbers and carpet layers).

HOW TO DIAGNOSE A KNEE COMPLAINT

1. *Note the patient's age and sex,* bearing in mind the following important distribution of the common knee conditions.

Age Group	Males	Females
0–12	Discoid lateral meniscus	Discoid lateral meniscus
12–18	Osteochondritis dissecans	First incident of recurrent dislocation of the patella
	Osgood–Schlatter's disease	Osgood–Schlatter's disease
18–30	Longitudinal meniscal tears	Recurrent dislocation of the patella
		Chondromalacia patellae
		Fat pad injury
30–50	Rheumatoid arthritis	Rheumatoid arthritis
40–55	Degenerative meniscus lesions	Degenerative meniscus lesions
45+	Osteoarthritis	Osteoarthritis

Infections are comparatively uncommon and occur in both sexes in all age groups. Reiter's syndrome occurs in adults of both sexes; ankylosing spondylitis nearly always occurs in male adults. Ligamentous and extensor apparatus injuries are rare in children.

2. *Find out if the knee swells.* An effusion indicates the presence of pathology which must be investigated. (Note, however, that the *absence* of effusion does not necessarily eliminate significant pathology.)

3. *Try to establish whether there is a mechanical problem* (internal derangement) accounting for the patient's symptoms. Do this by:

- *Obtaining a convincing history of an initiating injury*. Note the degree of violence, and its direction. The initial incapacity is important: for example, a footballer is unlikely to be able to finish a game with a freshly torn meniscus. Note whether there was bruising (not a feature of meniscal injuries) or swelling after the injury, and whether the patient was able to weight-bear.

- *Asking if the knee 'gives way'*. 'Giving way' of the knee on going down stairs or jumping from a height follows cruciate ligament tears, loss of full extension in the knee and quadriceps wasting. 'Giving way' on twisting movements or walking on uneven ground follows many meniscus injuries.

- *Asking if the knee 'locks'*. Patients often confuse stiffness and true locking. Ask the patient to show the position the knee is in if it locks. *Remember that the knee never locks in full extension.* Locking which is due to a torn meniscus generally allows the joint to be flexed fully or nearly fully, but the last 10° to 40° of extension are impossible. Attempts to obtain full extension are accompanied by pain. Ask what produces any locking. With long-standing meniscus lesions, a slight rotational force, such as the foot catching on the edge of a carpet, may be quite sufficient. In chronic lesions, weight-bearing is not an essential factor, locking not infrequently occurring during sleep. If the knee is not locked at the time of the patient's attendance, ask how it became free: unlocking with a click is suggestive of a meniscus lesion. Locking from a loose body may occur in various degrees of flexion; there may be deformity with locking from a dislocating patella.

- *Asking about pain.* Find out the circumstances in which it is present and ask the patient if he can localise it by pointing to the site with one finger.

Additional investigations

Occasionally a firm diagnosis cannot be made on the basis of the history and clinical examination alone. The following additional investigations are often helpful:

Suspected internal derangement

Arthroscopy: may give much useful information, and in conjunction with the clinical examination will permit a firm, accurate diagnosis to be made in the majority of cases. Incorrect diagnoses are most common in lesions involving the menisci in their posterior thirds. An increasing number of conditions are amenable to arthroscopic surgery which can often be performed after diagnostic arthroscopy as a follow-on procedure during the same session.

MRI scans: can be useful in diagnosing lesion of the menisci and ligaments where there is uncertainty. Although an accuracy of 90% is claimed, there is often an increase in the signal intensity in the region of the posterior third of the medial meniscus which can lead to false interpretations.

Arthrography: may be helpful, although interpretation of the radiographs is specialised and often difficult.

Examination under anaesthesia. If pain prevents full examination (e.g. by preventing flexion) anaesthesia may allow this to be performed. This may be followed up by arthroscopy.

Suspected acute infections
- Aspiration and culture of the synovial fluid.
- Blood culture.
- Full blood count, including differential white count, and estimation of the sedimentation rate and C-reactive protein.

Suspected tuberculosis of the knee
- Chest radiograph.
- Synovial biopsy, with specimens of synovial membrane being sent for both histological and bacteriological examination. At the same time, synovial fluid specimens are also sent for bacteriology and sensitivities.
- Mantoux test.

Suspected rheumatoid arthritis
- Examination of other joints.
- Estimations of rheumatoid factor.
- Full blood count and sedimentation rate.
- Serum uric acid.

Further investigation of poor mineralisation, bone erosions, etc.
- Estimation of serum calcium, phosphate and alkaline phosphatase.
- Estimation of rheumatoid factor.
- Serum uric acid.
- Full blood count and differential count.
- Skeletal survey and chest radiograph.
- Radioisotope scan.
- Bone biopsy.

Further investigation of chronic effusion, aspirate negative
- Tests as for suspected rheumatoid arthritis.
- Brucellosis agglutination tests.
- Radiography of the chest and sacroiliac joints.
- Arthroscopy and synovial biopsy.

Further investigation of severe undiagnosed pain
- X-ray examination of the chest, pelvis and hips.
- Arthroscopy or exploration.

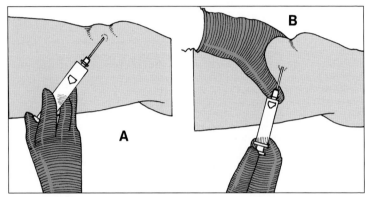

Aspiration of the knee joint. Indications include the presence of a tense haemarthrosis or to obtain specimens for bacteriology in suspected infections. Begin, using full aseptic precautions, by raising a skin weal with local anaesthetic just above and lateral to the patella (**A**). Infiltrate the tissues more deeply down to the level of the synovial membrane of the suprapatellar pouch. Unless the knee is very tense, squeeze fluid from the upper limits of the suprapatellar pouch to float the patella forwards before inserting the aspiration needle (**B**). Squeeze the superior aspect and sides of the joint during the terminal stages of aspiration.

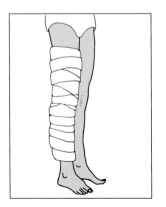

Unless other treatment is contemplated, after withdrawal of the needle and application of a sterile dressing, apply a Jones compression bandage. This consists of several layers (2–4) of wool in the form of wool roll, gamgee, or cotton wool sheets, each held in place with firmly, but not tightly, applied calico, domette or crepe bandaging. (Its main function is to comfortably limit flexion of the joint.)

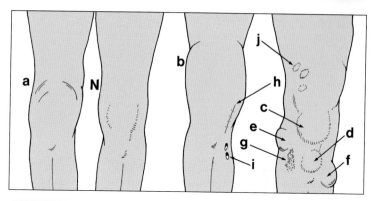

ASSESSMENT

Inspection

Swelling. If there is any swelling, note if it is confined to the limits of the synovial cavity and suprapatellar pouch (**a**), suggesting effusion, haemarthrosis, pyarthrosis or a space-occupying lesion in the joint. Note if any swelling extends beyond the limits of the joint cavity (**b**), suggesting infection (of the joint, femur or tibia), tumour or major injury. Examine any local swelling, e.g. (**c**) prepatellar bursitis (housemaid's knee); (**d**) infrapatellar bursitis (clergyman's knee); (**e**) meniscus cyst, occurring in the joint line; (**f**) diaphyseal aclasis (exostosis, often multiple and sometimes familial).

Skin appearance. Note any bruising (**g**) which suggests trauma to the superficial tissues, or knee ligaments. Bruising is not usually seen in meniscus injuries. Redness suggests inflammation. Note (**h**) scars of previous injury or surgery—the relevant history must be obtained; (**i**) sinus scars are indicative of previous infections, often of bone, and with the potential for reactivation; (**j**) evidence of psoriasis, with the possibility of psoriatic arthritis. In beat knee there is chronic bursal enlargement, with thickening of the overlying skin.

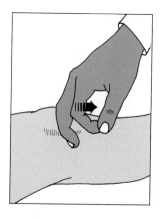

Temperature. Note any increased local heat and its extent, suggesting in particular rheumatoid arthritis or infection. There may also be increased local heat as part of the inflammatory response to injury, and in the presence of rapidly growing tumours. Always compare the two sides. A warm knee and cold foot suggest a popliteal artery block. Always make allowance for any warm bandage the patient may have been wearing just prior to the examination, and check the peripheral pulses.

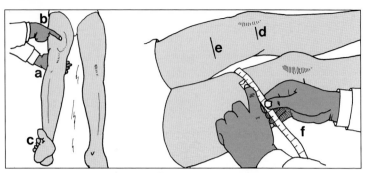

The quadriceps muscle. Slight wasting and loss of bulk are normally apparent on inspection. Proceed to examine the contracted quadriceps by placing a hand behind the knee (**a**) and ask the patient to press against it. The muscle tone may be felt with the free hand (**b**). Now ask the patient to dorsiflex the inverted foot (**c**), to show and feel the tone in the important vastus medialis portion of the muscle.

Substantial wasting may be confirmed by measurement, assuming the other limb is normal. This objective test may be valuable for repeat assessments and in medico-legal cases. Begin by locating the knee joint and marking it (**d**) with a ball-point pen. Make a second mark on the skin 18 cm above this (**e**). Repeat on the other leg. Compare the circumference of the legs at the marked levels (**f**). Wasting of the quadriceps occurs most frequently as the result of disuse, generally from a painful or unstable lesion of the knee, or from infection or rheumatoid arthritis.

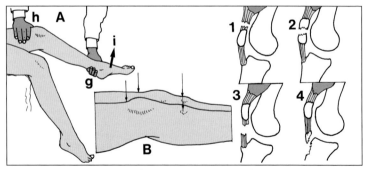

Extensor apparatus. With the patient sitting with his legs over the end of the examination couch (**A**), ask him to straighten the leg while you support the ankle with one hand (**g**). Feel for quadriceps contraction (**h**), and look for active extension of the limb (**i**). Loss of active extension of the knee (excluding paralytic conditions) follows (**1**) rupture of the quadriceps tendon; (**2**) many patellar fractures; (**3**) rupture of the patellar ligament; (**4**) avulsion of the tibial tubercle. The site of the pathology may be determined by looking for tenderness, palpable gaps in the components of the extensor apparatus, and proximal patellar displacement (**B**).

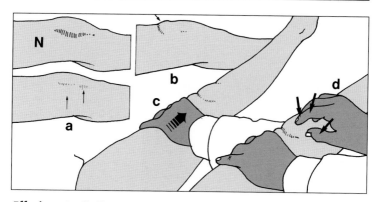

Effusion. Small effusions are detected most easily by inspection. The first signs are bulging at the sides of the patellar ligament and obliteration of the hollows at the medial and lateral edges of the patella (**a**). With greater effusion into the knee the suprapatellar pouch becomes distended (**b**). Effusion indicates synovial irritation from trauma or inflammation.

Patellar tap test. Squeeze any excess fluid out of the suprapatellar pouch with the index and thumb, slid firmly distally from a point about 15 cm above the knee to the level of the upper border of the patella (**c**). Place the tips of the thumb and three fingers of the free hand squarely on the patella, and jerk it quickly downwards (**d**). A click indicates the presence of effusion. N.B. If the effusion is *slight* or *tense*, the tap test will be *negative*.

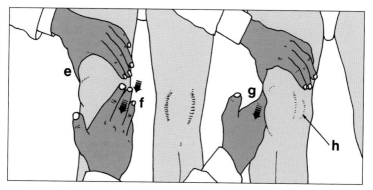

Fluid displacement test. Small effusions may be detected by this manoeuvre. Evacuate the suprapatellar pouch as in the patellar tap test (**e**). Stroke the medial side of the joint to displace any excess fluid in the main joint cavity to the lateral side of the joint (**f**). Now stroke the lateral side of the joint (**g**) while closely watching the medial. Any excess fluid present will be seen to move across the joint and distend the medial side (**h**). This test will be negative if the effusion is gross and tense. In a haemarthrosis, the joint has a doughy feel in the suprapatellar region, while in a pyarthrosis there is widespread tenderness.

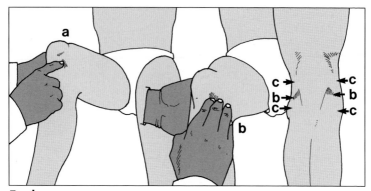

Tenderness

It is the first essential to identify the joint line quite clearly. Begin by flexing the knee and looking for the hollows at the sides of the patellar ligament; these lie over the joint line. Then confirm by feeling with the fingers or thumb for the soft hollow of the joint (**a**), with the firm prominences of the femur above and the tibia below. Begin by palpating carefully from in front and then back along the joint line on each side (**b**). Localised tenderness here is commonest in meniscus, collateral ligament and fat pad injuries. Now systematically examine the upper and lower attachments of the collateral ligaments (**c**). Associated bruising and oedema is a feature of acute injuries.

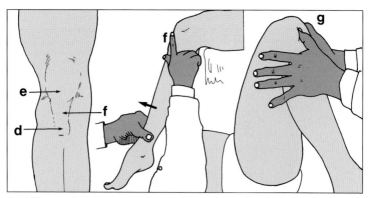

In children and adolescents, tenderness is found over the *tibial tubercle* (**d**) (which may be prominent) in Osgood–Schlatter's disease and after acute avulsion injuries of the patellar ligament and its tibial attachment. Tenderness over the *lower pole of the patella* (**e**) is found in Sinding–Larsen–Johansson disease. Where a problem with the patellar ligament is suspected in an athletic patient, look for *patellar ligament* tenderness (**f**), especially while the patient is attempting to extend the leg against resistance. In suspected osteochondritis dissecans, flex the knee fully and look for tenderness over the *femoral condyles* (**g**). Note that osteochondritis dissecans most frequently involves the medial femoral condyle.

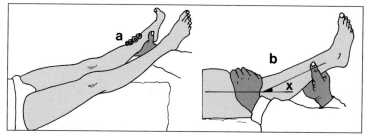

Movements

Extension (normal = 0°). Normally the line of the tibia and femur should coincide, with full extension being recorded as 0°. Loss of full extension may be described as 'the knee lacks X° of extension'. Try to obtain full extension if this is not obviously present (**a**). A springy block to full extension is very suggestive of a bucket handle meniscus tear. A rigid block (commonly described as a fixed flexion deformity) is often present in the arthritic knee. *Hyperextension* (genu recurvatum) is present if the knee extends beyond the point when the tibia and femur are in line (**b**), and is recorded as 'X° hyperextension'. It is often seen in girls associated with a high patella, chondromalacia patellae and recurrent dislocation of the patella. It sometimes accompanies tears of the anterior cruciate, medial ligament, or medial meniscus. If severe, look for other signs of joint laxity.

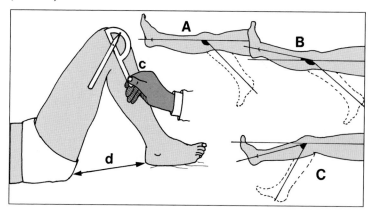

Flexion (normal = 135° or more). Measure the range of flexion using a goniometer (**c**). Flexion of 135° and over is regarded as normal, but compare the two sides. Loss of flexion is common after local trauma, effusion and arthritic conditions. Alternatively, measure the heel to buttock distance (**d**) with the leg fully flexed. (This can be a very accurate way of detecting small alterations in the range, with 1 cm = 1.5° approximately, and is useful for checking daily or weekly progress.) The range of movements in the examples would be recorded as follows: (**A**) 0–135° (normal range); (**B**) 5° hyperextension–140° flexion; (C) 10–60° (or 10° fixed flexion deformity with a further 50° flexion).

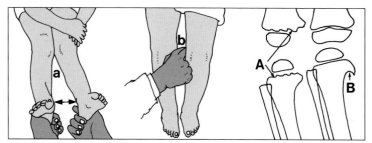

Genu valgum and varus

In children, note if any *genu valgum* (knock knee) is unilateral or bilateral. Assess by bringing the legs together, to touch lightly at the knees (**a**). Normally the knees *and* malleoli should touch. Make sure the patellae are pointing upwards. Measure the intermalleolar gap. In the older 10–16 age group, < 8 cm in females and < 4 cm in males is regarded as normal. *Genu varum* (bow leg) may be assessed by measuring the distance between the knees, using the fingers as a gauge (**b**). The patient should be weight-bearing, and the patellae should be facing forwards. In the 10–16 age group, < 4 cm in females and < 5 cm in males is regarded as being within normal limits. Radiographs may help. In (**A**) *rickets*, note the wide and irregular epiphyseal plates. In (**B**) *tibia vara*, note the sharply down-turned medial metaphyseal border. Note that radiological varus is normal till a child is 18 months old.

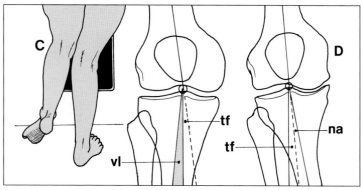

In adults, genu valgum deformity is seen most often in association with rheumatoid arthritis. It is also common in teenage girls. It is best measured by X-ray, and the films should be taken with the patient taking all his weight on the affected side (**C**) (and preferably in 30° flexion). The degree of valgus (**vl**) may be roughly assessed by measuring the angle formed by the tibial and femoral shafts and deducting the 'normal' tibiofemoral angle (**tf**), which is approximately 6° in the adult. The shaded area represents genu valgum. (Note that the tibiofemoral angle is virtually the same as the Q-angle used in the assessment of patellar instability.) *Genu varum* (**D**) may be assessed by adding the 'normal' tibiofemoral to the actual (negative) angle (**na**). It is seen most commonly in osteoarthritis and Paget's disease.

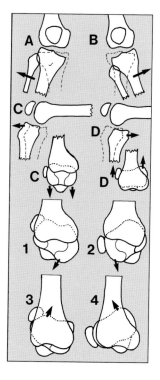

Knee instability

The following *potential* deformities may be looked for: **(A)** *valgus*, (when the medial ligament is torn: severe when the posterior cruciate is also damaged); **(B)** *varus*, (when the lateral ligament is torn: severe when the posterior cruciate is also torn); **(C)** *anterior displacement of the tibia* (anterior cruciate tears: worse if medial and/or lateral structures torn); **(D)** *posterior displacement of the tibia* (posterior cruciate ligament tears). *Rotatory:* **(1)** *the medial tibial condyle subluxes anteriorly* (anteromedial instability): this is usually due to combined tears of the anterior cruciate and medial structures; **(2)** *the lateral condyle subluxes anteriorly* (anterolateral instability): this is usually due to tears of the anterior cruciate plus the lateral structures; **(3)** *the lateral tibial condyle subluxes posteriorly* (posterolateral instability) or **(4)** *the medial tibial condyle subluxes posteriorly* (posteromedial instability); **(5)** combinations of these instabilities. Types **(3)** and **(4)** are mainly due to tears of the posterior cruciate and lateral or medial structures.

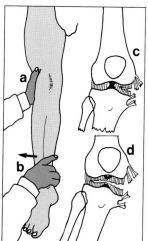

Examining for valgus stress instability.

Begin by examining the medial side of the joint, and the medial ligament in particular. Tenderness in injuries of the medial ligament is commonest at the upper (femoral) attachment and in the medial joint line. Bruising may be present after recent trauma, but haemarthrosis may be absent. Extend the knee fully. Use one hand as a fulcrum **(a)**, and with the other **(b)** attempt to abduct the leg. Look for the joint opening up, and the leg going into valgus. *Moderate* valgus is suggestive of a major medial and posterior ligament rupture **(c)**. *Severe* valgus may indicate additional cruciate (particularly posterior cruciate) rupture **(d)**. If in doubt, the thumb or index, placed over the joint line may be used to detect any opening up as it is stressed. If there is still some uncertainty, compare the two sides.

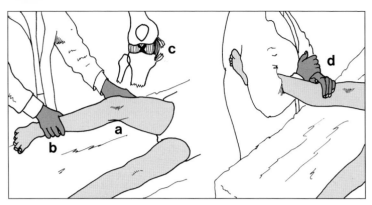

If no instability has been demonstrated with the knee fully extended, repeat the tests with the knee *flexed to 30°* (a) and the foot internally rotated (b). Some opening up of the joint is normal, and *it is essential to compare sides*. Demonstration of an abnormal amount of valgus suggests less extensive involvement of the medial structures (e.g. partial medial ligament tear (c)). If the knee is very tender and will not permit the pressure of a hand as a fulcrum, attempt to stress the ligament with a cross-over arm grip, with one hand placed over the proximal part of the tibia distal to the knee joint (d).

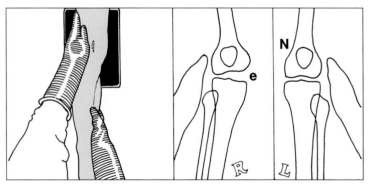

Stress films. If there is still some doubt, then compare radiographs of both knees, taken while applying a valgus stress to each. (In (e) there is evidence of opening up of the join, suggestive of a medial ligament tear when compared with the other side.) If a haemarthrosis is present (and this is not always the case), preliminary aspiration of the joint may allow a more meaningful examination of the joint.

Examination under anaesthesia. If the knee remains too painful to permit examination, the joint should be fully tested under anaesthesia; there should be provision to carry on with a surgical repair or with an arthroscopy should major instability be demonstrated (i.e. where there is the involvement of several major structures).

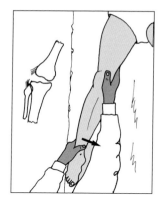

Examining for varus stress instability. First examine the lateral side of the joint, looking for tenderness over the lateral ligament and capsule: then attempt to produce a varus deformity by placing one hand on the medial side of the joint and forcing the ankle medially. Carry out the test as in the case of valgus stress instability, first in full extension and then in 30° flexion, and compare one side with the other. Varus instability in extension as well as flexion, suggests tearing of the posterior cruciate ligament as well as the lateral ligament complex. Check the common peroneal nerve. Stress films and examination under anaesthesia may be required.

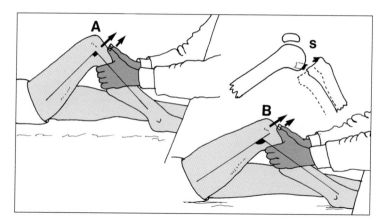

Anterior instability

The anterior drawer test. Flex the knee to 90°, with the foot pointing straight forwards, and steady it by sitting on or close to it. Grasp the leg firmly with the thumbs on the tibial tubercle (**A**). Check that the hamstrings are relaxed, and jerk the leg towards you. Repeat with the knee flexed to 70° (**B**), and compare the sides. Note that significant displacement (i.e. the affected side more than the other) confirms anterior instability of the knee. When the displacement is marked (say 1.5 cm or more), the anterior cruciate is almost certainly torn (**s**), and there is a strong possibility of associated damage to the medial complex (medial ligament and medial capsule) and even the lateral complex. If the displacement is less marked, and one tibial condyle moves further forward than the other, the diagnosis is less clear: it may suggest an isolated anterior cruciate ligament laxity or a tibial condylar subluxation (rotatory instability).

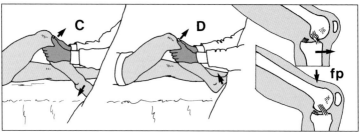

Repeat the test with the foot in *15° of external rotation* (**C**). Excess excursion of the medial tibial condyle suggests a degree of anteromedial (rotatory) instability, with possible involvement of the medial ligament as well as the anterior cruciate ligament. Now turn the foot into *30° of internal rotation*, and repeat the test (**D**). Anterior subluxation of the lateral tibial condyle suggests some anterolateral rotational instability, with possibly damage to the posterior cruciate and the posterior ligament as well as the anterior cruciate ligament. *Beware of the following fallacy:* a tibia *already* displaced backwards as a result of a *posterior cruciate ligament tear* may give a false positive (**fp**) in the drawer tests. This also applies to the following Lachman tests. Check by inspection of the contours of the knee prior to the examination.

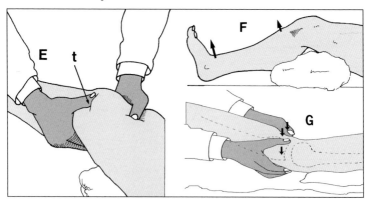

The Lachman tests. These are also used to detect anterior tibial instability. In the *manipulative Lachman test* (**E**), the knee should be relaxed and in about 15° flexion. One hand stabilises the femur while the other tries to lift the tibia forwards. The test is positive if there is anterior tibial movement (detected with the thumb in the joint (**t**)), with a spongy end point. Feagin and Cooke recommend that the test be performed with the patient prone with the thigh supported with a sandbag (**G**). In the *active Lachman test* (**F**) the relaxed knee is supported at 30° and the patient asked to extend it. If the test is positive, there will be anterior subluxation of the lateral tibial plateau as the quadriceps contracts, and posterior subluxation when the muscle relaxes. It is considered that this is best seen from the medial side. Repeat, resisting extension by applying pressure to the ankle.

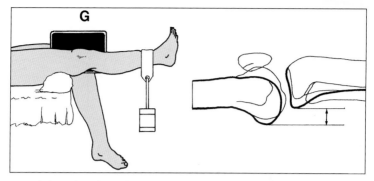

Radiological analysis of anterior cruciate function. The lower thigh is supported by a sandbag, and the leg extended against the resistance of a 7 kilo weight (**G**). The limb should be in the neutral position, with the patella pointing upwards, and the X-ray film cassette placed between the legs. On the films, draw two lines parallel to the posterior shaft of the tibia, with one tangent to the medial tibial plateau and the other tangent to the medial femoral condyle. Measure the distance between them. *Normal* = 3.5 mm ± 2 mm. *Ruptured anterior cruciate* = 10.2 mm ± 2.7 mm. The latter figure is slightly increased if the medial meniscus is also torn. The diagnostic reliability of this examination is high.

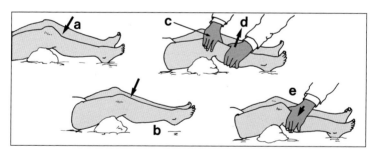

Posterior instability

Testing the posterior cruciate ligament. Rupture, detachment or stretching of the posterior cruciate ligament may permit the tibia to sublux backwards, often with a diagnostic deformity (**a**). (The knee should be flexed 20°, with a sandbag under the thigh.) Ask the patient to lift the heel from the couch, while observing the knee from the side. Any posterior subluxation should normally correct (**b**). Now place the thumb on one side of the joint line and the index on the other to assess any tibial movement (**c**). Try to pull the tibia forwards with the other hand (**d**). If the posterior cruciate ligament is torn, and the tibia subluxed posteriorly, the forward movement as the tibia reduces will be easily felt. If the posterior cruciate is lax or torn, but subluxation has not yet occurred (uncommon), then backward pressure on the tibia (**e**) will normally produce a detectable, excessive posterior excursion of the tibia (posterior drawer test).

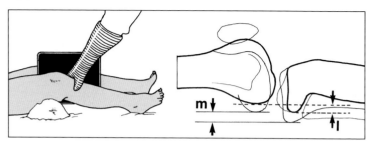

Radiological examination of posterior cruciate ligament function. A sandbag is placed behind the thigh, and the proximal tibia forcibly pressed backwards (with a force equivalent to 25 kilos). This is repeated, and after the second pre-loading cycle, radiographs are taken while the same force is maintained. The gap between the medial femoral and tibial condyles (**m**) is measured, along with that between the lateral condyles (**l**). A displacement in the order of 8 mm on each side is indicative of an uncomplicated posterior cruciate tear. Excessive movement on the lateral or medial sides indicates posterolateral or posteromedial instability. Note that MRI scans allow an accurate assessment of the state of the cruciate ligaments in 80% of cases, although this is inferior to clinical assessment. The cruciates may also be inspected by arthroscopy.

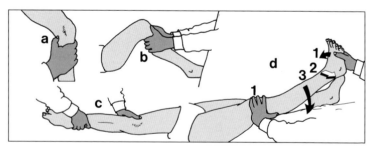

Rotatory instability. Begin by looking for bruising, tenderness (**a**) or oedema over the collateral ligaments. Perform the drawer tests (**b**), noting any variations. Test for laxity on valgus stress (**c**) (often positive in anterior subluxations of the medial tibial condyle), and on varus stress (usually positive when the lateral tibial condyle subluxes forwards or backwards).

Perform the *MacIntosh test* (**d**) for anterior subluxation of the lateral tibial condyle (the pivot shift test). Fully extend the knee while holding the foot in internal rotation (**1**). Apply a valgus stress (**2**). In this position, if instability is present, the tibia will be in the subluxed position. Now flex the knee (**3**): reduction should occur at about 30° with an obvious jerk. A positive test indicates an anterior cruciate abnormality, with or without other pathology.

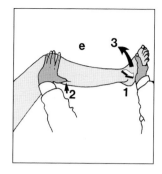

Alternatively, perform the *Losee pivot shift test* (e) (also for anterior subluxation of the lateral tibial condyle). The patient should be completely relaxed, with no tension in the hamstrings. Apply a valgus force to the knee (1), while at the same time pushing the fibular head anteriorly (2). The knee should be partly flexed. Now extend the joint (3). As full extension is reached, a dramatic clunk will occur as the lateral tibial condyle subluxes forwards (if rotatory instability is present). Note: the patient should relate this to the sensations experienced in activity.

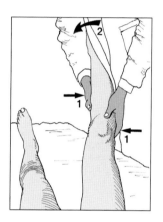

A further modification of the pivot shift or jerk test is preferred by some. To perform this, grasp the patient's foot between your arm and chest and apply a valgus force to the knee (1). Lean over to internally rotate the foot (2). Now flex the knee. If the test is positive (and because the tibia is firmly held), the lateral femoral condyle will appear to jerk anteriorly. Now extend the knee, and as the tibia subluxes, the femoral condyle will appear to jerk backwards.

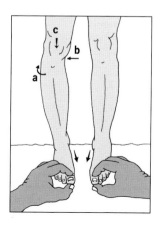

To check for *posterolateral instability*, begin by performing the posterior drawer test with the patient's foot in external rotation, looking for excessive travel on the lateral side. Then perform the *external rotation recurvatum test*. To do this, stand at the end of the examination couch (with the patient in the supine position) and lift the legs by the great toes. The test is positive if the knee falls into external rotation (a), varus (b), and recurvatum (c).

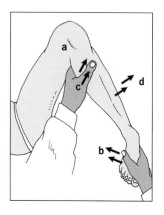

As a further check for *posterolateral instability*, Jakob's reverse pivot shift test may be employed. Begin by flexing the knee to 90° (**a**). Now externally rotate the foot (**b**), apply a valgus force (**c**) and extend the joint (**d**). If the test is positive, the posteriorly subluxed lateral plateau suddenly reduces, usually at about 20°.

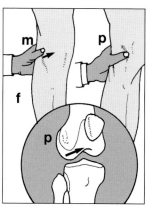

Alternatively, perform the *standing apprehension test for posterolateral instability* (**f**). The patient should be taking his weight through the slightly flexed knee. Grasp the knee, and with the thumb at the joint line press the anterior part of the lateral femoral condyle medially (**m**). The test is positive (**p**) if movement of the condyle occurs (allowing the tibia to slip posteriorly under it), and if this is accompanied by a feeling of giving-way.

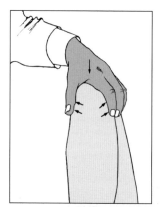

Examining the menisci

Look for tenderness in the joint line, and note if there is a springy block to full extension. These two signs, in association with evidence of quadriceps wasting, are the most consistent and reliable signs of a torn meniscus. In recent injuries, look for tell-tale oedema in the joint line. Bruising is *not* a feature of meniscal injuries.

Now fully flex the knee and place the thumb and index along the joint line. The palm of the hand should rest on the patella. This position is critical, as it allows you to localise the source of any clicks or other sensations emanating from the joint.

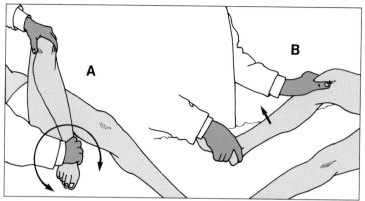

(A) *Posterior meniscal lesions.* Sweep the heel round in a U-shaped arc, looking and feeling for clicks, accompanied by pain, coming from the joint. Watch the patient's face, not the knee, while carrying out this test. (B) *Anterior meniscal lesions.* Press the thumb firmly into the joint line at the medial side of the patellar ligament. Now extend the joint. Repeat on the other side of the ligament. A click, accompanied by pain, is often found in anterior meniscal lesions.

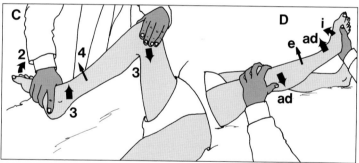

(C) *McMurray manoeuvre for the medial meniscus.* Place the thumb and index along the joint line to detect any clicks. First (**1**), flex the leg fully; then externally rotate the foot (**2**), and abduct the lower leg (**3**). Keeping up abduction pressure, extend the joint smoothly (**4**). A click in the medial joint line, accompanied by pain, suggests a medial meniscus tear. (D) *McMurray manoeuvre for the lateral meniscus.* Repeat the last test with the foot internally rotated (**i**) and the leg adducted (**ad**). Feel for any clicks accompanied by pain as the joint is extended (**e**). A grating sensation may be felt in degenerative lesions of the meniscus.

The normal limb should be examined to help eliminate symptomless, non-pathological clicks (e.g. from the patella clicking over the femoral condyles, or from soft tissues snapping over bony prominences). If a unilateral painful click is obtained, repeat the test with the sensing finger or thumb removed. The source of the click may be visible on close inspection of the joint line.

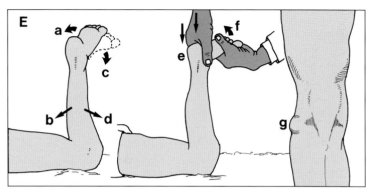

(E) *Apley's grinding tests.* In the tests, the suspect meniscus is subjected to compression and shearing stresses; sharp pain is suggestive of a tear. The patient is prone. The foot is externally rotated (a) and the knee flexed fully (b); then the foot is internally rotated (c) and the knee extended (d). The sides are compared. This demonstrates any limitation of rotation, or where any pain occurs. Then, while standing on a stool, the examiner throws his weight along the axis of the limb (e) and externally rotates the foot (f). Severe sharp pain is indicative of a medial meniscus tear. Repeat in a greater degree of flexion to test the posterior horn. To test the lateral meniscus, repeat the tests with the foot forcibly internally rotated.

Note the presence of any *meniscal cysts*. These lie in the joint line, feel firm on palpation and are tender on deep pressure. Cysts of the menisci may be associated with tears. Lateral meniscus cysts (g) are by far the commonest. Cystic swellings on the medial side are sometimes due to ganglions arising from the pes anserinus (insertion of sartorius, gracilis and semitendinosus).

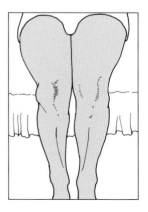

The patella

Examine both knees flexed over the end of the couch. This may show a torsional deformity of the femur or tibia, and a *laterally placed patella*, which will be predisposed to instability (e.g. recurrent dislocation) or chondromalacia patellae. Look for *genu recurvatum* and the position of the patella relative to the femoral condyles. A high-placed patella (*patella alta*) is a predisposing factor in recurrent lateral dislocation of the patella. Note if there is any *knock knee* deformity. Because this leads to an increase in the quadriceps angle (similar to the tibiofemoral angle and readily measured), it predisposes the knee to recurrent dislocation, anterior knee pain and chondromalacia patellae. These are particularly common in adolescent girls.

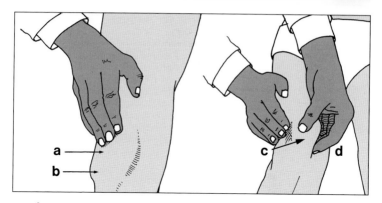

Tenderness. Look first for tenderness over the anterior surface of the patella (**a**), and note if a tender, bipartite ridge is present. Lower pole tenderness (**b**) occurs in Sinding–Larsen–Johannson disease. (Tenderness may also occur over the patellar ligament, quadriceps tendon and tibial tuberosity in other extensor apparatus traction injuries and variants of 'jumper's knee'.) Now displace the patella medially (**c**) and palpate (**d**) its *articular* surface. Tenderness is found when this is diseased, e.g. in chondromalacia patellae. Repeat the test, displacing the patella laterally. Two thirds of the articular surface is normally accessible in this way.

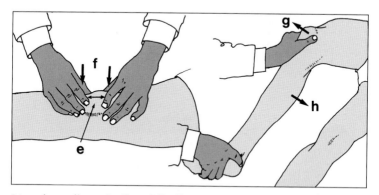

Move the patella proximally and distally (**e**), at the same time pressing it down hard against the femoral condyles (**f**). Pain is produced in chondromalacia patellae and retropatellar osteoarthritis. Also test side-to-side mobility of the patella; this is reduced in retropatellar osteoarthritis.

Apprehension test. Try to displace the patella laterally (**g**) while flexing the knee (**h**) from the fully extended position. If there is a tendency to recurrent dislocation, the patient will be apprehensive and try to stop the test, generally by pushing the examiner's hand away.

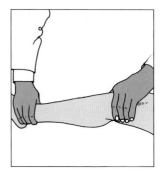

Articular surfaces. Place the palm of the hand over the patella, and the thumb and index along the joint line. Flex and extend the joint. The source of crepitus from damaged articular surfaces can then be detected. Compare one side with the other. If in doubt, auscultate the joint. Ignore single patellar clicks. Note also if there is any apparent broadening of the joint and palpable exostosis formation typical of osteoarthritis.

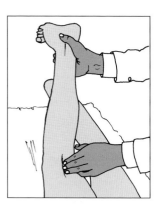

Popliteal region

All the previous tests have involved examination of the joint from the front. Do not forget to examine the back of the joint, both by inspection and palpation. If the knee is flexed the roof of the fossa is relaxed, and deep palpation becomes possible. Semi-membranosus bursae become obvious when the knee is extended. Compare the sides. A bursa may be small at the time of examination, and transillumination is worth trying although not always positive. Note that semimembranosus bursae may be secondary to rheumatoid arthritis or other pathology in the joint.

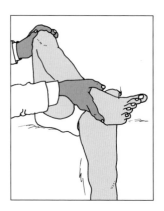

The hip

Always examine the hip, especially where there is complaint of severe knee pain without any obvious cause: remember that hip pain is often referred to the knee joint. The hip may be screened by testing rotation at 90° flexion, noting pain or restriction of movements.

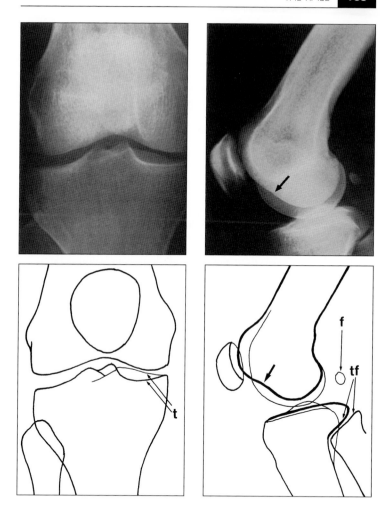

RADIOGRAPHS

In the AP the patellar shadow is faint. Medially, two tibial shadows (**t**) are formed by the anterior and posterior margins of the medial tibial plateau.

In the lateral note the condylopatellar sulcus (marked with an arrow): this helps identify the lateral femoral condyle which is large and flat; in the diagram it is drawn in bold. The lateral condyle of the tibia (also in bold) may be distinguished from the medial by the tibiofibular articulation (**tf**). The medial tibial condyle blends with the shadow of the tibial spines. Do not mistake the fabella (**f**), an inconstant sesamoid bone, for a loose body.

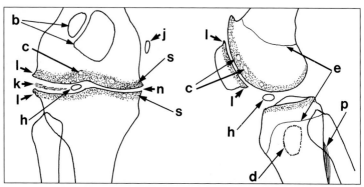

Representative pathology. Note joint space narrowing (indicating cartilage loss) (**n**), lipping (**l**), marginal sclerosis (**s**), cysts (**c**), loose bodies (**h**), varus or valgus (all common in osteoarthritis). Do not mistake a bipartite patella, which affects the upper and outer quadrant (**b**), or epiphyseal lines (**e**) for fracture. Note abnormal calcification as in (**j**) Pellegrini–Stieda disease, (**k**) calcified meniscus and pseudogout. Look for alterations in bone texture (e.g. in Paget's disease, rheumatoid arthritis, osteomalacia, infections). Note any bone defects (**d**) or periosteal reaction (**p**) such as may occur in tumours or infection.

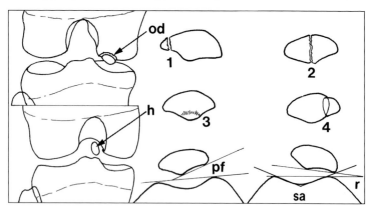

Other projections. *Intercondylar* radiographs often help in diagnosing osteochondritis dissecans (**od**) (as they show the common site of origin in the medial femoral condyle), and in locating loose bodies (**h**). Where the patella is suspect, a *tangential* (skyline) view may show (**1**) a marginal (medial) osteochondral fracture, common in recurrent dislocation of the patella, (**2**) other fractures, (**3**) occasionally, evidence of chondromalacia patellae, (**4**) bipartite patella. The lateral patellofemoral angle (**pf**), normally positive in a 20° radiographic projection, may be reduced to zero or reversed (**r**) in recurrent dislocation of the patella. Reduction of the sulcus angle (**sa**) — normal 132° to 144°— is highly significant in cases of suspected patellar instability.

Representative radiographs

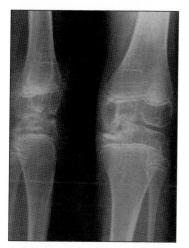

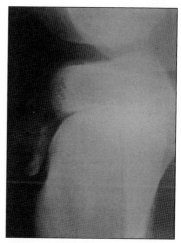

Left: Tuberculous arthritis with destruction of the medial joint compartment. Note the horizontal striations (Looser's zones) indicative of transient growth arrest. *Right:* Osgood–Schlatter's disease.

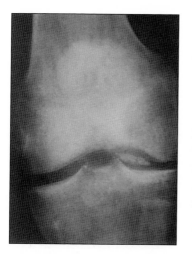

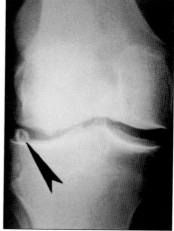

Left: Osteochondritis dissecans with involvement of a large portion of the medial femoral condyle. *Right:* The arrow indicates a loose body associated with osteoarthritis. Note the narrowing and irregularity of the lateral joint compartment.

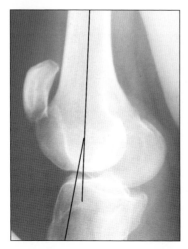 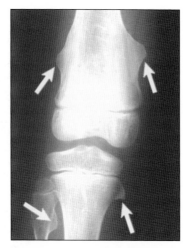

Left: Patella alta with a minor degree of genu recurvatum. *Right:* diaphyseal (metaphyseal aclasis). Note the prominent exostoses on both sides of the distal femur and of the upper tibia; there are also changes in the proximal fibula.

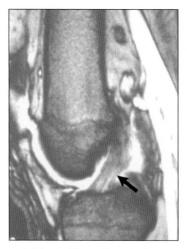 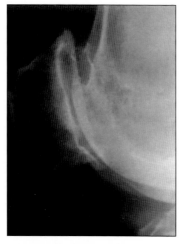

Left: The CAT scan shows an intact anterior cruciate ligament. *Right:* Gross patellofemoral osteoarthritis, with cyst formation both in the femur and the patella.

CHAPTER

11

The tibia

Common causes of pain in the anterior aspect of the lower leg 170

Common causes of pain in the posterior aspect of the lower leg 171

Deformities of the tibia 171

Guide to commoner causes of leg pain 171

Assessment 172

Radiographs 174

COMMON CAUSES OF PAIN IN THE ANTERIOR ASPECT OF THE LOWER LEG

Osteitis of the tibia

This occurs predominantly in children, with or without a history of previous trauma or sore throat. Pain is intense, tenderness is acute and initially well localised over the metaphyseal area, and there is inability to weight-bear. There is systemic upset with fever and tachycardia, and often but not always a polymorph leucocytosis. The sedimentation rate is elevated, but in children C-reactive protein levels rise more quickly (and fall more quickly in successfully treated cases). Admission and investigation with repeated blood cultures is essential. Radiographs of the tibia are initially normal. Cellulitis from insect stings, small wounds and abrasions and hair follicle infections may sometimes cause difficulty in diagnosis. Low grade osteitis of the tibia (Brodie's abscess) may give rise to chronic upper tibial pain.

Bone tumours

The tibia is a common site for many primary bone tumours, so that radiological examination of the tibia is essential in any case of undiagnosed leg pain.

Anterior tibial compartment syndrome

In this condition, pain in the front of the leg is usually preceded by intense (usually athletic) activity or as a complication of a tibial fracture. Oedema and swelling within the confines of the anterior compartment produce ischaemia and eventually necrosis of muscle. The leg is diffusely swollen and tender, and the skin has a glossy appearance. Tibialis anterior and extensor hallucis longus are first affected, with weakness and later inability to extend the ankle and great toe. The dorsalis pedis pulse may be absent, and there may be sensory loss in the first web space from ischaemic changes in the deep peroneal nerve.

Stress fracture of the tibia

Here the onset of leg pain may be sudden or less acute. There is sharply localised bone tenderness and overlying oedema. Initial X-rays may not reveal any underlying hairline fracture, and if pain persists, repeat examination is essential. A radioisotope bone scan may be helpful in diagnosing a local 'hot spot'. In many cases the diagnosis may not be firmly established until a small area of tell-tale callus is showing. The condition is also common in Paget's disease where, of course, there is an easily identifiable radiological abnormality.

Shin splints/Medial tibial syndrome

Pain on the medial side of the shin in sportsmen (shin splints) may be severe, and gives rise to tenderness along the posteromedial border of the lower part of the shin. It may result from interosseous membrane tears, periosteal avulsions, tendinitis, periostitis, muscle sprains or fascial hernias. In a number of cases the symptoms may arise from stress fractures of the tibia, but in the others the precise pathology is often difficult to determine.

Tabes dorsalis

Severe pain in the shins (lightning pains) is common in tabes dorsalis. Usually other criteria are present (e.g. Argyll–Robertson pupils) and serological tests will confirm the diagnosis.

COMMON CAUSES OF PAIN IN THE POSTERIOR ASPECT OF THE LOWER LEG

'Ruptured plantaris tendon'. Sudden pain in the calf during activity, with diffuse tenderness in the upper and outer part of the calf is now regarded as being due to tearing of muscle fibres of soleus or gastrocnemius, rather than injury to the plantaris muscle. Pain often persists for several months.

Thrombophlebitis. Thrombosis in the superficial veins of the calf with local inflammatory changes is a common cause of recurrent calf pain and the presence of tenderness and other inflammatory signs along the course of a calf vein make diagnosis easy. Thrombosis in the deep veins is often silent, and its importance in the postoperative situation is well known.

Other causes of posterior leg pain. Pain in the calf is common in patients suffering from prolapsed intervertebral discs. Claudication pain is a feature of vascular insufficiency and spinal stenosis. Lesions of the foot and ankle which lead to protective muscle spasm on standing and walking frequently give rise to marked calf and leg pain.

DEFORMITIES OF THE TIBIA

Alteration in the normal curvature of the tibia is not uncommon and may be a cause for complaint. The bone may curve convex laterally (tibial bowing), convex anteriorly (tibial kyphosis) or undergo a rotational deformity (tibial torsion). Deformities of these types are particularly likely to occur in infants and young children when the immature bone may yield under the weight of a relatively heavy child. In the majority of cases no other cause is apparent and spontaneous correction by the time the child reaches the age of 6 is the rule. Nevertheless, rickets and other osteodystrophies must be excluded.

Pseudarthrosis of the tibia is a rare congenital abnormality of the tibia which leads to progressive tibial kyphosis. The tibia becomes progressively thinner and undergoes spontaneous fracture which proceeds to non-union. It is particularly resistant to treatment. The diagnosis is made on the radiological findings.

In the adult, deformity of the tibia may be seen following rickets in childhood, malunited fractures, Paget's disease and syphilis.

GUIDE TO COMMONER CAUSES OF LEG PAIN

Children:
- Osteitis or other infections
- Bone tumour.

Adolescents and young adults:
- Stress fracture tibia
- Bone tumours (especially osteoid osteoma, osteoclastoma, osteosarcoma)
- Brodie's abscess
- Anterior compartment syndrome.

Adults:
- PID and spinal stenosis
- Vascular insufficiency
- Paget's disease
- 'Ruptured plantaris tendon'
- Painful conditions of the foot
- Syphilis
- Bone tumours.

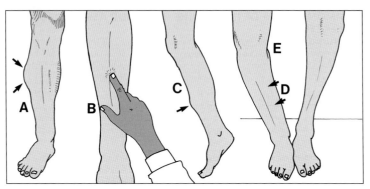

ASSESSMENT

Inspection

Note the site and extent of any *soft tissue swelling* (**A**). In the case of oedema, note particularly if bilateral (suggesting a general rather than a local cause). Unilateral leg oedema in women over 40 is a common sign of intrapelvic neoplasm. *Localised oedema* (**B**) is found over inflammatory lesions and stress fractures. *Local bone swelling* (**C**) is suggestive of neoplasm (e.g. osteoid osteoma) or old fracture. Multiple or single exostoses commonly occur in the tibia in diaphyseal aclasis. Thickening of the ends of the tibia is seen in rickets, and osteoarthritis. *Diffuse bone thickening* (**D**) is seen in chronic osteitis and Paget's disease (which is usually accompanied by a *bow-leg deformity* (**E**)).

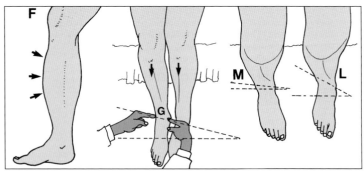

Tibial shape. Note any abnormal *anterior curvature* (**F**), possibly secondary to Paget's disease, malunited fracture, syphilis or rickets. Rickets affects the distal half of both tibia and fibula, and there are associated lateral and torsional deformities. *Tibial torsion*: flex the legs over the edge of the examination couch. The tibial tubercles must face directly forwards. Place the index fingers over the malleoli (**G**). Looking from above, the medial malleolus normally lies 20° in front of the lateral in the coronal plane. *Medial* torsional deformity (a decrease in the angle) (**M**) is associated with flat foot and intoeing. *Lateral* torsional deformity (an increase in the angle) (**L**) is seen in pes cavus.

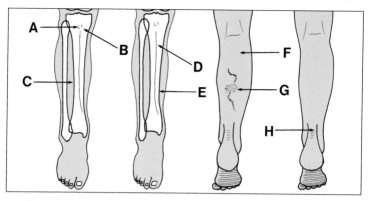

Tenderness

At the front of the leg, this is characteristically sited as indicated **(A)** in Osgood–Schlatter's disease; **(B)** Brodie's abscess and acute osteitis; **(C)** anterior tibial compartment syndrome; **(D)** stress fracture; **(E)** shin splints. *At the back of the leg,* in **(F)** 'ruptured plantaris tendon' syndrome; **(G)** over varicosities in superficial thrombophlebitis; and **(H)** over the tendocalcaneus in partial tears, complete ruptures and tendinitis.

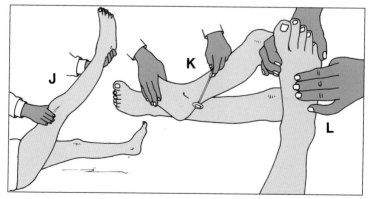

Screening tests

In the investigation of any case of leg pain, examine straight leg raising **(J)**, as in many cases pain in the leg below the knee is referred from the spine; elicit the lower limb reflexes **(K)**, and if indicated, test the pupils for reaction to light and accommodation (lower leg pain is a common symptom of late syphilis); assess the peripheral circulation and especially the distal pulses **(L)** as ischaemia is an extremely common cause of leg pain.

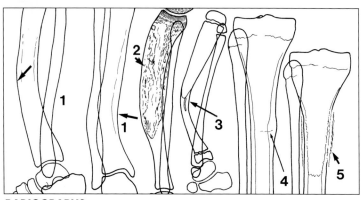

RADIOGRAPHS

The standard films are an AP and lateral, which should include both ends of tibia and fibula. Localised views and CAT and MRI scans are often of value, especially in evaluating cystic defects. Begin by noting the general shape of the bones, their texture and their mineralisation. In (late) *rickets* (1) there may be angulatory and torsional deformities; in *Paget's disease* (2) there is thickening and disturbance of bone texture, sometimes with sarcomatous change; in *pseudarthrosis of the tibia* (3) there is local thinning and angulation of the bone which progresses to tibial dissolution; in *stress fracture* (4) there may be localised subperiosteal new bone formation; greater new bone formation may occur in *tumours* and *infections* (5).

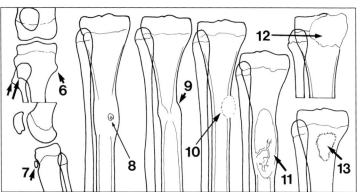

Note any localised deformity such as in *diaphyseal aclasis* (6); *Osgood–Schlatter's disease* (7); *osteoid osteoma* (often with a central nidus) (8); or *healed fracture* (9). Note any cortical bone destruction (10) suggesting a *lytic neoplasm* or *infection*. Examine the cavity and ends of the bone for space-occupying lesions such as a *unicameral bone cyst* in the shaft (11), an *osteoclastoma* occurring in the epiphysis (12), and a *Brodie's abscess* (13) in the metaphysis.

CHAPTER

12

The ankle

Common conditions about
the ankle 176
Guide to painful conditions
round the ankle 177
Assessment 178
Radiographs 183

COMMON CONDITIONS ABOUT THE ANKLE
For injuries to the ligaments and tendo calcaneus see Chapter 27.

Achilles tendon (tendo calcaneus)
Achilles tendinopathy. This generally results from excessive repetitive overload of the tendon to a degree that exceeds its capacity to recover. The preferred term 'tendinopathy' includes a number of conditions which may only be differentiated by direct inspection and histological examination of the tendon or surrounding structures. These include *tendinitis*, where there is a clear inflammatory process involving the tendon; *tendinosis*, where there is collagen degeneration within the tendon; *paratendinitis*, when there are inflammatory changes in the sheath of the tendon; and *insertional tendinitis*, which affects the tendon at its calcaneal insertion (and tends to occur most often in middle aged and overweight patients).

The condition is common in athletes, particularly runners and jumpers, but also in footballers, tennis players and ballet dancers. It gives rise to localised pain which is related to lower limb activity. In severe cases of tendinopathy there may be progressive weakness of plantar flexion, accompanied by impaired function, and in some cases, spontaneous rupture of the tendon.

Acute traumatic Achilles tendon rupture. See Chapter 28.

Tenosynovitis
Inflammatory changes in the tendon sheaths behind the malleoli may give rise to pain at the sides of the ankle joint. Tenosynovitis may follow excessive activity, or be associated with degenerative changes, flat foot or rheumatoid arthritis. There is puffy swelling in the line of the tendons, with tenderness often extending for several centimetres along their length. Tibialis posterior and peroneus longus are most frequently involved, and stretching these structures by forced inversion and eversion of the foot gives rise to pain. Spontaneous rupture may occur.

Footballer's ankle
Ill-localised pain in the front of the ankle may follow repeated incidents of forced plantar flexion of the foot, which result in tearing of the anterior capsule of the ankle joint. This often occurs in footballers, where this form of stress is common. Calcification in the resulting areas of avulsion and haemorrhage leads to the appearance of characteristic exostoses in lateral radiographic projections of the ankle. These may lead to mechanical restriction of dorsiflexion.

Osteochondritis of the talus
Although rather uncommon, this condition (which is seen most frequently in adolescents and young men) may give disabling pain in the ankle and sometimes mechanical problems secondary to loose body formation. The diagnosis is made on the X-ray findings, although the site of the pain and local tenderness over the upper articular surface of the talus may lead one to suspect it. CAT and MRI scans are invaluable in doubtful cases.

Snapping peroneal tendons
This is an uncommon cause of ankle pain and is due to tearing of the superior peroneal retinaculum. The patient complains of a clicking sensation in the ankle

and is usually able to demonstrate the peroneal tendons riding over the lateral malleolus. The treatment is by surgical reconstruction of the retinaculum.

Osteoarthritis
Primary osteoarthritis of the ankle is rare. Secondary osteoarthritis is sometimes seen after ankle fractures, avascular necrosis of the talus or osteochondritis of the talus.

Rheumatoid arthritis
Rheumatoid arthritis of the ankle is not uncommon, but is seldom seen as a primary manifestation of the disease, so that diagnosis seldom presents difficulty.

Tuberculosis
Tuberculous infections of the ankle joint are rare in the UK. When they occur there is swelling of the joint, wasting of the calf and the usual signs of inflammation. The patient develops a painful limp, and as the joint is superficial, sinus formation is common at a comparatively early stage.

Shortening of the Achilles tendon (tendo calcaneus)
Shortening of the Achilles tendon results in plantar flexion of the foot and clumsiness of gait as the heel fails to reach the ground. The more severe degrees of shortening are accompanied by a tendency to flat foot. In many cases, flexion of the knee, by taking the tension off the gastrocnemius, will permit dorsiflexion of the foot. Shortening of the Achilles tendon may occur as an apparently isolated condition with no obvious predisposing cause, but in a great many cases it is associated with congenital deformities of the foot or neurological disorders—of which subclinical poliomyelitis is one of the commonest. On occasion it may result from ischaemic contracture of the calf muscles.

GUIDE TO PAINFUL CONDITIONS ROUND THE ANKLE
History of recent injury:

- Sprain of lateral ligament
- Complete tear of lateral ligament, ankle fracture, fracture of the fifth metatarsal base
- Tibiofibular diastasis
- Ruptured Achilles tendon (tendo calcaneus).

History of past injury:

- Complete tear of lateral ligament
- Secondary osteoarthritis (e.g. from previous ankle fracture).

No history of injury:

- Osteochondritis tali
- Rheumatoid arthritis
- Primary osteoarthritis
- Footballer's ankle
- Achilles tendinopathy
- Secondary osteoarthritis (e.g. osteochondritis tali)
- Tenosynovitis
- Snapping peroneal tendons.

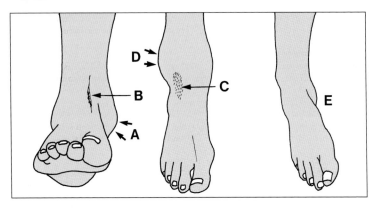

ASSESSMENT

Inspection

Look for deformity of shape (**A**), suggesting recent or old fracture, and sinus scars (**B**), suggesting old infection, particularly tuberculosis. Look for bruising (**C**), swelling (**D**) or oedema. If there is any swelling, note if it is diffuse or localised. Note also if oedema is bilateral, suggesting a systemic rather than a local cause. Look for deformity of posture (**E**) (e.g. plantar flexion from a short tendo calcaneus, talipes deformity, ruptured tendo calcaneus or drop foot).

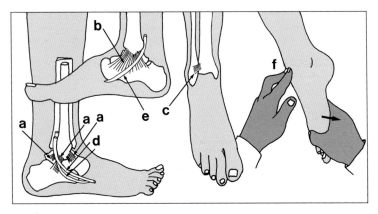

Tenderness

Diffuse tenderness may be found over the fasciculi of the lateral ligament (**a**), over the deltoid ligament (**b**) or over the inferior tibiofibular ligament (**c**) in chronic strains of these structures. Tenderness distal to the malleoli occurs in tenosynovitis of the peroneal tendons (**d**) or of tibialis posterior (**e**). In osteochondritis of the talus (**f**), local tenderness may be elicited when the foot is plantarflexed. (Note that when there is tenderness localised over the malleoli following injury, an X-ray examination to exclude fracture is essential.)

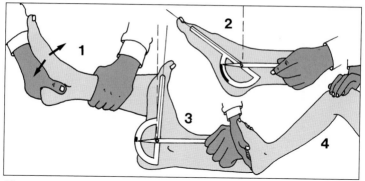

Movements

First confirm that the ankle is mobile and that any apparent movement is not arising in the midtarsal or more distal joints. To do so, firmly grasp the foot *proximal* to the midtarsal joint and try to produce dorsiflexion and plantar flexion (**1**). **Plantar flexion (normal = 55°) (2). Dorsiflexion (normal = 15°) (3).** Both are measured from the neutral position when the foot is at right angles to the leg. If dorsiflexion is restricted, *bend the knee* (**4**). If this restores a normal range, the Achilles tendon is tight. If it makes no difference, joint pathology (such as OA, RA or infection) is the likely cause. If there is loss of active dorsiflexion (drop foot), a full neurological examination is required. The commonest causes are stroke, old polio, PID and common peroneal nerve palsy.

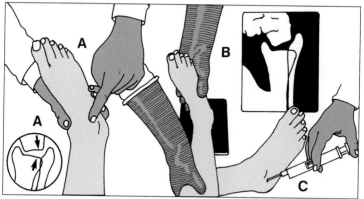

Instability

Whole lateral ligament lesions: stress testing. Grasp the heel and forcibly invert the foot, feeling for any opening-up of the lateral side of the ankle between tibia and talus (**A**). If in doubt, have a radiograph taken while the foot is forcibly inverted (**B**). If tilting of the talus in the ankle mortice is demonstrated, repeat the examination on the other side and compare the films. If pain prevents a satisfactory examination, the area of the lateral ligament may be infiltrated with 15–20 ml of 0.5% lignocaine (**C**).

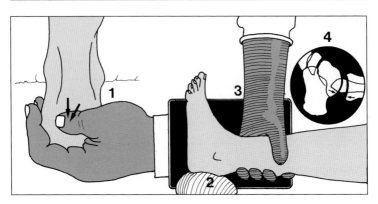

Anterior talofibular component of the lateral ligament: stress testing. Instability may sometimes follow tears of this part of the lateral ligament. With the patient prone, press downwards on the heel (**1**), looking for anterior displacement of the talus which is often accompanied by dimpling of the skin on either side of the tendo calcaneus. Anterior displacement may be confirmed by radiographs taken in the prone position. Alternatively, with the patient supine, (and preferably with local anaesthesia), support the heel on a sandbag (**2**) and press firmly downwards on the tibia (**3**) for 30 seconds up to when the plate is exposed. A gap between the talus and tibia on the resulting film of > 6 mm is regarded as pathological (**4**).

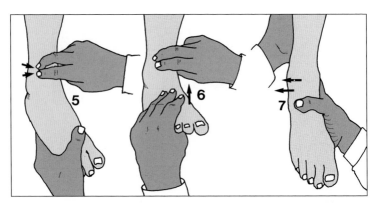

Inferior tibiofibular ligament. Where tears of this ligament (which has anterior and posterior components) are suspected, check first for tenderness over the ligament just above the line of the ankle joint (**5**). Dorsiflex the foot (**6**); this displaces the fibula laterally, and the production or exacerbation of pain is suggestive of ligament involvement. Now grasp the heel and try to move the talus directly laterally in the ankle mortice (**7**). Lateral displacement indicates a tear of the ligament.

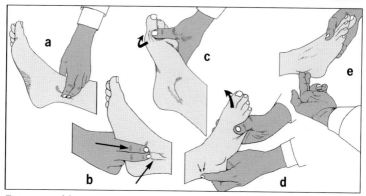

Tenosynovitis

Look for medial tenderness (usually diffuse) along the line of the long flexor tendons (**a**), and the site and extent of any local thickening. Check for an associated synovitis; excess synovial fluid may often be milked in a proximal direction (**b**). Plantarflex and evert the foot (**c**); this may produce pain when tibialis posterior is involved, and feel for any gaps in the tendon. On the lateral side, examine the peroneal tendons for tenderness and the presence of excess synovial fluid in their sheaths (**d**). Also feel for crepitus along their line as the foot is swung backwards and forwards between inversion and eversion; confirm by auscultation. Ask the patient to evert the foot against light resistance while palpating the tendons (**e**). In cases of 'snapping peroneal tendons' sudden displacement of the tendons may be felt (and often seen).

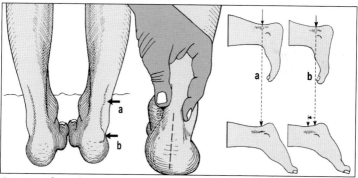

Suspected tendinopathy

In the prone patient, look for local redness or diffuse swelling (**a**), or a Haglund deformity (lateral calcaneal exostosis) (**b**), often found in insertional tendinitis. Feel for any swelling. Pain on gently squeezing the tendon is found in tendinosis with associated paratendinitis. If tenderness is found, see if the site changes with dorsiflexion and plantar flexion. If secondary to paratendinitis it will remain fixed (**a**), but if associated with tendinosis it will move with the tendon (**b**).

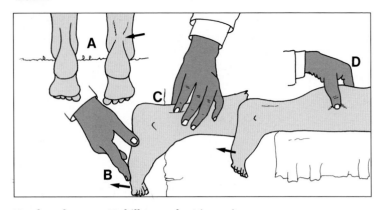

Tendo calcaneus (Achilles tendon) integrity

The patient should be prone, with the feet over the edge of the couch. Defects in the contour of the tendon may be obvious (**A**). Note any enlargement of the bursae related to the tendon. Test the power of plantar flexion by asking the patient to press the foot against your hand (**B**). Compare one side with the other, noting the shape of each calf and the prominence of each tendon. Palpate the tendon while the patient continues resisted plantar flexion, when any gap should be obvious (**C**). *Thomson test.* Normally when the calf is squeezed the foot moves as the ankle plantarflexes (**D**).

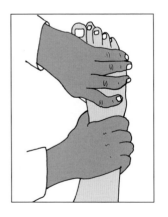

Articular surfaces

Place a hand across the front of the ankle and passively dorsiflex and plantarflex the foot. Crepitus, which may be confirmed by auscultation, suggests articular surface damage.

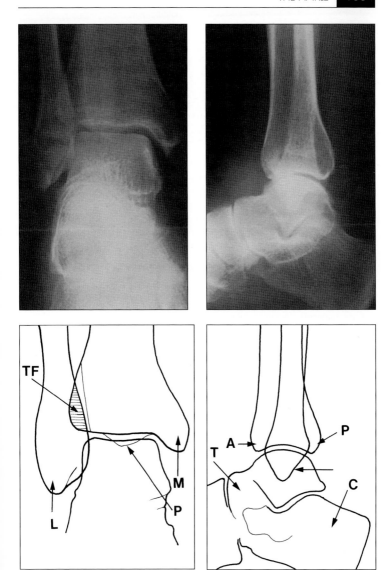

RADIOGRAPHS

These are standard AP and lateral projections of the ankle. Note lateral (**L**), medial (**M**), and so-called posterior (**P**) and anterior (**A**) malleoli. Note normal tibiofibular overlap (**TF**), head of talus (**T**) and calcaneus (**C**).

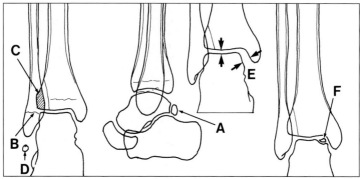

In the standard AP and lateral projections do not mistake the common os trigonum accessory bone (**A**) and the epiphyseal line of the fibula (**B**) for fractures. The amount of tibiofibular overlap (**C**) is dependent on positioning and any diastasis. The os fibulare (**D**) is now thought to represent an avulsion of the anterior talofibular ligament, and may be associated with instability. Note any widening of the gap (**E**) between talus and medial malleolus: this is suggestive of diastasis (compare its size with the one between the upper surface of talus and the tibia—both should normally be equal). Note the presence of any defects in the articular surface of the talus (**F**), suggestive of osteochondritis tali. A CAT scan may help in the doubtful case.

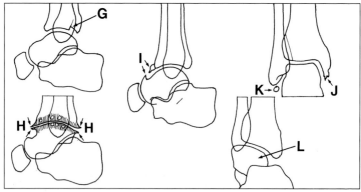

Note any irregularity in the joint surfaces which may suggest previous fracture, e.g. of the posterior malleolus (**G**). Examine the articular margins for exostoses: these are a feature of osteoarthritis (**H**), where there may be other signs such as joint space narrowing and cystic change, and footballer's ankle (**I**), where there may be corresponding changes in the talus. Look at the malleoli, where deformity (**J**) or rounded shadows (**K**) suggest previous avulsion injuries. Distortion of the talus occurs in association with talipes deformities (**L**) and after injuries which have resulted in avascular necrosis where there may be increases in bone density.

CHAPTER

13

The foot

Conditions commencing or
    first seen in childhood
    186
Conditions affecting the
    adolescent foot 187
Conditions affecting the
    adult foot 188
Diagnosis of foot complaints
    190
Infant club foot 191
Examination of the mature
    foot 192
Radiographs 204

CONDITIONS COMMENCING OR FIRST SEEN IN CHILDHOOD

Talipes equinovarus

This is the commonest of the major congenital abnormalities affecting the foot. The deformity is a complex one; characteristically there is varus of the heel and adduction of the forefoot, accompanied by some degree of plantar flexion and supination. In untreated cases the primary soft tissue anomaly is followed by alteration in the shape and development of the tarsal bones. Where correction is incomplete, the commonest residual deformities are adduction of the forefoot, shortening of the Achilles tendon and some stunting of overall growth of the foot.

Talipes calcaneus

This is a much less common congenital abnormality in which the dorsum of the child's foot lies against the shin. There are frequently associated deformities of the subtalar and midtarsal joints, with the heel lying in the varus or valgus position (talipes calcaneovarus, talipes calcaneovalgus).

Intoeing

After walking has commenced, parents may seek advice because the child is walking with the feet turned inwards (intoeing, hen-toed gait). When severe the child may repeatedly trip and fall. Sometimes this may be due to torsional deformity of the tibiae (which must be excluded), but more often it is the result of a postural deformity of the hips (internal rotation) or excessive anteversion of the femoral neck. The condition generally corrects spontaneously by the age of six.

Flat foot

The arches of the foot do not start to appear until a child starts walking, and they are not fully formed until about the age of ten; *the young child's foot is normally flat*. Failure of establishment of the arches is rare, but if this occurs it can lead to awkwardness of gait, rapid, uneven wear and distortion of the shoes, but seldom pain or other symptoms. Persistent flat foot may be associated with valgus deformities of the heel, knock knees, torsional deformities of the tibiae and shortening of the Achilles tendon. Rarely, it may result from an abnormal talus (vertical talus) or neuromuscular disorders of the limb.

Pes cavus

Abnormally high longitudinal arches are produced by muscle imbalance which disturbs the forces controlling the formation and maintenance of the arches. In many cases there is a varus deformity of the heel and a first metatarsal drop. Two distinct groups are seen: those in which subtalar mobility is maintained, and those in which subtalar movements are decreased or absent. A neurological abnormality should always be sought, and sometimes this may be obvious (e.g. spastic diplegia or old poliomyelitis). Many cases are associated with spina bifida occulta, which may be confirmed by clinical and radiological examination. Rarely, fibrosis of the muscles of the posterior compartment of the leg from ischaemia may be the cause. In the more severe cases there is weakness of the intrinsic muscles of the foot, with clawing of the toes; the abnormal distribution of weight in the foot leads to excessive callus formation under the metatarsal heads and the heel.

Kohler's disease
This is an osteochondritis of the navicular occurring in children between the ages of 3 and 10. Pain of a mild character is centred over the medial side of the foot. Symptoms settle spontaneously over a few months and are not influenced by treatment.

Sever's disease
Chronic pain in the heel in children in the 6 to 12 age group generally arises from the calcaneal epiphysis, which radiologically often shows increased density and fragmentation. The condition is usually referred to as Sever's disease, which although originally considered to be an osteochondritis, is now believed to be due to an Achilles tendon traction injury.

CONDITIONS AFFECTING THE ADOLESCENT FOOT
Hallux valgus
In adolescence, and particularly in girls where there is competition between the rapidly growing foot, tight stockings and often small, high-heeled, unsuitable shoes, valgus deformity of the great toe first appears. In some cases, a hereditary short and varus first metatarsal (metatarsus primus varus) may contribute to the problem. As the deformity progresses, the drifting proximal phalanx of the great toe uncovers the metatarsal head, which presses against the shoe and leads to the formation of a protective bursa (bunion), often associated with recurrent episodes of inflammation (bursitis). The great toe may pronate, and further lateral drift results in crowding of the other toes. The great toe may pass over the second toe, or more commonly the second toe may ride over it. The second toe may press against the toe cap of the shoe where there is little room for it and develop painful calluses. Later it may dislocate at the metatarsophalangeal joint. The sesamoid bones under the first metatarsal head may sublux laterally, leading to sharply localised pain under the first metatarsophalangeal joint. In the late stages of the condition, arthritic changes may develop in the metatarsophalangeal joint. More commonly, there is associated disturbance of the mechanics of the forefoot, leading to anterior metatarsalgia.

Peroneal (spastic) flat foot
In adolescents (boys in particular), a painful flat foot may be found in association with apparent spasm of the peroneal muscles. The foot is held in a fixed, everted position. Inversion of the foot is not permitted, and there is often marked disturbance of gait. The condition is frequently associated with ossification in a congenital cartilaginous bar bridging the calcaneus and navicular (tarsal coalition).

Exostoses
The commonest exostoses to cause symptoms are of the first metatarsal head (in hallux valgus), the calcaneus, the cuneiforms (especially the medial), the fifth metatarsal head and the fifth metatarsal base.

CONDITIONS AFFECTING THE ADULT FOOT

Hallux rigidus

Primary osteoarthritis of the MP joint of the great toe often commences in adolescence and ultimately gives rise to pain and stiffness in this joint. It is commoner in males and is not associated with hallux valgus. Sometimes the toe is held in a flexed position (hallux flexus), and there is circumferential exostosis formation involving the proximal phalanx and metatarsal head.

Adult flat foot

Gradual flattening of the medial longitudinal arch (incipient flat foot) may occur in those who spend much of the day on their feet. It is often associated with an increase in body weight and the degenerative changes of ageing in the supporting structures of the arch. When these changes are rapid, they give rise to pain ('medial foot strain'). Secondary (tarsal) arthritic changes may also give rise to pain in long-standing flat foot and are associated with loss of movement in the foot (rigid flat foot). Nevertheless, in two thirds of cases of flat foot, mobility is preserved in the ankle and subtalar joints (flexible or mobile flat foot). Dysfunction or rupture of the tendon of tibialis posterior may also cause flat foot. Flat foot associated with forefoot adduction is known as *skew foot*.

Splay foot

Widening of the foot at the level of the metatarsal heads is known as splay foot. This may occur as a variation of normal growth, causing no difficulty apart from that of obtaining suitable footwear. Splay foot may also be seen in association with metatarsus primus varus, hallux valgus, pes planus and pes cavus.

Anterior metatarsalgia

In anterior metatarsalgia there is often pain under the metatarsal heads. The condition is common in the middle-aged woman and is often associated with some forefoot splaying. Symptoms may be triggered off by periods of excessive standing or increase in weight, and there is often a concurrent flattening of the medial longitudinal arch. Weakness of the intrinsic muscles is usually present, so that there is a tendency to clawing of the toes; hyperextension of the toes at the MP joints leads to exposure of the plantar surfaces of the metatarsal heads which give high spots of pressure against the underlying skin. In turn this produces pain and callus formation in the sole. This pathological process is by far the commonest cause of forefoot pain, but in every case, March fracture, Freiberg's disease, plantar digital neuroma and verruca pedis should be excluded.

Freiberg's disease

This is an osteochondritis of the second metatarsal head associated with palpable deformity and pain. Pain may persist for 1 to 2 years, and in severe cases surgery may be indicated.

Plantar (digital) neuroma (Morton's metatarsalgia)

A neuroma situated on one of the plantar digital nerves just prior to its bifurcation at one of the toe clefts may give rise to piercing pain in the foot. It most often affects the plantar nerve running between the third and fourth metatarsal heads to the third web space, but any of the digital nerves may be involved. It is commonest in women, particularly in the 25 to 45 age group.

Verruca pedis (plantar wart)

Verrucae, thought to be viral in origin, are common in the region of the metatarsal heads, the great toe and the heel. They must be differentiated from calluses.

Plantar fasciitis

Pain in the heel is a common complaint in the middle-aged and may be due to tearing of the calcaneal attachment of the plantar fascia following degenerative changes in its structure.

Mallet toe, hammer toe, claw toe, curly toe

In a *mallet* toe, there is a fixed flexion deformity of the DIP joint of the toe; in a *hammer* toe there is a fixed flexion deformity of the PIP of a toe: the DIP and MP joints are extended; in a *claw* toe both IP joints are flexed, and the MP joint extended; and in a *curly* toe, all three joints are flexed. All may develop corns where the deformed toe presses against the footwear.

The nail of the great toe

Ingrowing of the great toenail gives rise to pain and a tendency to recurrent infection at the nail fold. In *onychogryphosis* there is gross thickening and deformity of the nail. *Subungual exostoses* are often a source of great pain, especially when pressure is applied to the upper surface of the nail. Deformities of the nails may result from *mycelial infections* and are very resistant to treatment. Irregularity of nail growth is a common feature of *psoriasis* and is usually associated with skin lesions elsewhere. There may be an accompanying psoriatic arthritis.

Rheumatoid arthritis

The foot is commonly involved in rheumatoid arthritis, and the deformities are often multiple and severe. They frequently include pes planus, splay foot, hallux valgus, clawing of the toes and subluxation of the toes at the MP joints. Anterior metatarsalgia is often marked, and the metatarsal weight-bearing pad is frequently displaced anteriorly, uncovering the inferior surfaces of the MP joints.

Gout

Gout classically affects the MP joint of the great toe, but in severe cases the other MP joints and even the tarsal joints are involved in the arthritic process.

Tarsal tunnel syndrome

The posterior tibial nerve may become compressed as it passes beneath the flexor retinaculum into the sole of the foot, giving rise to paraesthesia and burning pain in the sole of the foot and in the toes. The superficial peroneal nerve may also be compressed as it runs under the extensor retinaculum on the dorsum of the foot, giving paraesthesia in the area of distribution of the nerve.

DIAGNOSIS OF FOOT COMPLAINTS
The commonest foot disorders related to age

Age group	Heel pain	Pain on dorsal and medial side of foot	Great toe pain	Forefoot pain
Children	Sever's disease	Kohler's disease	Tight shoes and stockings, ingrowing toenail	Verruca
Adolescents	Calcaneal exostosis, bursitis	Cuneiform exostosis, peroneal spastic flat foot	Early hallux rigidus, bunion, hallux valgus, nail problems	March fracture, Freiberg's disease, pes cavus, verruca
Adults	Plantar fasciitis	Flat foot, osteoarthritis, rheumatoid arthritis, cuneiform exostosis	Hallux valgus and bunion, hallux rigidus, gout, nail problems	Anterior metatarsalgia, plantar neuroma, pes cavus, rheumatoid arthritis, gout, verruca, tarsal tunnel syndrome

Assessment of pes planus and pes cavus

Age group	Factors in pes planus	Factors in pes cavus
Infants	'Normal foot', vertical talus	In all age groups this is due to muscle imbalance, often from a neurological disorder, e.g. spastic diplegia, poliomyelitis, Freidrich's ataxia, peroneal muscle atrophy, spina bifida (usually occulta). Many cases are associated with varus heels
Children	Knock knee, valgus heels, neurological disturbances, torsional deformities of the tibia	
Adolescents	Continuation of childhood factors, peroneal flat foot	
Adults	Continuation of childhood factors, overweight, excessive standing, degenerative processes, rupture of tibialis posterior	

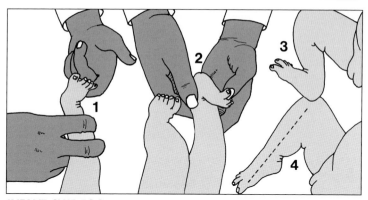

INFANT CLUB FOOT

The new born child often holds the foot in planter flexion and inversion, giving a false impression of deformity. Watch the child as it kicks. If it maintains the foot in the inverted position, support the leg and lightly scratch the side of the foot (1). Normally the child will respond by dorsiflexion of the foot, eversion and fanning of the toes. This reaction does not take place if there is a talipes deformity. If there is no response, gently dorsiflex the foot (2). In the normal child, the foot can be brought either into contact with the tibia or very close to it. Note that in the less common talipes calcaneus deformity, the foot is held in a position of dorsiflexion (3), and that in the normal infant the foot can be plantarflexed to such a degree that the foot and tibia are in line (4).

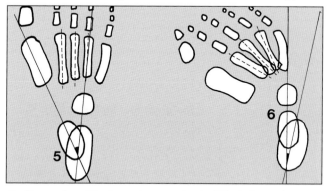

Radiographs: AP view. Interpretation is difficult due to the incompleteness of ossification. Centres for the talus, calcaneus, metatarsals, phalanges and often the cuboid are present at birth. Lines through the long axes of the talus and calcaneus normally subtend an angle of 30–50° (5). The axis of the calcaneus passes through or close to the fourth metatarsal, and the axes of the middle three metatarsals are roughly parallel. In club foot, these relations are altered (6) due to forefoot adduction. (There are other constructions for the lateral projection, and MRI scans can give a more accurate assessment.)

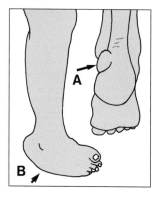

EXAMINATION OF THE MATURE FOOT

The key stages, not necessarily performed in the following order, are: (1) inspection of the foot in recumbency; (2) inspection of the weight-bearing foot; (3) palpation of the foot, noting any tenderness, increased local heat or circulatory disturbance; (4) assessment of joint movements; (5) observation of the gait, and if necessary, examination of the CNS, other joints, the foot print and shoes; (6) other investigations (e.g. X-ray examination).

Inspection

The heel. Note first if the foot is normally proportioned; then if there is (**A**) a calcaneal prominence ('calcaneal exostosis'), or deformity suggesting old fracture, or (**B**) a talipes deformity.

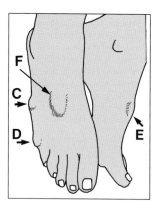

The dorsum. Note if there is any prominence of the fifth metatarsal base (**C**), or the fifth metatarsal head (**D**) ('bunionette'). Both can be a source of local pressure symptoms. Note if there is a cuneiform exostosis (**E**) or a dorsal ganglion (**F**). Observe the general state of the skin and nails. If there is any evidence of ischaemia, a full cardiovascular examination is required. In all cases, the presence of the dorsalis pedis pulse should be sought routinely.

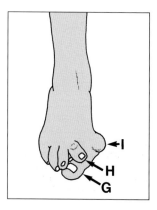

The great toe: hallux valgus. Note any valgus deformity of the great toe (**G**). If this is severe, the great toe may pronate and under-ride (**H**) or over-ride the second. The second toe may sublux at the MP joint. Always re-assess any valgus deformity with the foot weight bearing. Note too the presence of any *bursa* over the MP joint (bunion) (**I**) and whether active inflammatory changes are present (from friction or infection).

Discoloration of the joint with acute tenderness is suggestive of gout.

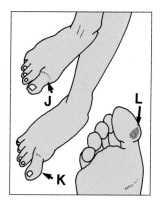

Hallux rigidus (osteoarthritis of the first metatarsophalangeal joint).

When this is present, the great toe may be thickened at the MP joint (**J**) or held in a flexed position (hallux flexus, **K**). Note too the presence of excess callus under the great toe (**L**). This finding on its own is highly suggestive of a degree of hallux rigidus.

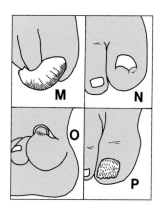

Great toenail.

Note if the great toenail is *deformed* (onychogryphosis, **M**), *ingrowing* (**N**), possibly with accompanying inflammation, *elevated* (suggesting subungual exostosis, **O**), or of *uneven texture* and growth (suggesting fungal infection or psoriasis, **P**).

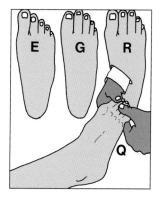

Lesser toes

Lengths. Inspect the foot and note the length of the toes. (In the so-called *Egyptian* foot (**E**), the commonest, the great toe is longest; in the *Greek* foot (**G**) the second toe is the longest; while in the *rectangular* foot (**R**) the great and second toes are of equal length). A second toe longer than the first may become clawed or throw additional stresses on its MP joint. To assess the relative lengths of the *metatarsals*, flex the toes, thereby throwing the MP joints into prominence (**Q**). Abnormally short first or fifth metatarsals are a potential cause of forefoot imbalance and pain. When both are short, there is often painful callus under the second metatarsal.

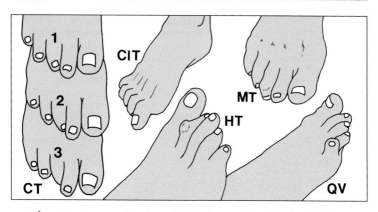

Deformities. In cases of *curly toe* (**CT**), a degree of fixed flexion develops in both IP joints and the MP joint. It is generally caused by interosseous muscle weakness. In **Grade 1**, the toe is mildly flexed, with or without some adduction; in **Grade 2**, there is a degree of under- or over-riding; and in **Grade 3**, the nail is not visible from the dorsum. *Claw toes* (**ClT**) are extended at the MP and flexed at both IP joints. If all the toes are involved, this suggests that there may be an associated pes cavus or some other cause of intrinsic muscle insufficiency (the lumbricals and interossei flex the MP joints and extend the IP joints). In *hammer toe* (**HT**) the PIP joint is flexed, and the MP and DIP joints extended. The second toe is most commonly affected, often due to an associated hallux valgus deformity. There is usually callus over the prominent interphalangeal joint as a result of shoe pressure. In a *mallet toe* (**MT**) the DIP joint is flexed, and there is usually callus under the tip of the toe or deformity of the nail. In *quinti varus deformity* (**QV**), which is often congenital, the little toe overlaps the adjacent toes.

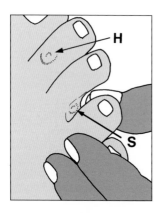

Callosities. Note the presence of *hard corns* (**H**). These are areas of hyperkeratosis which occur over bony prominences and are generally caused by pressure against the shoes. *Soft corns* (**S**) are macerated hyperkeratotic lesions occurring between the toes. They are not associated with pressure or friction.

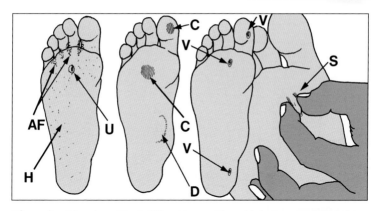

The sole. Note *hyperidrosis* (H); evidence of fungal infection or *athlete's foot* (**AF**); *ulceration of sole* (**U**) (e.g. in diabetes, pes cavus or other neurological disturbances). Note the presence of *callus* (**C**), indicating an uneven or restricted area of weight bearing. Be careful to distinguish between abnormal *local* thickenings and *diffuse* moderate thickenings at the heel and under the metatarsal heads (which are normal). Note any localised fibrous tissue masses in the sole, typical of *Dupuytren's contracture* of the feet (**D**). These tissue thickenings arise from the plantar fascia and are attached to the skin. Always inspect the hands, as both the upper and lower limbs are often simultaneously involved. Note the presence of a *verruca* (plantar wart, **V**). These occur in three classical sites: at the heel, under the great toe and in the forefoot in the region of the metatarsal heads. In the sole they are situated between the metatarsal heads: unlike calluses, they *do not occur in pressure areas*. However, a verruca is exquisitely sensitive to side to side pressure (**S**). Calluses are much less tender and only to direct pressure. When in doubt, use a magnifying lens to see if the central papillomatous structure characteristic of a verruca is present.

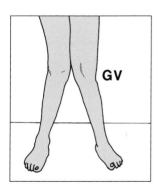

Posture
Limb posture. Examine the patient standing. Begin by observing the presence of any general abnormality of the lower limbs. *Genu valgum* (**GV**) is frequently associated with valgus flat foot and in turn is most commonly seen as a result of a growth disturbance about the knee or as a complication of rheumatoid arthritis. If *intoeing* is present, examine for torsional deformity of the tibiae, increased internal rotation of the hips and anteversion of the femoral neck, or adduction of the forefoot.

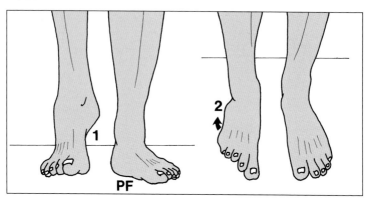

Foot posture. Check that both the heel and forefoot are capable of contacting the ground at the same time (*plantigrade foot*, **PF**). If the heel does not touch the ground (1), examine for shortening of the leg or of the tendo calcaneus. If the foot is *everted* (2), this suggests peroneal spastic flat foot, a painful lesion on the lateral side of the foot or, if less marked, pes planus.

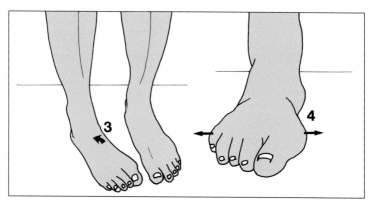

If the foot is *inverted* (3), this suggests muscle imbalance from stroke or other neurological disorder, hallux flexus or rigidus, pes cavus, residual talipes deformity or a painful condition of the forefoot. Broadening of the forefoot (*splaying*, 4) is often the result of intrinsic muscle weakness and may be associated with pes cavus, callus under the metatarsal heads, hallux valgus, anterior metatarsalgia and trouble with shoe fitting.

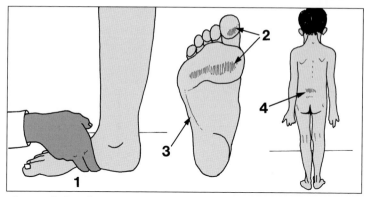

The medial arch. With the patient weight-bearing, look at the medial longitudinal arch and try to assess its height. Try to slip the fingers under the navicular (1). In *pes cavus*, the fingers may penetrate a distance of 2 cm or more from the medial edge of the foot. A high arch suggests a degree of pes cavus. Look for clawing of the toes, callus (2) or ulceration under the metatarsal heads, narrowing of the lateral weight-bearing part of the sole (3) (reflected in the foot-print). If pes cavus is present, carry out a full neurological examination. Look at the lumbar spine for dimpling of the skin, a hairy patch (4) or pigmentation suggesting spina bifida or neurofibromatosis. Radiological examination of the lumbar spine is desirable.

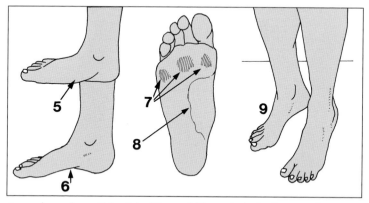

In *pes planus,* the medial arch is obliterated. The navicular is often prominent (5), and the fingers cannot be inserted under it. Ask the patient to attempt to arch the foot (6), as in mobile flat foot the arch can often be restored voluntarily. Check the sole for confirmatory evidence of callus under the metatarsal heads (7) and an increase in the lateral part of the sole involved in weight bearing (8). Note any knock-knee deformity. Re-assess the mobility of the foot by (a) asking the patient to stand on the toes (9), while examining any alteration in the shape of the arch by sight and feel, and (b) by noting the range of inversion and eversion.

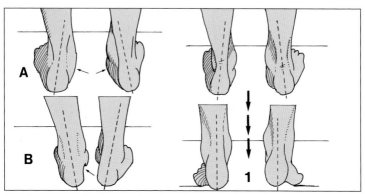

Heel posture. Look at the foot from behind, paying particular attention to the slope of the heels. Note that valgus heels (**A**) are associated with pes planus, and varus heels (**B**) with pes cavus. Again, ask the patient to stand on the toes, observing the heels. If the heel posture corrects (**1**), this indicates a mobile subtalar joint. Where the heel is valgus it may suggest shortening of the tendo calcaneus.

Gait. Watch the patient walking, first bare-footed and then in shoes, to assess the gait. Examine from behind, from in front and from the side. A child should also be made to run. A reluctant child can usually be coaxed to walk holding a mother's hand.

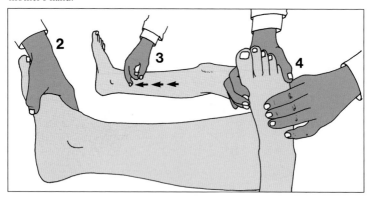

Circulation
Skin temperature. Grasp the foot (**2**) and assess the skin temperature, comparing one side with the other. Take into account the effects of local bandaging and the ambient temperature. A warm foot is particularly suggestive of rheumatoid arthritis or gout. If the foot is cold, note the temperature gradient along the length of the limb (**3**). Proceed to examine the *peripheral pulses* (**4**). Observe the skin colour, the nutrition of the skin and nails, and any trophic changes. Note any cyanosis of the foot when it is dependent, and blanching on elevation, suggestive of marked arterial insufficiency.

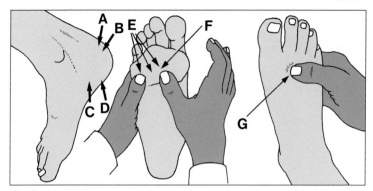

Tenderness

Heel. This is found in Sever's disease (**A**); superior calcaneal exostosis and tendo calcaneus tendinopathy (**B**); plantar fasciitis (**C**) and inferior calcaneal exostosis; and pes cavus (**D**).

Forefoot. Diffuse tenderness under *all* the metatarsal heads (**E**) is common in anterior metatarsalgia, pes cavus, pes planus, gout and rheumatoid arthritis. Tenderness *under* the second metatarsal head (**F**) and *over* the second MP joint is found when the second toe subluxes as a sequel to hallux valgus or rheumatoid arthritis. Puffy, localised swelling on the dorsum of the foot, palpable thickening of the second MP joint (**G**), pain on plantar-flexion of the toe and joint tenderness are diagnostic of *Freiberg's disease*.

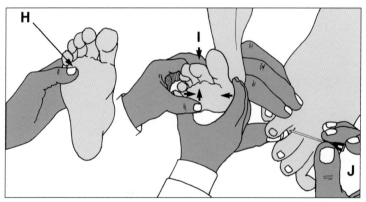

Plantar neuroma (Morton's metatarsalgia). Sharply defined tenderness between the metatarsal heads (**H**), most commonly between the third and fourth, is found in plantar digital neuroma. Occasionally the neuroma may be felt to move by compressing the metatarsal heads with one hand while simultaneously pressing from the sole towards the dorsal surface and back again (**I**). Sometimes the patient complains of paraesthesia in the toes, and sensory impairment should be sought on both sides of the web space involved (**J**).

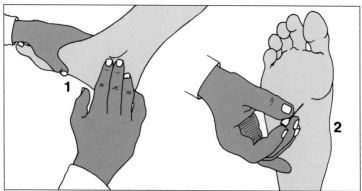

Tarsal tunnel syndrome. Tenderness may be found over the tibial nerve (1) in the tarsal tunnel syndrome, and tapping over it may give rise to paraesthesia in the sole of the foot (Tinel's sign). Test sensation over the whole of the sole of the foot and the toes (2) in the area of the distribution of the nerve, and compare the feet. In doubtful cases, apply a tourniquet to the calf and inflate to just above the systolic blood pressure. If this brings on the patient's symptoms in 1–2 minutes, the diagnosis is confirmed. Pain and paraesthesia on the *dorsum* of the foot may be encountered in the much rarer *superficial peroneal nerve compression syndrome.*

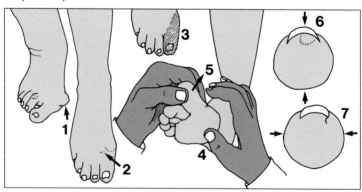

Great toe. In *hallux valgus*, tenderness is often absent or confined to the bunion (1), while in *hallux rigidus* there is usually tenderness over the exostoses (2) which form on the dorsal, medial and *lateral* surfaces of the joint. In gout, tenderness is often most acute but is diffusely spread (3) round the metatarsophalangeal joint, and often the entire toe which is a reddish blue in colour. In *sesamoiditis* there is tenderness over the sesamoid bones (4) situated under the first metatarsal head. Pain is produced if the toe is dorsiflexed (5) while pressure is maintained on the sesamoid bones. In *subungual exostosis*, pain is produced by squeezing the toe in the vertical plane (6). In *ingrowing toenail*, there is pain on side-to-side pressure (7).

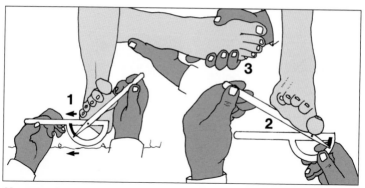

Movements

In assessing foot movements, remember that the total range of supination and pronation in the foot is made up of movements which occur in the subtalar joint, the midtarsal joint, and the tarsometatarsal joints.

(1) Supination (normal = 35°). Ask the patient to turn the soles of the feet towards one another. The patellae should be vertical and the legs parallel to the side of the couch; the angle may be measured using the edge of the couch as a guide.

(2) Pronation (normal = 20°). If supination and pronation are restricted, fix the heel with one hand and with the other assist the patient to repeat these movements **(3)**. No reduction in the range means a stiff subtalar joint.

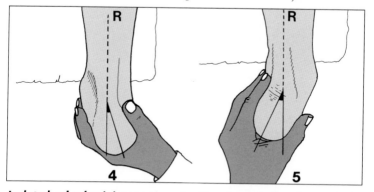

Isolated subtalar joint movements. Turn the patient face down with the feet over the edge of the examination couch. Grasp and move the heel, observing the presence and range of movements in the subtalar joint.

(4) Eversion of the heel (normal = 10°). Repeat, forcing the heel into inversion.

(5) Inversion of the heel (normal = 20°). Loss of movement indicates a stiff subtalar joint (e.g. old calcaneal fracture, rheumatoid or osteoarthritis, spastic flat foot). In idiopathic pes cavus and pes cavus secondary to neuromuscular disease, the subtalar joint is generally mobile; in pes cavus secondary to congenital talipes equinovarus, the subtalar joint is often stiff.

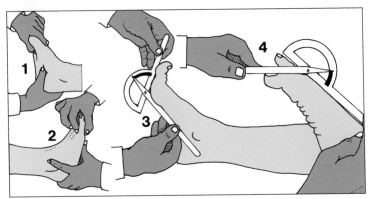

Movements: tarsometatarsal joints. Roughly assess mobility in the first (**1**), fourth and fifth (**2**) tarsometatarsal joints by steadying the heel with one hand and attempting to move the metatarsal heads individually in a dorsal and plantar direction.

Great toe: metatarsophalangeal joint. Check the range with a goniometer.
  Dorsiflexion (normal = 65°) (**3**).
  Plantarflexion (normal = 40°). (**4**) MP joint movements are severely restricted and painful in hallux rigidus. There is often little impairment in hallux valgus unless secondary arthritic changes are quite severe.

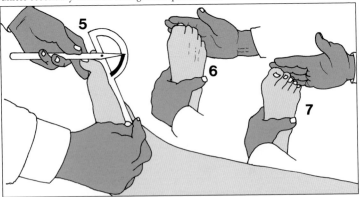

Great toe: interphalangeal joint. Check the range with a goniometer. **Flexion (normal = 60°)** (**5**). **Extension (normal = 0°)**. Restriction is common after fractures of the terminal phalanx.

Lesser toes. Overall mobility may be roughly assessed by alternately curling (**6**) and straightening (**7**) the toes. Accurate measurement of individual ranges is seldom needed. Restriction is often seen in gout, rheumatoid arthritis, Sudeck's atrophy and ischaemic conditions of the foot and leg.

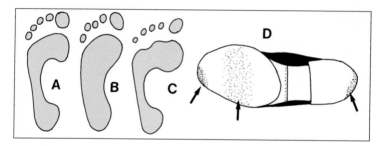

Other tests

Footprint. It is sometimes helpful to see the pattern of weight distribution in the foot, and there are many means of obtaining this. At the simplest level, note the imprint of the sweaty foot on a vinyl floor, or apply olive oil to the sole, and after weight-bearing, dust the imprint with talc. **Typical patterns:** (A) *Normal foot*; (B) *Pes planus:* note the increase in area of the central part of sole taking part in weight-bearing; (C) *Pes cavus:* note the decrease in area of contact in the mid-sole and the splaying of the anterior part of the foot. In extreme cases the lateral weight-bearing strip may disappear.

Shoes. The patient's only complaint may be abnormal shoe wear. Inspection is expected and may be helpful. In the normal sole (**D**), wear is fairly even, being maximal across the tread and at the tip (to the lateral side). At the back of the heel, maximum wear is also lateral.

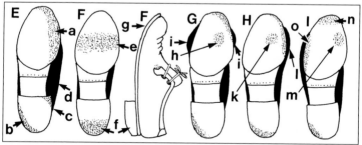

Pes planus (**E**). Note wear on medial side of the sole extending to the tip (**a**); wear on the outer side of heel (**b**); in severe cases, wear on the diagonal corner of heel (**c**). The upper bulges over the sole on the medial side (**d**) and the quarter bulges away from the foot. *Pes cavus* (**F**). Note excessive wear under the metatarsal head region (**e**); excessive wear at the back of the heel (**f**). The anterior part of the sole may become elevated and lose contact with the ground (**g**). *Splay foot* (**G**). Note excess wear in the region of the first or second metatarsal heads (**h**); the upper bulges over the sole anteriorly (**i**). *Hallux valgus* (**H**). There is often excess wear due to splay foot under the area of the first and second metatarsal heads (**k**). In addition, the upper may bulge (**l**) to accommodate the prominent first metatarsal head. *Hallux rigidus* (**I**). There may be excessive wear under the first metatarsal head (**m**), the tip (**n**) and lateral side (**o**) of the sole. The toe of the shoe may be up-turned.

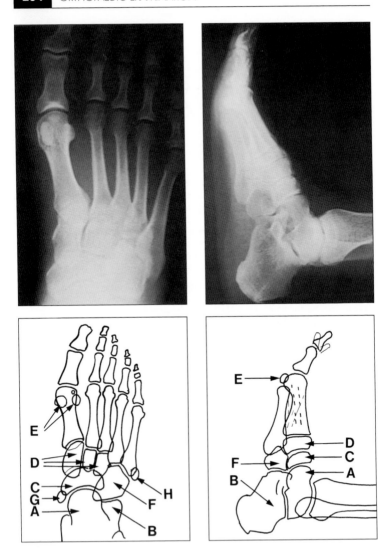

RADIOGRAPHS

The standard projections are an AP along with a lateral or oblique. Note talus
(**A**); calcaneus (**B**); navicular (**C**); cuneiforms (**D**); sesamoids (**E**) (often bi- or tripartite); cuboid (**F**). Accessory bones if present (e.g. os tibiale externum (**G**), or
os Vesalianum (**H**)) should not be mistaken for fracture or loose bodies. In the
lateral, it is often difficult to trace the outline of individual metatarsals due to
bony superimposition, although the first and fifth are usually quite clear.

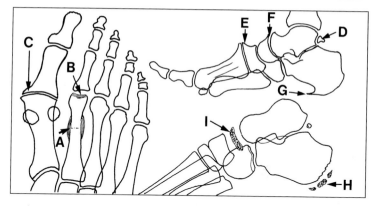

In the AP view, note the bone texture and typical anomalies such as march fracture (**A**), with periosteal reaction occurring in the healing stages; Freiberg's disease (**B**); osteoarthritic changes with exostosis formation (hallux rigidus) (**C**). Note if present the accessory os trigonum (**D**) (often mistaken for a fracture); a cuneiform exostosis (**E**); narrowing of the midtarsal joint (**F**) and other changes suggestive of midtarsal rheumatoid or osteoarthritis; a calcaneal spur (**G**), sometimes associated with plantar fasciitis. In the child, note increased density and fragmentation of the calcaneal epiphysis (**H**) (seen in Sever's disease), and increased density of the navicular typical of Kohler's disease (**I**).

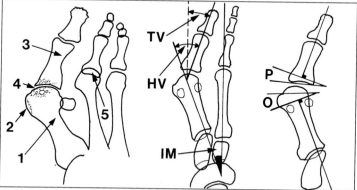

Hallux valgus.   Note, if present, metatarsus primus varus (**1**); first metatarsal 'exostosis' (**2**); hallux valgus (**3**); joint space narrowing or cyst formation (**4**) (also seen in rheumatoid arthritis and gout); metatarsophalangeal joint subluxation (**5**) (also common in rheumatoid arthritis). In assessing hallux valgus, note that (**IM**) the *intermetatarsal angle* (the so-called '{1/2} angle') is normally 9° or less—more suggests metatarsus primus varus. The so-called *hallux valgus angle* (**HV**) is normally 16° or less (*true valgus* (**TV**) of the hallux is HV–IM). The normal *distal metatarsal articular* and *proximal phalangeal articular angles* (**O&P**) are respectively 15° and 5° or less.

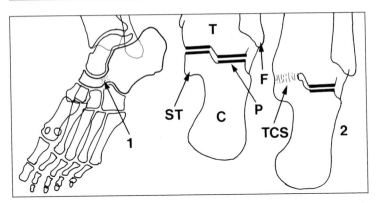

Tarsal coalitions. *Calcaneonavicular bar or synostosis* (1), the commonest of the tarsal coalitions, is best seen in oblique projections of the foot. It is often associated with spastic flat foot. *Talocalcaneal synostosis* (2) is best shown by CAT scan or by axial radiographs of the heel; the latter is also of value in assessing the subtalar joint. In an axial projection, note the talus (T); calcaneus (C); posterior talocalcaneal joint (P); sustentaculum tali and related anterior talocalcaneal joint (ST); base of fifth metatarsal (F); any talocalcaneal synostosis (TCS).

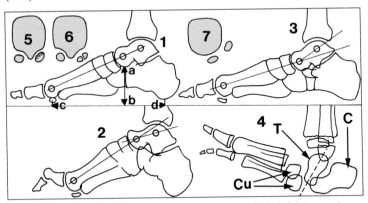

The arches. A weight-bearing lateral projection may be helpful in assessing the medial longitudinal arch and the toes. The axes of the talus and first metatarsal normally coincide, and the height of the arch may be assessed by noting the *ratio ab/cd*: normal (1), pes cavus (2), pes planus (3). In the child, congenital vertical talus (4), which is associated with dislocation of the talonavicular joint, has a classical radiographic appearance. Note the direction of the long axis of the talus (talus (T), calcaneus (C), both centres of ossification of the cuboid (Cu)). *The sesamoids:* a tangential projection may show (5) osteochondritic changes; (6) stress fracture; (7) dislocation and loss of the crista, seen most commonly in association with advanced hallux valgus.

Representative radiographs

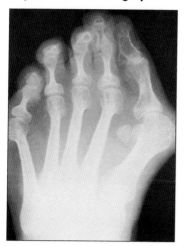 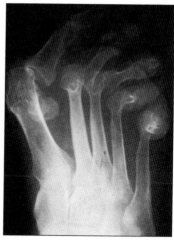

Left: metatarsus primus varus; hallux valgus; splayed forefoot; subluxed sesamoids; pronation of the great toe. *Right:* rheumatoid arthritis, with valgus deformities of all toes including the great toe; dislocation of the lesser toes at the metatarsophalangeal joints.

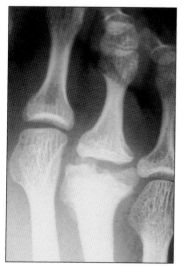 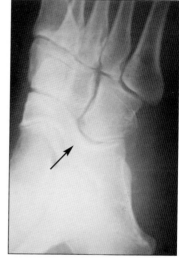

Left: Freiberg's disease, with gross deformity of the metatarsal head. *Right:* tarsal coalition, associated clinically with a peroneal spastic flat foot. The arrow points to a calcaneonavicular bar.

FRACTURES AND DISLOCATIONS

CHAPTER

14

Fractures: basic terminology

Fracture patterns and their significance 212
Describing fractures 215
Fracture healing 219
The classification of fractures 220

Definitions

- **Fracture.** A fracture is present when there is loss of continuity in the substance of a bone. The term covers all bony disruptions, ranging from hairline fractures at one end of the scale to multifragmentary (or comminuted) fractures at the other.
- **Closed and open fractures.** In a *closed fracture* the skin is either intact, or if there are any wounds these are superficial or unrelated to the fracture. In an *open fracture* there is a wound in continuity with the fracture, and the potential exists for organisms to enter the fracture site from outside. In addition, blood loss from external haemorrhage may be significant. (Note: the term 'compound' is still frequently used to describe a fracture which is open; the term 'simple', to describe a closed fracture, may lead to confusion and is now seldom employed.)
- **Dislocations and subluxations.** In a dislocation there is complete loss of contact between the articulating surfaces of a joint. In a subluxation, the articulating surfaces of a joint are no longer congruous, but loss of contact is not complete.
- **Sprains.** A sprain is an incomplete tear of a ligament or a complex of ligaments supporting a joint, and is not normally associated with instability (as distinct from a complete ligament tear). The term is also applied to incomplete tears of muscles and tendons.

Causes of fracture

Fractures are caused by the application of stresses which exceed the limits of strength of a bone. In the case of *direct violence*, a bone may be fractured by being struck by a moving or falling object, or if the bone itself strikes a resistant object. In the case of *indirect violence*, a twisting or bending stress applied to a bone results in its fracture at some distance from the application of the causal force. Indirect violence is also the commonest cause of dislocation. *Fatigue fractures* may result from stresses applied to a bone with excessive frequency. A *pathological fracture* is one which occurs in an abnormal or diseased bone. If the osseous abnormality reduces the strength of the bone then the force required to produce the fracture is reduced and may even become trivial. *The commonest causes of pathological fracture are osteoporosis and osteomalacia.*

FRACTURE PATTERNS AND THEIR SIGNIFICANCE

Hairline fractures. These result from minimal trauma and are not severe enough to produce any significant displacement of the fragments. *Stress fractures* are generally of this pattern. They may be difficult to detect on the radiographs, and where there are reasonable clinical grounds for suspecting a fracture, the rules are quite clear: (1) additional oblique radiographic projections of the area may be helpful; (2) do not accept poor quality films; (3) films repeated after 7–10 days may show the fracture quite distinctly (due to decalcification at the fracture site).

Greenstick fractures. Greenstick fractures occur in children, but not all children's fractures are of this type. The less brittle bone of the child tends to buckle on the side opposite the causal force. Tearing of the periosteum and of the surrounding soft tissues is often minimal, and this facilitates manipulative reduction. However, the elastic spring of the periosteum may lead to recurrence of angulation, so that particular attention must be taken over plaster fixation and after-care. Because of this, some surgeons deliberately overcorrect the initial deformity, tearing the periosteum on the other side of the fracture. Healing in all greenstick fractures is rapid.

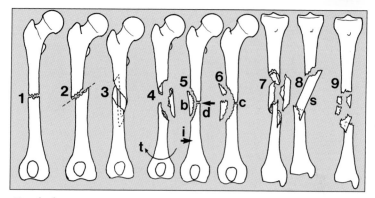

Simple fractures. (1) *Simple transverse fractures* run either at right angles to the long axis of a bone or with an obliquity of less than 30°. The inherent stability of this type of fracture reduces the risks of shortening and displacement in conservatively managed cases, so that in the tibia weight-bearing may often be permitted at an relatively early stage. However, the area of bony contact is small, requiring very strong union before external supports can be discarded. (*Note:* the term 'simple' used to describe this and the following fractures means that the fracture runs circumferentially round the bone with the formation of only two main fragments.) (2) *Simple oblique fractures* run at an oblique angle of 30° or more. (3) *Simple spiral fractures* have the line of the fracture spiralling round the bone and result from indirect torsional forces. Union can be rapid as there is often a large area of bone in contact. In both oblique and spiral fractures, unopposed muscle contraction or premature weight-bearing readily lead to shortening, displacement and sometimes loss of bony contact.

Multifragmentary (comminuted) fractures. In these fractures there are more than two fragments. The *spiral wedge fracture* (4) is produced by torsional forces (**t**), and the *bending wedge fracture* (5) by direct (**d**) or indirect (**i**) violence. (**b**) Because of its shape this is often called a butterfly fragment: if it fractures, the result is termed a *fragmented (comminuted) wedge fracture* (6). [All these fractures are of Type B in the AO Classification (see later) and their characteristic is that after reduction there is still bony contact between the main fragments (**c**)].

Multifragmentary complex fractures. In these there is no contact between the main fragments after reduction. In *complex spiral fractures* (7) there are two or more spiral elements; in *complex segmental fractures* (sometimes called double fractures) (8) there is at least one quite separate complete bone fragment(s). In *complex irregular fractures* (9) the bone lying between the main elements is split into many irregular fragments. [All these fractures are classified as Type C in the AO Classification.] Multifragmentary fractures are usually the result of great violence and are not infrequently open. There is an increased risk of damage to neighbouring blood vessels and nerves, the fractures tend to be unstable and difficult to reduce, and delayed union and joint stiffness are common. Reduction of segmental fractures by closed methods is often difficult, and direct exposure may threaten the precarious blood supply to the central segment.

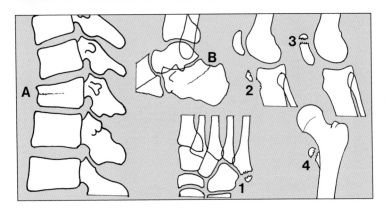

Compression (or crush) fractures. These occur in cancellous bone which is compressed beyond the limits of its tolerance. Common sites are the vertebral bodies **(A)** (as a result of flexion injuries) and the heels **(B)** (following falls from a height). If the deformity is accepted, union is invariably rapid. In the spine, if correction is attempted, recurrence is almost invariable.

Avulsion fractures. These may be produced by a sudden muscle contraction—the muscle pulling off the portion of bone to which it is attached. Common examples include: **(1)** the base of fifth metatarsal (peroneus brevis); **(2)** the tibial tuberosity (quadriceps); **(3)** upper pole of patella (quadriceps); **(4)** lesser trochanter (iliopsoas). (These are all AO Type A fractures.) Avulsion fractures may also result from traction on a ligamentous or capsular attachment and are often witness of *momentary dislocation*.

Impacted fractures. These occur when one fragment is driven into the other. Cancellous bone is usually involved and union is often rapid. The *stability* of these fractures varies and is more implied than real.

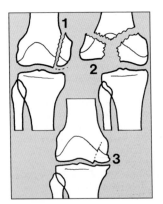

Fractures involving the articular surfaces of a joint. In *partial articular fractures* (1) part of the joint surface is involved, but the remainder is intact and solidly connected to the rest of the bone. (AO Type B fracture.) In *complete articular fractures* (2) the articular surface is completely disrupted and separated from the shaft. (AO Type C fracture.) When a fracture involves the articular surfaces, any persisting irregularity may cause secondary osteoarthritis (3). *Fractures close to a joint* may cause stiffness through muscle tethering. *In a fracture–dislocation*, a dislocation is complicated by a fracture of one of the bony components of the joint. There may be problems with reduction and stability, stiffness and avascular necrosis.

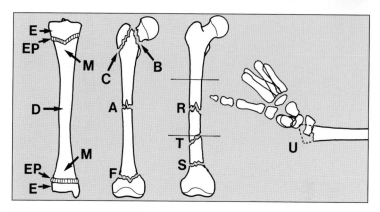

DESCRIBING FRACTURES

The level of a fracture

The *anatomical divisions* of a long bone include the epiphysis (**E**), the epiphyseal plate (**EP**) and the diaphysis or shaft (**D**). Between the latter two lie the metaphyses (**M**). A fracture may be described as lying within these divisions, or involving a distinct anatomical part, e.g. (**A**) fracture of the femoral diaphysis; (**B**) fracture of the femoral neck; (**C**) fracture of the greater trochanter; (**F**) supracondylar fracture of the femur.

For descriptive purposes a bone may be divided arbitrarily into thirds. In this way (**R**) may be described as a fracture of the mid third of the femur; (**S**), a fracture of the femur in the distal third; (**T**), a fracture of the femur at the junction of the middle and distal thirds. An eponym may be used to describe the level of a fracture: e.g. a Colles' fracture (**U**) involves the radius, and occurs within an inch (2.5 cm) of the wrist.

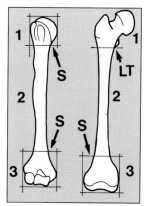

In *AO terminology*, long bones are divided into three unequal segments: (**1**) *a proximal segment*, (**2**) a central *diaphyseal segment* and (**3**) a *distal segment*. The boundaries between these segments are obtained by erecting squares (**S**) which accommodate the widest part of the bone ends; in the special case of the femur the diaphysis is described as commencing at the distal border of the lesser trochanter (**LT**).

The deformity

If there is no deformity—i.e. if the violence which has produced the fracture has been insufficient to cause any movement of the bone ends relative to one another—then the fracture is said to be in anatomical position. Similarly, if a perfect position has been achieved after manipulation of a fracture, it may be described as being in anatomical position.

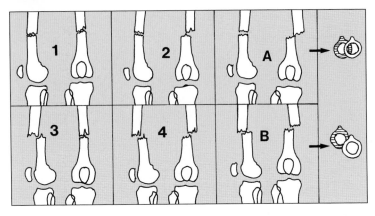

Displacement. Displacement (or translation) is present if the bone ends have shifted relative to one another. The *direction* of displacement is described in terms of *movement of the distal fragment*. For example, in these fractures of the femoral shaft there is (**1**) no displacement, (**2**) lateral displacement, (**3**) posterior displacement, (**4**) both lateral and posterior displacement. The *degree* of displacement must also be considered. A rough estimate is usually made of the percentage of the fracture surfaces in contact, e.g. (**A**) 50% bony apposition, (**B**) 25% bony apposition. Good bony apposition encourages stability and union. Where *none* of the fracture surfaces is in contact, the fracture is described as having 'no bony apposition' or being 'completely off-ended'. These fractures are potentially unstable and liable to shortening. They may be hard to reduce (sometimes due to trapping of soft tissue between the bone ends), and delayed or non-union is not uncommon. Displacement of spiral, oblique or off-ended transverse fractures will result in shortening. Speaking generally, however, displacement, whilst undesirable, is of much less significance than angulation.

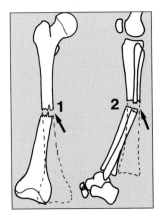

Angulation. The long accepted method of describing angulation is in terms of the position of the *point of the angle*, e.g. (**1**) fracture of the femur with medial angulation, (**2**) fracture of the tibia and fibula with posterior angulation. This method can on occasion give rise to confusion, especially as *deformity* is always described in terms of the distal fragment. Equally acceptable, and perhaps less liable to error, would be to describe these fractures as (**1**) a fracture of the middle third of the femur with the distal fragment tilted laterally; (**2**) a fracture of the tibia and fibula in the middle thirds, with the distal fragment tilted anteriorly.

Significant angulation must always be corrected for several reasons. Deformity of the limb will be conspicuous and regarded (often correctly) by the patient as a sign of poor treatment. In the upper limb, function may be seriously impaired, especially in forearm fractures where pronation and supination may be badly affected. In the lower limb, alteration of the plane of movements of the hip, knee or ankle may lead to abnormal joint stresses, encouraging the onset of secondary osteoarthritis. (Note that persistent *displacement* is seldom conspicuous or the source of any other problem.)

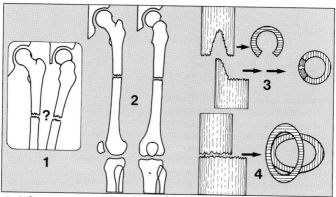

Axial rotation. This is a third deformity which may be present. It results from one fragment rotating on its long axis relative to the other, with or without accompanying displacement or angulation. It is easily overlooked, especially if the radiographs do not show both ends of the bone (1). When both ends are fully visualised on one film, rotation may be obvious (2). The moral is that in any fracture *both the joint above and the one below should be included* in the examination. Axial rotation may also be detected in the radiographs by noting (3) the position of interlocking fragments (a displaced fracture with 90° of axial rotation is illustrated). If a bone is not perfectly circular in cross-section at the fracture site, differences in the relative diameters of the fragments may also be suggestive of axial rotation (4). Axial rotation is of particular importance in forearm fractures.

Open fractures

Open (compound) fractures are of two types: those which are open from within out, and others which are open from without in. In fractures which are *open from within out*, the skin is broached by the sharp edge of one of the bone ends. This may occur at the time of the initial injury, or later from unguarded handling of a closed fracture. When first seen, the bone may be exposed or it may have reduced spontaneously. The risks of infection are much less in open from within out fractures than those from without in. Fractures *open from without in* are caused by direct violence. The violence may be severe, resulting in fractures which are often comminuted and difficult to manage. Besides skin itself, other important structures including muscles, nerves and blood vessels may be affected. Haemorrhage and shock may be greater than in corresponding within out fractures.

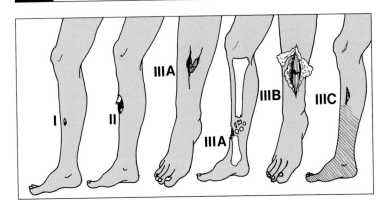

Gustilo classification of open fractures

Type I. An open fracture with a wound which is less than 1 cm and is clean.

Type II. An open fracture with a wound which is more than 1 cm long and which is not associated with extensive soft tissue damage, avulsions or flaps.

Type IIIA. An open fracture where there is adequate soft tissue coverage of bone in spite of extensive soft tissue lacerations or flaps; or irrespective of the size of the wound, high energy trauma has been responsible.

Type IIIB. An open fracture with extensive soft tissue loss, with periosteal stripping and exposure of bone. Massive contamination is usual.

Type IIIC. An open fracture associated with an arterial injury requiring repair.

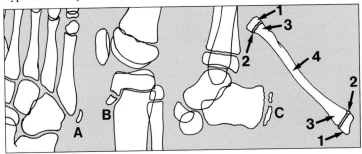

Epiphyseal injuries

Note that there are two types of epiphyses. *Traction epiphyses* lie at muscle insertions, are non-articular and do not contribute to the longitudinal growth of the bone. Avulsion is the commonest injury. The sites most affected include: **(A)** the base of the fifth metatarsal, **(B)** the tibial tuberosity and **(C)** the calcaneal epiphysis. Traction injuries are probably the basic cause of Osgood–Schlatter's and Sever's disease **(B & C)**. Other common sites include the lesser trochanter, ischium and the anterior iliac spines. *Pressure epiphyses* are situated at the ends of the long bones and take part in the articulations. The corresponding epiphyseal plates are responsible for longitudinal growth of the bone. (Circumferential growth is controlled by the periosteum.) *Note again:* **(1)** epiphysis; **(2)** epiphyseal plate; **(3)** metaphysis; **(4)** diaphysis.

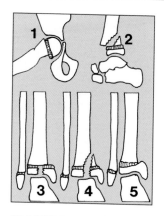

Classification of epiphyseal plate injuries (Salter and Harris classification). Type 1: the whole epiphysis is separated from the shaft. **Type 2:** the epiphysis is displaced, carrying with it a small, triangular metaphyseal fragment (the commonest injury). **Type 3:** separation of part of the epiphysis. **Type 4:** separation of part of the epiphysis, with a metaphyseal fragment. **Type 5:** crushing of part or all of the epiphysis. Note that in epiphyseal separations, the active region of growth remains with the epiphysis rather than the metaphysis, and that epiphyseal displacement may lead to avascular necrosis or growth arrest.

FRACTURE HEALING

As a result of the injury, there is tearing of the periosteum and disruption of the Haversian systems. A fracture haematoma forms and is rapidly vascularised: fibrovascular tissue replaces the clot, collagen fibres are laid down and mineral salts are deposited. Cells derived from the periosteum form new subperiosteal bone. (If the blood supply is poor or if it is disturbed by excessive mobility at the fracture site, cartilage may be formed instead and remain until a better blood supply is established.) This *primary callus response* remains active for a few weeks only, while the ability of the medullary cavity to form new bone remains indefinitely throughout the healing of the fracture.

It the periosteum is incompletely torn, with no significant loss of bony apposition, the primary callus response may result in establishing external continuity of the fracture ('bridging external callus'). If the gap is more substantial, fibrous tissue formed from the organisation of the fracture haematoma will lie between the advancing collars of subperiosteal new bone. This fibrous tissue may be stimulated to form bone ('tissue induction'), again resulting in bridging callus. If the bone ends are offset, the primary callus from the subperiosteal region may unite with medullary callus. The net result is that the fracture becomes rigid, function in the limb returns and the situation is rendered favourable for endosteal bone formation and remodelling.

Endosteal new bone formation, with re-establishment of the Haversian systems, cannot occur if fibrous tissue remains between the bone ends. If present there it must be removed and replaced with woven bone. This is generally achieved by ingrowth of medullary callus. Where the bone ends are supported by rigid internal fixation, there is no functional requirement for external bridging callus: as a result external bridging callus may not be seen, or be minimal. Healing of the fracture occurs slowly, and it is therefore essential that internal fixation devices are retained until this process is complete.

After the fracture has united, remodelling occurs. This is greatest in children, where most or all traces of fracture displacement will disappear. There is also some power to correct angulation, although this becomes progressively less as the child approaches adolescence. As any axial rotation is likely to remain, this should always be corrected. In the adult, remodelling is less good; there is virtually no correction of axial rotation or angulation, and it is therefore particularly important that these deformities are corrected.

THE CLASSIFICATION OF FRACTURES

There is no fracture of any bone which has escaped an attempt at classification. Sometimes this has been done on the basis of region and pattern, sometimes through a concept of the stresses to which the bone has been subjected, and usually with an eye on some understanding of the severity of the injury and its prognosis. Unfortunately, not everyone has the same ideas regarding the relative importance of the various factors concerned, and as time progresses and knowledge expands the number of classifications that exist has been continuing to grow.

The result is that in nearly every area there is a wealth of classifications, usually with grades, degrees or numbers attached to the originator's name. This bewilders the newcomer, and causes much confusion in those who are attempting to assess the results of various treatments, as the injuries classified by one author may not be easily compared with those described by another. There is too the problem of how to ascribe certain fractures which have been inconsiderate enough to adopt a pattern that does not quite fit within the classification.

No surgeon is able to master the wealth of classifications outside his own specialist area, and for purposes of communication, as far as single injuries are concerned, a fracture is described mainly by its site and pattern, along the lines already detailed. The AO Group (ASIF)[1] have sought a universal classification which is aimed to encompass all fractures, and after many years' work have published full details of their system for the major long bones.

The AO Classification of fractures of the long bones

Details are given overleaf, but the following general points should be noted:

- It is not a classification of injuries; it is a classification of fractures.
- It does not include dislocations, unless they have an associated fracture.
- It does not differentiate between undisplaced and displaced fractures of the shafts of the long bones (although it does so in the case of certain fractures of the bone ends).
- It does not give any indication of the relative frequency of particular fractures.
- The sorting of fractures (beyond the area of the bone involved) depends on the AO Group's assessment of the severity of the fracture; this they define as 'the morphological complexity, the difficulty in treatment and the prognosis'. In areas this may reflect a preference for the use of internal fixation rather than conservative methods of treatment.
- The classification results in an alpha-numeric code which is suitable for computer sorting, and which allows for research purposes (e.g. in assessing the results of any treatment, wherever carried out) and the comparison of like with like.
- Because of the format, it is not descriptive in a verbal sense and is not suitable for conveying information about the nature of an individual fracture (e.g. over the telephone).

---

[1]AO/ASIF, Arbeitsgemeinschaft für Osteosynthesefragen/Association for the Study of Internal Fixation.

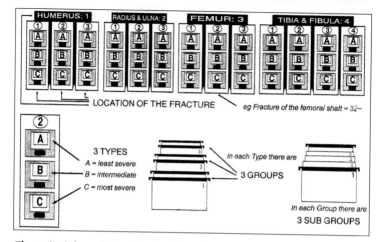

The principles of the AO classification. The AO classification for long bone fractures may be grasped by likening it to an X-ray storage system, with numbered blocks of filing cabinets: one block for each bone.

Within each block, each filing cabinet (which is also numbered) represents a particular area of each bone: cabinet number 1 stores fractures of the proximal segment, number 2 the diaphysis or shaft, and number 3 the distal segment. In the case of the tibia, there is a fourth cabinet to deal with fractures of the malleoli. (The method of determining the junction between the segments has been described.) When a fracture bridges the junction between two segments, the segment under which it is classified is determined by the site of the mid-point of the line of the fracture. In practice, therefore, a two-digit code determines the *location* of a fracture, e.g. under 22 would be stored all fractures of the shafts of the radius, or the ulna, or of both these bones.

In each cabinet all the radiographs for a single location of fracture are divided into fracture *types* (represented by the three drawers): the least severe go in drawer A (type A), those of intermediate severity in B (type B) and the most severe in C (type C).

Any type of fracture can be put in one of three *groups* (represented by folders and numbered 1–3). Within each group, fractures may be further sorted into *subgroups* (represented by partitions). Each of these subgroups has a numerical representation (.1, .2, .3).

[If an even more detailed classification is needed, fractures within each subgroup can have added qualifications. These can be described by a single number (or two numbers separated by a comma) added in parentheses after the main coding. The first digit in the range 1–6 is used to amplify the description of a fracture's location and its extent, while the second is purely descriptive. The number 7 is reserved to describe partial amputations, 8 for total amputation and 9 for loss of bone stock.]

As an example of the AO classification, a simple oblique fracture of the proximal part of the femoral shaft would be coded 32–A2.1:

3 = THE BONE: the femur.

2 = THE SEGMENT: the diaphysis.

– = Separator between location and type.

A = THE TYPE: A is the least severe type of fracture, with two bone fragments only.

2 = THE GROUP: Group 2 includes all oblique fractures.

.1 = SUBGROUP: Subgroup .1 includes fractures in the proximal part of the diaphysis where the medullary cavity is wider than in the more central part of the bone.

15

The diagnosis of fractures and the principles of treatment

History 224
Diagnosis 224
The treatment of fractures
    226

HISTORY

In taking the history of a patient who may have a fracture, the following points may prove to be helpful:

- What activity was being pursued at the time of the incident?
- What was the nature of the incident?
- What was the magnitude of the applied forces? (For example, in a fall it is helpful to know the height fallen, if the fall was broken, the manner of the landing and the nature of the surface on which the patient landed.)
- What was the point of impact and the direction of the applied forces?
- Is there any significance to be attached to the incident itself? For example, if there was a fall, was it precipitated by some underlying medical condition (such as a hypotensive attack) which requires separate investigation?
- Where is the site of any pain, and what is its severity?
- Is there loss of functional activity? For example, walking is seldom possible after any fracture of the femur or tibia; inability to weight-bear after an accident is of great significance.

DIAGNOSIS

In some cases the diagnosis of fracture is unmistakable, e.g. when there is gross deformity of the central portion of a long bone or when the fracture is visible as in certain open injuries. In others, begin by looking for any asymmetry of contour or posture, local bruising or skin damage (suggesting a point of impact or, for example in the case of pattern bruising, a run-over injury), or swelling, which initially may be well-localised and later becomes diffuse. Tenderness is usually well localised and follows the line of the fracture (i.e. in a long bone fracture it runs round the circumference of the bone). If the fracture is mobile, inadvertent movement of the limb will result in great pain, deformity and sometimes crepitus from the bone ends rubbing together. In virtually all cases, a fracture is *suspected* from the history and clinical examination, and *confirmed* by appropriate radiographs.

Radiographic examination

In every case of suspected fracture, radiographic examination of the area is mandatory. This will generally give a clear indication of the presence of a fracture and provide a sound basis for planning treatment. Where there is some clinical doubt, radiographs will reassure both patient and surgeon, and help avert any later medicolegal criticism regarding the initial management of the case. Stress films may be helpful in elucidating ligament injuries, and in children where the epiphyses present a confusing picture it may be helpful to obtain films of the uninjured side for comparison. In certain cases, CAT or MRI scans may be helpful in providing additional information: this is especially so in spinal injuries where it is important to assess the state of the spinal canal. Bone scans may assist in the detection of hairline fractures.

It is essential in every case that the radiographer is given unambiguous information on the request form. At its simplest, this must state *both the area to be visualised and the bone suspected of being fractured*, and it need hardly be stressed that this should be preceded by a thorough clinical examination.

The following table gives some of the commonest errors in requesting (diagnostic errors have been excluded):

Area suspected of fracture	Typical request	Error	Correct request
Scaphoid	'X-ray wrist, ? fracture'	Fractures of the scaphoid are hard to visualise: a minimum of three specialised views is required. A fracture may not show on the standard wrist projections	'X-ray scaphoid, ? fracture'
Calcaneus	'X-ray ankle, ? fracture' 'X-ray foot, ? fracture'	A tangential projection, with or without an additional oblique (along with the usual lateral), is necessary for satisfactory visualisation of the calcaneus. These views are not taken routinely when an X-ray examination of the foot or ankle is called for	'X-ray calcaneus, ? fracture'
Neck of femur	'X-ray femur, ? fracture'	Poor centring of the radiographs may render the fracture invisible	'X-ray hip ? fracture neck of femur' or 'X-ray to exclude fracture of femoral neck'
Tibial table or tibial spines	'X-ray tibia, ? fracture'	Poor centring may render the fracture invisible, or the area may not be included on the film	'X-ray upper third tibia to exclude fracture of tibial table'

Pitfalls

A number of fractures are missed with great regularity and you should always be on the lookout for the following:

- An elderly patient who is unable to weight-bear after a fall must be examined most carefully. The commonest cause by far is a fracture of the femoral neck, and this must be eliminated in every case. If the femoral neck is intact, look for a fracture of the *pubic rami*.
- If a car occupant suffers a fracture of the patella or femur from dashboard impact, always eliminate a patellar fracture on the other side, and most importantly, a silent dislocation of the hip.
- If a patient fractures the calcaneus in a fall, examine the other side most carefully. Bilateral fractures are extremely common.

- If a patient complains of a 'sprained ankle' always examine the foot as well as the ankle. Fractures of the base of the fifth metatarsal frequently result from inversion injuries and are often overlooked.
- In the unconscious patient, injuries of the cervical spine are frequently overlooked. It pays to have routine screening films of the neck, chest and pelvis in the unconscious patient.
- Impacted fractures of the neck of the humerus are often missed, and conversely, in children, the epiphyseal line is often wrongly mistaken for fracture.
- Posterior dislocation of the shoulder may not be diagnosed at the initial attendance. This is because the humeral head may come to lie directly behind the glenoid and may appear quite normal if only an AP projection is taken. If there is a strong suspicion of injury, and especially if there is deformity of the shoulder, a second projection is *essential* if no abnormality is noted on the AP film.
- The diagnosis of an isolated fracture of either the radius or ulna should be made with caution. The Monteggia and Galeazzi fracture–dislocations are still frequently missed. In the same way, it is unwise to diagnose a fracture of the tibia only until the whole of the fibula has been visualised; fracture of the tibia close to the ankle is, for example, often accompanied by a fracture of the fibular neck.
- At the wrist, greenstick fractures of the radius in children are often overlooked due to lack of care in studying the radiographs.
- In adults, fractures of the radial styloid or Bennett's fracture may be missed or treated as suspected fractures of the scaphoid. Complete tears of the ulnar collateral ligament of the MP joint of the thumb are frequently overlooked, sometimes with severe resultant functional disability.

THE TREATMENT OF FRACTURES
Primary aims
The primary aims of fracture treatment are:

1. The attainment of sound bony union without deformity.
2. The restoration of function, so that the patient is able to resume his former occupation and pursue any athletic or social activity he wishes.

To these might be added 'as quickly as possible' and 'without risk of any complications, whether early or late'. These aims cannot always be achieved, and in some situations are mutually exclusive. For example, internal fixation of some fractures may give rapid restoration of function but at the expense of occasional infection. The great variations that exist in fracture treatment are largely due to differences in interpretation of these factors and their relevance in the case under consideration.

Priorities of treatment/multiple injuries
If a fracture is a patient's sole injury, it is usually possible to proceed with its treatment without undue delay (although unfitness for anaesthesia may sometimes upset this ideal). If, however, a fracture is complicated by damage to other structures or involvement of other systems, treatment of the fracture usually takes second place. Immediate action must be taken to correct any life-endangering situation which may be present or anticipated. Therefore, when the patient is first seen, a rapid examination must be made to assess the need for

resuscitation and to detect any condition which merits priority in treatment. In cases of multiple injury, especially when the patient is unconscious, routine screening films of the skull, cervical spine, chest and pelvis should be carried out, along with an ultrasound examination of the abdomen.

The following situations may require consideration.

Resuscitation

The mnemonic 'A, B, C' may serve as a guide through this vital area, whose successful management is not as easy as the letters suggest.

A = Airway

Any blood, mucus or vomit must be removed from the upper respiratory passages by suction or swabbing, and dentures should be looked for and removed. In the more minor situations, respiratory obstruction may be avoided by support of the jaw, a simple airway and turning the patient on his side.

An endotracheal tube may have to be passed:

- in the unconscious patient with an absent gag reflex
- where inhalation of mucus or vomit has already taken place (or is suspected), so that the respiratory passages may be cleared under vision
- where there is bleeding from the upper airway
- to allow the more effective management of cases where there is respiratory difficulty or evidence of hypoxia—e.g. in cases of flail chest.

Where there is need for intubation in a patient when a cervical spine injury is suspected, the procedure should be carried out with great care, avoiding excessive cervical spine extension; nasotracheal intubation should be used. Confirm correct placement of the tube by auscultation (and/or by a radiograph). After any intubation assess the arterial blood gas levels so that appropriate steps may be taken to deal with any persistent impairment.

B = Breathing

- Administer 100% oxygen and check the breath sounds.
- Any open chest wound must be immediately covered to reduce the risks of tension pneumothorax. A vaseline gauze dressing, covered with a swab and firmly secured to the skin with broad adhesive tape is usually quite adequate in the emergency situation.
- If there is evidence of a tension pneumothorax (hyper-resonance and decreased breath sounds on the affected side, or tracheal shift to the other), or of pneumothorax or haemothorax, the appropriate chest cavities should be drained by intercostal catheters connected to water seal drains. A routine radiograph of the chest will usually confirm the diagnosis, but if this remains in doubt, the chest should be tapped in the fifth interspace in the midaxillary line.
- If there is evidence of paradoxical respiration due to flail rib segments, blood gas levels should be estimated. Normal values are:

pO_2	75–100 mm Hg
pCO_2	35–45 mm Hg
pH	7.38–7.44
Oxygen content	15–23%
Oxygen saturation	95–100%
Bicarbonate	22–25 millequivalent/l

- Slight impairment of respiratory function may be managed by giving oxygen by inhalation and analgesics with caution. When the blood gas levels are seriously disturbed, and especially in the presence of a concurrent head injury, some form of assisted respiration is usually the best method of management.

C = Circulation

Immediate treatment. Any severe external haemorrhage must be brought under rapid control. This can almost always be achieved with local padding or packing along with firm bandaging. The use of a tourniquet is best avoided except in the rarest of circumstances; then one should be used only in circumstances where its retention for excessive periods cannot occur. A tourniquet must be properly applied; too little pressure will increase the blood loss by preventing venous return, and too great a pressure will endanger underlying nerves. A pneumatic tourniquet should always be applied in preference to any other type. Remove blood for grouping and crossmatching, and the establishment of base-line parameters including haemoglobin and haematocrit.

Estimate the blood loss. The following list gives a crude guidance in anticipating potential blood loss:

- Closed fracture of the femoral shaft: 1 litre.
- Open book fractures of the pelvis: 2–3 litres (potentially much greater where there is a sacroiliac disruption).
- Intra-abdominal haemorrhage: 2–3 litres.
- Haemothorax: 1–2 litres.
- Closed head injury: blood loss is insubstantial and hypotension does not occur unless the patient is close to death.

Classify the haemorrhage. A 70 kilo male has a circulatory volume of 5 litres of blood (equivalent to 25 units of packed red blood cells).

- *Class I.* Loss of up to 15% of blood volume (equivalent to 4 units of packed red cells) normally does not cause a change in blood pressure or pulse.
- *Class II.* Loss of 15%–30% of blood volume (equivalent to 4–8 units of packed red cells) normally leads to tachycardia, but no significant disturbance of the blood pressure.
- *Class III.* Loss of 30%–40% of blood volume (about 2 litres in a 70 kilo man) results in tachycardia and lowering of the blood pressure.
- *Class IV.* Loss of more than 40% of blood volume leads generally to severe tachycardia and lowering of the blood pressure.

Assess the need for replacement. Initially the blood pressure and pulse are the most useful familiar guides to the state of the circulation, but note that tachycardia and a low blood pressure may sometimes be absent in those suffering from hypovolaemic shock, requiring the exercise of clinical judgement. The need for replacement depends on an assessment of loss and the circulatory state. The amount and type of replacement is dependent on the nature and extent of the loss. The rate of infusion is largely determined by the response to replacement.

If a substantial replacement is anticipated, set up two large bore (14–16 Gauge) intravenous lines, performing if necessary a rapid cut-down and insertion of a large bore intravenous cannula under vision.

If there is blood loss accompanied by tachycardia or hypotension, rapidly run in crystalloids (such as normal saline or Ringer-lactate). (In children, give 20 ml/kg body weight initially, and up to 60 ml/kg). Use of warmed solutions has been shown to reduce mortality and help preserve the haemostatic mechanisms and should be routine. (Note that crystalloids are poorly retained in the intravascular space. Some prefer the use of plasma or synthetic colloids which do not suffer from this disadvantage, but others claim that these have no superiority in the trauma setting. Fresh frozen plasma does have the advantage of covering any tendency to hypofibrinogenanaemia and factor V and factor VII deficiencies, but takes 20–30 minutes to thaw. Two units of fresh frozen plasma should be given where bleeding is continuing and there are coagulation factor deficiencies present.)

Assess the response to replacement. There is varying opinion on the best methods of assessing the stability of the circulation and the success of resuscitation. In all, the degree and maintenance of a positive response to treatment is more importance than the reading of isolated values which include the following:

1. *Pulse and blood pressure.* In spite of some unreliability, these remain the most valuable guides. The initial aim should be to restore the pulse rate to less than 140, and to obtain a blood pressure in excess of 90 mm systolic and rising.
2. *Urinary output.* Aim at 0.5 ml/kg body weight per hour in an adult (i.e. 6 ml every ten minutes in a 70 kilo man) and 1.0 ml/kg body weight in a child (i.e. twice the rate per kg).
3. *Central venous pressure (CVP).* This allows the monitoring of atrial filling pressures (normal value = less than 10 mm Hg).
4. *Haemoglobin.* If the Hb level reaches 10 g/dl and remains there, further blood is not usually required. (Below 9 g/dl, blood will usually be required and virtually invariably below 7 g/dl. When the Hb lies between 7 and 10 g/dl, and there is doubt, the PvO_2 and ER may be helpful in defining transfusion requirements). In the absence of continued bleeding, one unit of packed red blood cells would be expected to raise the Hb level by 1g/dl.

Dealing with persisting circulatory instability. If the patient fails to be stabilised by the administration of crystalloids, then blood will be needed. Normally, blood will also be required if the haemoglobin falls below 9 g/dl; note the following points:

- If the patient is exsanguinated and will die unless blood is administered immediately, give two units of Group O Rhesus negative blood pending supply of cross-matched blood which should ideally become available not more than 20 minutes after the patient's blood sample is submitted to the blood bank. Thereafter, or if the situation is less acute, administer cross-matched packed red cells. If bleeding continues, then whole blood becomes more appropriate. *The volume of the replacement required can vary enormously, and therefore must be judged by the response.* Where rapid, appropriate transfusion fails to control the situation, the commonest cause is continued bleeding. In most cases the site is obvious.
- External haemorrhage accompanying limb injuries should be readily controlled if this has not already been done.
- Continuing blood loss from intrathoracic injuries should be obvious. Assuming that a haemothorax has been diagnosed and treated by the insertion

of a chest drain, the quantity and rate of loss may be evaluated by monitoring the volumes in the collection bottle(s). This may be used to assess the need for exploration to control persisting haemorrhage.

- Massive bleeding from within the abdominal cavity (see later for diagnostic guides) usually requires immediate laparotomy, but it is essential to be sure that the bleeding is not from the pelvis. (An unstable fracture of the pelvis and a negative abdominal ultrasound would be a contraindication for laparotomy.)
- The commonest causes of intra-abdominal haemorrhage are tearing of the liver, spleen or mesentery, and all are potentially amenable to surgery.
- Haemorrhage accompanying fractures of the pelvis is most common in unstable fractures involving the sacroiliac joints; the bleeding may be from the pelvic plexus of veins or from damage to the iliac arteries. In the first instance, especially if there is little sacroiliac disruption, an external pelvic fixator should be employed, and replacement efforts renewed. If the sacroiliac joint is disrupted and the situation fails to resolve, a (posterior) C-clamp or sacroiliac screws should be used. If circulatory instability persists, then exploration may be needed as a last resort. Diffuse bleeding from the pelvic venous plexus is generally best controlled by packing. On rare occasions selective embolisation or ligature of the iliac arteries may be necessary.
- Haemorrhage from the urinary tract is seldom very severe, but nevertheless may be a problem. It should be suspected if there is a haematuria or some other indication (such as the presence of a fracture of the pelvis of appropriate pattern). The diagnosis may be clarified by an intravenous pyelogram, a cystogram or a urethrogram.

Other measures in assessing the severely injured patient

The alphabetic summary of the measures used in assessing the severely injured patient may be usefully expanded by the following.

- **D = drugs, allergies, disabilities.** Carry out a rapid screening of the patient and note any information (e.g. on warning cards, bracelets or lockets, or from relatives) of any relevant problem.
- **E = eating and exposure.** Obtain if possible information on the patient's intake of fluids and solids in case general anaesthesia is required. Where applicable, remove clothing to allow inspection of the entire patient to avoid overlooking any additional injuries.
- **F = Foley catheter.** In cases of multiple injury, and where no urinary tract damage is suspected, insert a catheter to allow monitoring of urinary output (and hence the adequacy of the blood pressure in maintaining renal function).

Head injury

Where there is a head injury the following procedures should be followed:

1. The unconscious patient should be intubated to minimise the risks of cerebral hypoxia.
2. A complete neurological examination must be carried out and the results charted, using the Glasgow Coma Scale; the examination should be repeated at regular intervals. Of particular significance is:
   - a history of a post-traumatic lucid interval
   - a history of progressive deterioration in the level of consciousness
   - focal neurological signs

- a rising blood pressure and falling pulse rate.
3. Where there is evidence of increased intracranial pressure or an increasing neurological deficit, further investigation by CAT scan and neurological referral are essential.

Glasgow Coma Scale

A patient is defined as being comatose if he does not open his eyes, if he does not obey commands, and if he does not utter recognisable words. The severity of the coma may be assessed by assigning a value to the eye, motor and verbal responses, and summing these. By repeating the examinations at regular intervals, progress may be monitored, and any deterioration (suggesting intracranial complications) recognised at an early stage.

Eye-opening (E)		Best motor response (M)		Verbal response (V)	
Variable	*Score*	*Variable*	*Score*	*Variable*	*Score*
Spontaneous	4	Obeys	6	Oriented	5
To speech	3	Localises	5	Confused conversation	4
To pain	2	Withdraws	4	Inappropriate words	3
Nil	1	Abnormal flexion	3	Incomprehensible sounds	2
		Extensor response	2	Nil	1
		Nil	1		

The coma score = E+M+V, with a value of 3 being the worst possible response and 15 the best. A value of less than 7 indicates severe coma, 8–12 moderate and 13–14 mild. Severe injuries are infrequent, and most patients who develop haematomas requiring surgery are classified as moderate or minor on admission.

Where there is a head injury in which the immediate prognosis is hopeless, any temporary splintage of the fracture should be retained but no fresh treatment planned. Where no active neurosurgical treatment is contemplated and the prognosis regarded as very poor but not absolutely hopeless, it is usually possible to devise some simple measures to give reasonable support to the injured part but at the same time permitting more definitive treatment in the near future should unexpected improvement occur.

Cardiac tamponade: intrathoracic rupture of the aorta

Widening of the thoracic mediastinum requires further investigation (echocardiography, angiography). Prompt drainage of an intrapericardial haematoma may be a life-saving measure. Aortic rupture may not be immediately fatal, and if confirmed by investigation, arrangements should be made without delay for exploration. As bypass facilities will be required, in some cases this will require transfer of the patient to a specialist unit. Thoracotomy may also be indicated where there is a tracheal, bronchial or oesophageal injury, or a penetrating injury to the mediastinum.

Visceral complications

Injury to the liver, spleen and kidneys may cause severe intra-abdominal haemorrhage. Haemorrhage may also follow mesenteric tears and ruptures of the stomach and intestine, with which the problems of perforation are also associated. Apart from initial ultrasound examination, suspected intra-abdominal injuries may be investigated by:

- peritoneal lavage, where the presence of blood, bile or digestive contents may be diagnostic
- MRI or CAT scans
- in the case of the urinary tract, examination of the urine for blood, retrograde cystography and intravenous pyelography. Abdominal exploration takes priority over fracture treatment.

In the evaluation of patients with multiple injuries several systems have been developed in an attempt to assess the overall severity (e.g. Abbreviated Injury Scale (AIS) and the Hospital Trauma Index (HTI)). These may be used as an alert for the need for prompt and expert treatment, and they may give an indication of the prognosis. Over a period they may be used statistically to evaluate the performance of a team, unit or hospital, or to draw attention to some injury pattern where treatment efforts might be profitably concentrated. Their use is not as yet widespread.

Treatment of the fracture itself
The *initial* stages are clear:

- Undue movement at the fracture site should be prevented by the use of temporary splintage till radiographic and any other examination is complete. This will reduce pain and haemorrhage, and minimise the chances of a closed fracture becoming open.
- If the deformity is so great that the viability of the skin overlying a fracture or dislocation is seriously endangered, it is usually advisable to do something to correct this. In many cases, gentle repositioning of the distal part of the limb is sufficient; the use of Entonox may be required.
- If the fracture is an open one, a bacteriological swab should be taken and the wound covered with sterile dressings. Appropriate antibiotic therapy should be commenced immediately.
- The fracture should be fully assessed by clinical and X-ray examination: the site, pattern, displacement and angulation should be noted. Involvement of the skin and damage to related structures, such as important nerves or blood vessels, should be determined.

With this information, a number of key decisions must be made:

1. Does the fracture require reduction? If a fracture is only slightly displaced, reduction may nevertheless be highly desirable, as for example in fractures involving the ankle joint, where even slight persisting deformity may lead to the development of osteoarthritis. In other situations, some displacement may often be accepted, depending on the site involved: where good remodelling may be anticipated (especially in children), and if the patient is very old, when the risks (anaesthesia, etc.) may be considered to outweigh an improvement which may be problematic. If the fracture is appreciably angled or rotated, reduction is generally essential for cosmetic and functional reasons.

2. If the fracture requires reduction, how is it planned to carry this out? The commonest method is by the *application of traction*, followed by *manipulation* of the fracture under general anaesthesia. General anaesthesia has most to offer in terms of muscle relaxation, duration and overall versatility, but for minor procedures regional anaesthesia and intravenous diazepam are popular and useful measures, with the advantage that waiting time may be reduced.

Continuous traction may be used to achieve a reduction, especially in the case of fractures of the femur and fracture dislocations of the cervical spine.

Open reduction of the fracture is carried out:

- as an obvious part of the treatment of an open fracture—i.e. debridement of the wound exposes the fracture which may then be reduced under vision
- where conservative methods have failed to give a satisfactory reduction
- where it is considered that the best method of supporting the fracture involves internal fixation, and exposure of the fracture is a necessary part of that procedure.

3. What support is required until union of the fracture occurs?

- *Non-rigid methods of support.* Arm slings, bandages and adhesive strapping may be used, and serve some of the following purposes:
  (i)   Firm support may help to limit swelling and oedema, and restrict the spread of haematoma.
  (ii) Arm slings are often employed to gain the benefits of elevation.
  (iii) Restriction of movement may relieve pain and may be enough to prevent displacement of the fracture.
- *Continuous traction.* Traction may be maintained for several weeks to maintain a reduction until healing is advanced. Fractures of the femoral shaft are frequently treated by this method.
- *Plaster fixation.* Plaster of Paris, generally in the form of plaster-impregnated bandages, is the commonest method of supporting a fracture. The plaster is carefully moulded to fit the contours of the limb, and its quick-setting properties allow the limb to be held without undue strain in the correct position until setting has occurred.
- *Internal fixation.* Internal fixation is indicated:
  (i)   Where a fracture cannot be reduced by closed methods.
  (ii) Where a reduction can be achieved but cannot be satisfactorily held by closed methods (e.g. fractures of the femoral neck).
  (iii) Where a higher quality of reduction and fixation is required than can be obtained by closed methods (e.g. some fractures involving articular surfaces).
  (iv) In the case of multiple injuries involving the lower extremities, the risks of respiratory distress syndrome, fat embolism and other complications are considerably reduced by early operative stabilisation of lower extremity fractures and by rapid mobilisation. The present tendency in dealing with multiple injuries is to stabilise all major lower limb fractures as soon as the patient's general condition will allow, and preferably as part of the initial treatment on the day the injuries are sustained.
  (vi) In addition, there is a controversial area where the risks of internal fixation in a particular set of circumstances are outweighed, in the experience and opinion of the surgeon in charge, by the advantages.
- *External skeletal fixation.* With this method the bone fragments are held in alignment with pins inserted percutaneously. Such systems are often of value in the management of open fractures where the state of the skin and other factors may make the use of internal fixation devices undesirable. The use of

external fixators is sometimes followed, even in the case of closed fractures, by pin track infections. The quality of the fixation is also dependent on the pins remaining tight in the bone, and there is some risk of non-union.

- *Cast bracing.* Cast-bracing techniques are sometimes employed some weeks after the initial conservative management of a fracture. The method is used particularly in the treatment of fractures of the femur and tibia, and permits early ambulation and mobilisation of the knee.

4. If the fracture is open, how will this influence treatment? The following points will require separate consideration:

- As debridement of the wound will almost certainly be needed, general anaesthesia and theatre facilities are essential.
- In every case, potential difficulty in skin cover must be anticipated. It is usual practice to carry out a secondary wound closure once good healing has become established.
- If wound contamination is judged to be slight, and if good cover of the fracture can be expected, internal fixation is often carried out where it is felt to contribute to the chances of union and a successful outcome. If wound contamination is more marked and the skin damage substantial, the use of large implants is discouraged. Where there is much tissue damage and the risks of infection are high, the use of an external fixator should be considered.
- Open fractures are usually associated with greater damage to surrounding soft tissues than is found in closed fractures. Postoperative swelling is invariable, is often severe and may lead to circulatory impairment in the limb. Admission for observation is almost always required. In some cases there is a serious elevation of pressure within the closed fascial compartments of the limb, and this may require prompt surgical decompression.
- As a rule, open fractures are associated with greater violence, more initial deformity and more direct soft tissue damage. Neurological and vascular involvement is more common and should be looked for.
- The majority of open fractures have microbial contamination which may be of both gram-negative and gram-positive organisms. The risk of the development of infection is closely related to the degree of soft tissue injury and the nature of any contamination. Swabs are taken from wounds on admission, and as a rule the administration of an appropriate broad-spectrum antibiotic is advised. Attention should also be paid to tetanus prophylaxis.
- In the most severe open injuries, where there is perhaps much comminution of bone, extensive crushing of muscle, gross wound contamination and neurological damage, primary amputation may have to be considered. Such an irrevocable line of treatment should not of course be suggested to a patient without the backing of a second, independent and senior opinion. In coming to a decision it may be helpful to consider the Mangled Extremity Severity Score (Johansen et al). This scheme has been devised to give a quantitative assessment of the severity of injury to a limb, and to offer a guide in making the difficult decision as to whether it is worth striving to save a limb or to minimise losses and advise a primary amputation. Its value is somewhat controversial.

5. Does the patient require admission to hospital? In most cases the decision is an easy one, being related to the seriousness of the injury, the nature of the treatment and the need for continuous observation. The main criteria for admission very frequently overlap and include the following:

- Admission dictated by treatment.
- Admission for observation.
- Admission for general nursing care.
- Admission for mobilisation.
- Admission for social reasons.
- Admission in the case of suspected child abuse.

Admission in the case of suspected child abuse. Where this is a possibility, admission is mandatory. About 80% of cases are under the age of three, and other factors which might alert you to this possibility include the following:

1. The presence of a fracture with no history of injury, or a vague history which is not in keeping with the nature or the extent of the injury.
2. The presence of multiple fractures or other injuries, especially when these are at different stages of healing.
3. The presence of multiple soft tissue injuries, including swellings, bruises, burns, welts, lacerations, scars and hand infections secondary to local burns.
4. If there is a head injury, radiographs of the skull may show evidence of fracture or widening of sutures in about 25% of child abuse victims.
5. Evidence of failure to thrive, growth retardation, fever, anaemia or seizures. The commonest fractures that are found, in order of frequency, are of the ribs, humerus, femur, tibia and skull, and in the average case 3–4 fractures are present. The presence of multiple lesions in varying states of healing is pathognomonic.

In the metaphyseal region the fractures may be impacted with copious new bone formation; there may be buckling of the bone without much in the way of new bone formation; or there may be irregular deformity with new bone appearing in layers as a result of repeated trauma. Injuries to the epiphyses and the growth plates are very uncommon in cases of child abuse (whereas this pattern of injury is seen frequently in other forms of trauma).

Apart from admission and the carrying out of treatment appropriate to the fractures or other injuries, further investigations should usually include the following:

- review of the records of previous admissions
- observations of the child's weight and height
- obtaining an X-ray skeletal survey, including the skull
- obtaining clinical photographs
- *most importantly,* informing the Social Services so that the child's home background can be looked into, and the appropriate action taken to safeguard the child should the diagnosis of child abuse seem likely.

Basic reduction techniques
238
Application of plaster casts
239
After-care of patients in
plasters 245
Polymer resin casts 247

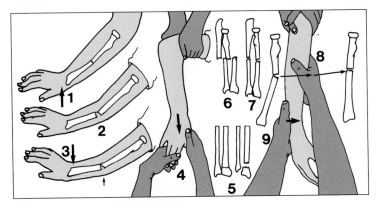

BASIC REDUCTION TECHNIQUES

The direction and magnitude of the causal force **(1)** and the deformity **(2)** are related, and may be worked out from the history, the appearance of the limb and the radiographs. Any force required to correct the displacement of a fracture is applied in the opposite direction **(3)**. The first step in most closed reductions is to apply traction—generally in the line of the limb **(4)**. Traction will lead to the disimpaction of most fractures **(5)** and this may occur almost immediately in the relaxed patient under general anaesthesia. Traction will also lead to reduction of shortening **(6)**, and in most cases to reduction of the deformity **(7)**. Any residual angulation following the application of traction may be corrected by using the heel of the hand under the fracture **(8)** and applying pressure distally with the other **(9)**. (In some fractures difficulty in reduction may be due to prominent bony spikes or soft tissue interposition, and may be aided by initially *increasing* the angulation prior to manipulation. This method must be pursued with care to avoid damage to surrounding vessels and nerves.)

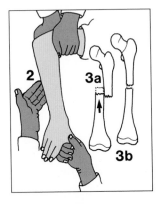

The *effectiveness of reduction* may be assessed by **(1)** noting the appearance of the limb; **(2)** by palpation, especially in long bone fractures; by checking for the presence **(3a)** or absence **(3b)** of telescoping (i.e. axial compression along the line of the limb leading to further shortening); and **(4)** by check radiographs.

After reduction of the fracture it must be prevented from redisplacing until it has united. The methods include plaster fixation, skin and skeletal traction, application of a Thomas splint, cast bracing, rigid external fixation (and various forms of internal fixation).

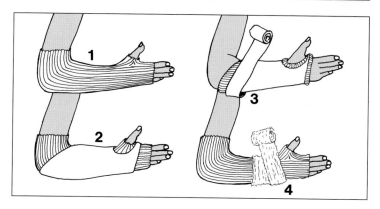

APPLICATION OF PLASTER CASTS

Protecting the skin

Stockingette. A layer of stockingette is usually applied next to the skin (**1**). This helps prevent the limb hairs becoming caught in the plaster, facilitates the conduction of perspiration, protects the skin from plaster rough edges and may aid in the removal of the plaster. After the plaster has been applied (**2**), the stockingette is turned back. Excess is removed, leaving 3–4 cm only at each end, and the loose edges are then secured with a turn or two of a plaster bandage (**3**).

Wool roll. A layer of wool should be used to protect bony prominences (**4**). In complete plasters, where swelling is anticipated, several layers of wool may be applied over the length of the limb; the initial layer of stockingette may be omitted. Wool roll is also advisable where an electric saw is used for plaster removal.

Felt. Where friction is likely to occur over bony prominences, protection may be given with felt strips or felt cut-outs, fashioned to isolate the area to be relieved (e.g. the vertebral and iliac spines, the pubis and manubrium in plaster jackets). Adhesive felt should not be applied directly to the skin if skin eruptions are to be avoided.

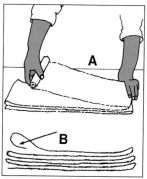

Plaster slabs

These consist of several layers of plaster bandage and may be used for the treatment of minor injuries or where potentially serious swelling is anticipated. Pre-formed slabs from a dispenser may be used. A single slab of six layers of bandage will usually suffice for a child. In a large adult, two slab thicknesses may be necessary. In a small adult, one slab thickness with local reinforcement may suffice. Alternatively, manufacture a slab by repeated folding of a plaster bandage (**A**). Turn in the end of the bandage (**B**) so that when the slab is dipped in water the upper layer does not fall out of alignment.

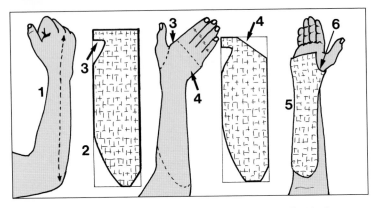

Tailoring plaster slabs. Ideally the slab should be trimmed with plaster scissors so that it will fit without being folded over. For example, a slab for an undisplaced greenstick fracture of the distal radius should stretch from the metacarpal heads to the olecranon. It may be measured (1) and trimmed as shown (2), with a tongue (3) to lie between the thumb and index. If being prepared for a Colles' fracture, where the hand should be placed in a position of ulnar deviation (4), the slab should be trimmed to accommodate this position. An *anterior* slab (5) may be used as a foundation for a scaphoid plaster, or to treat an injury in which the wrist is held in dorsiflexion (measuring from a point just distal to the elbow crease with the elbow at 90° to the proximal skin crease in the palm). The proximal end is rounded while the distal lateral corner (6) is trimmed for the thenar mass.

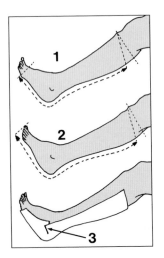

For the ankle (1) a plain untrimmed slab may be used, measuring from the metatarsal heads to the upper calf, 3–4 cm distal to a point behind the tibial tubercle. For the foot (2) where the toes require support, choose the tips of the toes as the distal point. Owing to the abrupt change in direction of the slab at the ankle, the slab requires cutting on both sides so that it may be smoothed down with local overlapping (3). (The same technique of side-cutting is required for long arm plaster slabs. These are measured from the upper arm to the metacarpal heads, with a cut-out at the thumb as in a Colles' plaster slab.)

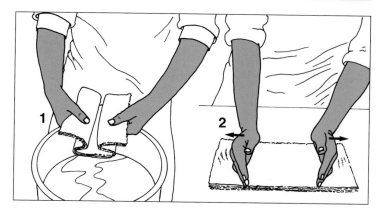

Wetting plaster slabs. Hold the slab carefully at both ends (1) and immerse it completely in *tepid* water. (Plaster setting time is decreased by both hot and soft water.) Lift it out and momentarily bunch it up at an angle to expel excess water. Now consolidate the layers of the slab. If a plaster table is available, quickly place the slab on the surface and, with one movement with the heels of the hands (2), press the layers firmly together. (Retained air, if not expelled, reduces the ultimate strength of the plaster and leads to cracking or separation of the layers).

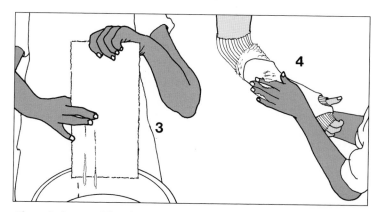

Alternatively, consolidate the layers by holding the plaster at one end, and pulling it between two adducted fingers (3). Repeat the procedure from the other edge of the slab.

Applying plaster slabs. Carefully position the slab on the limb and smooth out with the hands (4) so that the slab fits closely to the contours of the limb without rucking or forming sore-making ridges on its under surface.

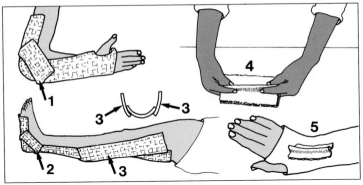

Reinforcing plaster slabs. At this stage any weak spots should be reinforced. Where there is a right-angled bend in a plaster—for example at the elbow (**1**) or the ankle (**2**)—two small slabs made from 10 cm (4″) plaster bandages may be used as triangular reinforcements on either side. A similar small slab may be used to reinforce the back of the wrist. In the case of a long leg plaster slab, additional strengthening at the thigh and knee is always necessary, and this may be achieved by the use of two additional 15 cm (6″) slabs (**3**). Where even greater strength is required, the plaster may be girdered. For example, for the wrist, make a small slab of six thicknesses of 10 cm bandage and pinch up in the centre (**4**). Dip the reinforcement, apply and smooth down to form a T-girder over the dorsum (**5**).

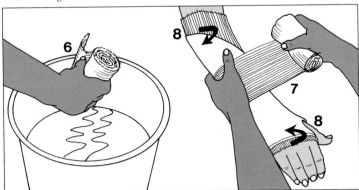

Securing plaster slabs. Bandages used to secure plaster slabs should be of open weave (cotton or muslin) and be thoroughly wetted (to avoid tightening from shrinkage after contacting the slab.) Secure the end of the bandage between the thumb and fingers (**6**) and squeeze several times under water. Apply to the limb firmly (**7**), but without too much pressure. Do not use reverse turns which tend to produce local constrictions. The ends of the underlying stockingette may be turned back and secured with the last few turns of the bandage (**8**). On completion, secure the bandage with a small piece of wetted plaster bandage.

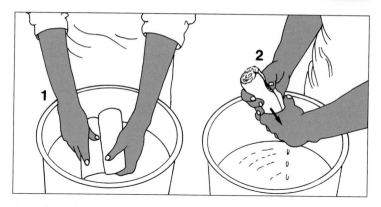

Complete plaster casts
Protection of skin. The skin should be protected as previously described, using where applicable stockingette, wool roll and felt.

Size of bandages. The following sizes of plaster bandage are recommended for normal application: upper arm and forearm, 15 cm (6″); wrist, 10 cm (4″); thumb and fingers, 7.5 cm (3″); trunk and hip, 20 cm (8″); thigh and leg, 20 cm; ankle and foot, 15 cm.

Wetting. Plaster bandages should be dipped in tepid water (1). Secure the end of the bandage with one hand to prevent the end becoming lost in the mass of wet bandage. Hold the bandage lightly with the other *without compression*. Immerse at an angle of 45° and keep under water until the bubbles stop rising. Remove excess water by gently compressing in an axial direction and twisting slightly. Alternatively, pull the bandage through the encircled thumb and index while lightly gripping the bandage (2).

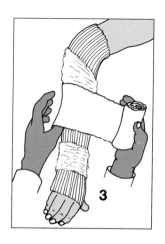

Application. It is often useful to apply the more proximal parts first, so that moulding can be more profitably carried out against a set or nearly set cuff of plaster (i.e. start a forearm plaster just below the elbow, and a below knee plaster at the tibial tubercle).

Roll each bandage without stretching if there is no wool beneath; if there is a layer of wool, and no swelling is anticipated, a little even pressure may be applied to compress the wool to half thickness. Plain tucks may be used (3) to ensure a smooth fit, but figure-of-eight or reverse turns should be avoided. Smooth the layers down to exclude trapped air. The distal part may then be completed, and the hand or foot portion moulded before setting is complete.

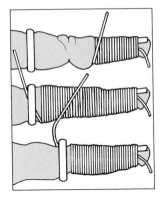

Reducing the risks of circulatory complications

Removal of rings. Wherever possible, rings should be removed to reduce the risks of finger gangrene. A tight ring can generally be coaxed from a finger if it is well coated with olive oil or a similar lubricant. If this fails, the finger may sometimes be sufficiently compressed by binding it with fine string and then unwinding as shown. Otherwise a ring cutter may be used. If one is not available, use a fine hacksaw while protecting the skin with a spatula slipped under the ring. After the cut has been made, the ring may be sprung open.

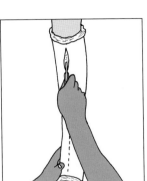

Plaster precautions. After an acute injury, if much swelling is anticipated use a plaster slab in preference to a complete plaster. If a slab does not give sufficient support, then allow for swelling with a generous layer of wool beneath the plaster and consider splitting it. This should be done *routinely* after any operative procedure when swelling may be considerable. Use a sharp knife and cut down through the plaster to the underlying wool. This should be done immediately after application of the plaster before it has had time to dry out. Be sure the plaster has been *completely* divided down to the wool along its whole length.

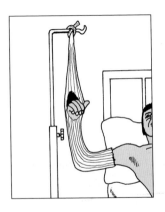

Elevation. Wherever possible, the injured limb should be elevated. In the case of the hand and forearm in a patient who has been admitted, the limb may be secured in stockingette (or in a roller towel using safety pins) attached to a drip stand at the side of the bed. In the case of the ambulant patient a sling may be used, provided the arm is kept high enough: if the sling is too slack the arm will hang down, encouraging oedema. In the case of the lower limb, the leg may be elevated on pillows and the end of the bed raised. The ambulant patient should be advised to keep the foot as high as possible on a couch or chair whenever he is at rest.

Instructions for patients in plaster of Paris splints

A (1) If fingers or toes become swollen, blue, painful or stiff, raise limb.

(2) If no improvement in half an hour call in doctor or return to hospital immediately.

B (1) Exercise all joints not included in plaster—especially fingers and toes.

(2) If you have been fitted with a walking plaster, walk in it.

(3) If plaster becomes loose or cracked—report to hospital as soon as possible.

AFTER-CARE OF PATIENTS IN PLASTER

The patient who is being allowed home must be given clear warnings to return should the circulation appear in any way to be impaired. Inform the patient, or where appropriate, a relative who will be looking after the patient. It is also useful to reinforce this by pasting an instruction label (such as the one illustrated) directly to the plaster. The importance of exercising those joints which remain free should be stressed (e.g. the fingers and shoulder in the case of a Colles' fracture), and the instructions should include the frequency with which the exercises should be performed.

At review, note the following:

- *Is there swelling?* Be careful to distinguish between moderate swelling which is a normal response to trauma (and which should respond to elevation), and severe swelling which may be associated with circulatory impairment.
- *Is there discoloration of the toes or fingers?* Compare one side with the other and assess whether swelling of the limb within the plaster has reached such a level as to impair the venous return (which will necessitate measures similar to those employed when there is evidence of arterial obstruction).
- *Is there in fact any evidence of arterial obstruction?* Note the five Ps: intense *pain*, *paralysis* of finger or toe flexors, *paraesthesia* in fingers or toes, *pallor* of the skin with disturbed capillary return and *'perishing cold'* feel of the fingers and toes. Arterial obstruction requires immediate, positive action. Treatment: Elevate the limb and in the case of a plaster slab, cut through the encircling bandages and underlying wool until the *skin is fully exposed*, and ease back the edges of the plaster shell until it is apparent that it is not constricting the limb in any way. Where the plaster is a complete one, split the plaster throughout its entire length. *Ease* back the edges of the cast to free the limb on each side of the midline. *Divide* all the overlying wool and stockingette and turn it back till skin is exposed. The same applies to any dressing swabs hardened with blood clot. If the circulation has been restored, gently pack wool between the cut edges of the plaster and firmly apply an encircling crepe bandage. If this is not done, there is risk of extensive local skin ('plaster') blistering. If the circulation is not restored, re-appraise the position of the fracture and suspect major vessel involvement. *On no account adopt an expectant and procrastinating policy.*
- *Can the plaster be completed?* If the plaster consists of a back-slab or shell, completion depends on your assessment of the present swelling and your prediction of any further swelling. Most plasters may be completed after 48 hours; but if swelling is very marked completion should be delayed for a further 2 days, or until it is showing signs of subsiding.
- *Is the plaster intact?* Look for evidence of cracking, especially in the region of the joints. In arm plasters, look for anterior softening, especially in the palm. In the leg, look for softening of the sole piece, the heel and calf. Any weak areas should be reinforced by the application of more plaster locally.

- *Is the plaster causing restriction of movement?* If so, trim the plaster accordingly.
- *Is the plaster too short?* Extend the defective plasters where appropriate.
- *Has the plaster become too loose?* A plaster may become loose when swelling recedes and muscles waste. To assess this, grasp the plaster and attempt to move it proximally and distally, while noting its excursion. If looseness is found, a plaster should be changed unless union is nearing completion (and risks of slipping are minimal), or the fracture is in a good position and the risks of it slipping while the plaster is being changed are thought to be greater than if left).
- *Is the patient complaining of localised pain?* Localised pain, especially over a bony prominence, may indicate inadequate local padding, local pressure and pressure sore formation. In a child it may sometimes suggest a foreign body pushed in under the plaster. In all cases, the affected area should be inspected by cutting a window in the plaster and replacing it after examination.

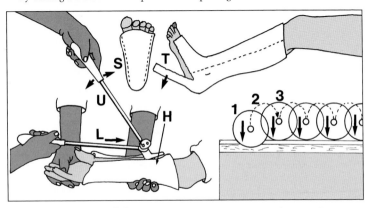

Removing plaster slabs. This is easily done by cutting the encircling open weave bandages. To help avoid nicking the skin use Böhler scissors.

Removing complete plasters. Using shears: the heel of the shears (**H**) must lie between the plaster and the limb. Choose a line of cut which avoids subcutaneous bony prominences (such as the shaft of the ulna) and any concavity. (At the ankle, it is often helpful to make two vertical cuts down through the sole piece (**S**) and turn it down (**T**) before cutting proximally on either side. Always keep the lower handle (**L**) parallel to the plaster, or even a little depressed. Lift up the upper handle (**U**); push the shears forward with the lower handle so that the plaster fills the throat of the shears. Maintaining a slight pushing force, all the cutting action may be performed with the upper handle, moving it up and down like a beer pump. Using a plaster saw: treat with respect and only use if there is a layer of wool between the plaster and the skin. Avoid using over bony prominences, or if the blade is bent, broken or blunt, or if a patient has a cardiomyopathy. (*Note:* the blade does not rotate but oscillates.) Reassure the apprehensive patient and a child should be given ear protectors. Cut down through the plaster at one level (**1**); the note will change as soon as it is through; remove the saw (**2**) and shift it laterally about an inch (2.5 cm) and repeat **(3)**. *Do not* slide the saw laterally in shallow cuts; the cutting movement should be up and down.

POLYMER RESIN CASTS

Plaster of Paris is the most frequently used casting material, although there are alternatives. Most use bandages of cotton (e.g. Bayer's Baycast®) or fibreglass (Smith & Nephew's Dynacast XR®), impregnated with a resin which hardens on contact with water. *Advantages* include: strength combined with lightness; rapid setting (5–10 minutes) and curing, reaching maximum strength in 30 minutes (cf. plasters whose slow 'drying out' period of about 48 hours may lead if unprotected to cracking); water resistance combined with porosity; and radiolucence. Disadvantages include: high item cost—but their durability reduces demands on staff and transport; they mould less well than plaster and are unyielding.

After acute injuries, where further swelling is likely, plaster is generally more suitable; it can be carefully moulded to the part, giving particularly good support; and where necessary it can be applied in the form of a slab. When swelling subsides and the stability of the fracture is not in doubt, a resin cast may be substituted. Where little swelling is anticipated in a stable fresh fracture, a resin cast may be used from the outset. Where wet weather or other factors are likely to test a plaster cast, there is much to be said for using polymer resin, and of course it is possible to reinforce an ordinary plaster cast with an outer resin bandage.

Application

(1) Apply conforming stockingette to the limb: ensure that it extends 3–5 cm (1–2″) beyond the proposed limits of the cast itself. Next, apply a layer of padding, paying particular care to protect the bony prominences. Where it is necessary to resist exposure to water or to moisture, a synthetic water-resistant padding may be used (e.g. Smith & Nephew's Soffban®).

(2) Open each bandage pack only as required, to avoid premature curing. Wear gloves to prevent the resin adhering to your skin or causing sensitisation. Immerse the bandage in warm water for 2–5 seconds, squeezing it two to four times to accelerate setting. Fewer bandages will be required than with plaster— e.g. a below-knee cast in an adult may be applied with two 7.5 cm (3″) and one to two 10 cm (4″) bandages. Use the smaller sizes for the areas requiring a high degree of conformity (e.g. the ankle).

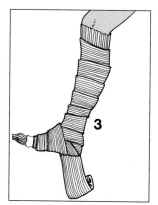

(3) Apply each turn so that it overlaps the one beneath by half a width. It is permissible to use a figure-of-eight round the ankle, elbow and knee to assist conforming to the limb. Turn back the stockingette before applying the top layers of the bandage and make quite certain that there will be no sharp or hard cast edges which can cause ulceration of the skin.

(4) In some cases, close moulding of the cast may be encouraged by the temporary application of a firm cotton or crepe bandage applied on top. This is first wetted, and then wrapped tightly round the limb. (It also helps to retain the last turn or two of the resin bandages, which tend to lift before setting has occurred.) Remove the wet overbandage once the cast has set.

Removal of resin casts

Because of their inherent springiness, resin casts cannot be cracked open after they have been cut down one side as can plasters. In most cases it is necessary to bivalve them by cutting down both sides. In the case of leg casts, it is best to turn down the sole piece first. Either shears or an oscillating saw may be used; in the latter case, a dust extractor should be employed to avoid the inhalation of resin dust. Resin casts are less likely to break after windowing than plasters.

Assessment of union

Elapsed time. Union in a fracture cannot be expected until a certain amount of time has elapsed, and it is pointless to start looking too soon. (See individual fractures for guidelines.) When it is reasonable to assess union, the limb should be examined out of plaster.

Oedema. Persistent oedema at the fracture site suggests union is incomplete.

Tenderness. Examine the limb carefully for tenderness. Persistent tenderness localised to the fracture site is again suggestive of incomplete union.

Mobility at the fracture site. Persistent mobility at the fracture site is certain evidence of incomplete union. Support the limb close to the fracture with one hand, and with the other attempt to move the distal part in both the anterior and lateral planes. In a uniting fracture this is not a painful procedure.

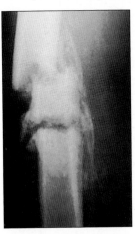

Radiographs. Although clinical assessment is often adequate in many fractures of cancellous bone, it is advisable in the case of the shafts of the femur, tibia, humerus, radius and ulna to have up-to-date radiographs of the region. The illustration is of a double (segmental) fracture of the femur at 14 weeks. In the proximal fracture, the fracture line is blurred and there is external bridging callus of good quality; union here is fairly far advanced. In the distal fracture, the fracture line is still clearly visible and bridging callus is patchy. Union is incomplete, and certainly not sufficient to allow unprotected weight-bearing. In assessing radiographs for union, be suspicious of unevenly distributed bridging callus, of a persistent gap, and of sclerosis or broadening of the bone ends. Note that where a particularly rigid system of internal fixation has been employed, bridging callus may be minimal or absent, and endosteal callus may be very slow to appear. If in doubt regarding the adequacy of union, continue with fixation and re-examine in 4 weeks.

Remember that in all cases you must assess whether the forces the limb is exposed to will result in displacement or angulation of the fracture, or cause such mobility that union will be prevented: you must balance the following equation:

The *degree of union + the support supplied by any internal fixation device and/or external splintage* must exceed *any external forces the limb will be subjected to.*

17

Open fractures/ gunshot wounds/ internal fixation

Open fractures 250
Gunshot wounds 251
Principles of internal fixation 252

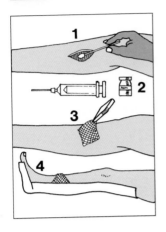

OPEN FRACTURES
Immediate care

When the case first presents, ensure that the following procedures are carried out in every case: (i) take a bacteriology swab from the wound; (ii) commence a course of appropriate antibiotics; (iii) cover the wound with care, using sterile dressings (to reduce the risks of secondary (hospital) infection); (iv) apply temporary splintage (e.g. a plaster back shell or if appropriate, an inflatable splint). Subsequent treatment is dependent on:

- the grading of the wound and the viability of the limb
- the nature of the fracture
- how it is planned to support the fracture.

Subsequent treatment on day of injury: general principles

Debridement. This must be meticulous, with removal of any foreign material and excision of all non-viable tissue; there should be a thorough lavage of the wound, first with saline and then with a solution of an appropriate antibiotic. Regimes change but Gustilo recommends for Type I fractures a single dose of 2.0 g of cephalosporin on admission followed by 1.0 g every 6–8 hours for 48–72 hours. For Type II or Type III injuries, gram-negative and gram-positive prophylaxis is necessary; as well as cephalosporin in the previously recommended dosage, the patient should be given aminoglycosides (tobramycin), 1.5 mg per kg body weight on admission and 3.0–5.0 mg per kg body weight daily thereafter in divided doses. This must be adjusted if there is renal insufficiency. If there is risk of clostridial infection, 10 million units of penicillin should also be given. If any secondary procedure (e.g. internal fixation, delayed wound closure) is being performed, the antibiotic courses should be repeated. Attention should also be paid to tetanus prophylaxis. As a general principle the wound should be left open, being lightly packed with dressings which will keep it moist.

Fixation of the fracture. The method used is dependent on the site, the quality of the fixation required and the risks of infection. Where the risks of infection are particularly high, an external fixator may be preferred. Intramedullary nailing is often employed in the tibia and femur. Where contamination is more than slight, caution should be exercised over reaming, especially in the case of the femur. Where the fracture is in good position, a plaster cast may be used, with windowing to permit inspection and dressing of the wound.

Treatment of associated vascular or neurological injuries. If there is a major arterial injury this must be repaired and the circulation restored within 4–6 hours if the limb is to survive. The commonest treatment is an interpositional graft, and before this is carried out the fracture must be fixed. If there is a nerve division and the ends can be approximated without tension, the best results follow immediate repair, and this may be carried out provided the wound is not badly contaminated.

Treatment after first day

General principles. The wound should be inspected on the second or third day. In Type I and II injuries it may be closed by secondary suture or split grafting if it is clean. If there is some infection with the presence of necrotic tissue, a further debridement should be carried out and the wound redressed. This is especially likely in Type III injuries, and the process of dressing and inspection may have to be repeated several times. The aim is to obtain skin cover as early as possible, and certainly within two weeks. A number of plastic surgical procedures are available, including split skin grafts, fasciocutaneous flaps, musculocutaneous flaps and microvascular free flaps. Their use is dependent on the circumstances and the facilities available.

Degloving injuries. In a degloving injury, an extensive area of skin is torn from its underlying attachments and thereby deprived of its blood supply. In the hand or arm it is commonly caused by the limb being crushed between rollers, and in the leg it may result from the shearing effect of a vehicle wheel passing over the limb in a run-over accident. The skin may remain unbroken, in which case the limb feels like a bag of fluid owing to the presence of an extensive haematoma between the skin and fascia. If the skin is torn the effect is the creation of a large flap of full-thickness skin. In either case, massive sloughing is likely unless the injury is properly managed. A number of plastic surgical procedures are available, including excision and storage of the flap, with its replacement after 1–2 weeks as a graft after the deeper layers have been removed.

Note: In any open injury it is vital to keep in mind the risks of serious, life-threatening infections, particularly tetanus and gas gangrene, and the appropriate protective measures must be taken.

GUNSHOT WOUNDS

The pattern of injury and the treatment required is dependent on the type of missile, but as a general rule there should be delayed wound suture and early split skin grafting.

Low velocity gunshot wounds (e.g. handgun wounds). The principles of treatment of uncomplicated wounds are as follows:
The margins of the entry and exit wounds should be excised.

- The track should be thoroughly irrigated with saline.
- A saline-soaked gauze swab should, if possible, be passed through and through and then removed.
- The track should be lightly packed open with Vaseline gauze.
- The wound should then be covered with saline-soaked dressings, dry gauze and wool, and secured with crepe bandages.
- The wound should be inspected at about 5 days and, if clean, sutured.

If there is a bullet in the tissues, the need for its removal should be carefully balanced against the risks of exploration. It should be noted that if a bullet remains in a joint, the toxicity of its metallic elements will have a disastrous effect on the articular cartilage. It is strongly advised that the affected joint should be thoroughly irrigated and every attempt made to remove the foreign body.

Plastic bullets. These tend to produce localised blunt injuries and seldom cause fractures.

High velocity gunshot wounds. These are characterised by small entry and large exit wounds. Shock waves may cause extensive tissue destruction and even fracture at a distance from the direct tract of the missile. A temporary wave of negative pressure may suck in clothing and other debris. If bone is struck, a multifragmentary (comminuted) fracture results.

These injuries must be treated with great respect along the lines of other Type IIIB open fractures. A full exploration with removal of all devitalised tissues is essential, and primary closure is contraindicated. In many cases, prophylactic compartmental fasciotomies are advisable. The fracture is often best fixed with an external fixator. If it is likely that a myocutaneous or other flap will be required, the fixator pins must be positioned so that this is possible.

Explosions. The severity of the injuries is inversely proportional to the distance between the victim and the source; the initial shock wave is followed by a short-lived fireball, but the accompanying blast wave causes most of the damage. There may also be accompanying respiratory and auditory damage, and falling masonry or flying debris may cause crush or other injuries. Where there are multiple casualties, Major Incident or Disaster Routines are generally followed, and the initial triage would normally be carried out by the most experienced surgeon present. Resuscitative procedures precede definitive treatment.

PRINCIPLES OF INTERNAL FIXATION

Implants—basic criteria
- They should not cause any significant tissue reaction.
- They should not corrode to any extent.
- They should satisfy the purposes for which they are intended, and be of sound mechanical design.

Devices and systems. Fractures vary enormously in pattern; bones vary in their size, texture and strength. To cope with even the most common situations and be a match for every subtle variation of circumstance requires an impressive range of equipment. The AO system of internal fixation devices and tools for their insertion is able to satisfy most criteria. They have been designed so that in most cases external splintage can be discarded at an early stage, permitting joint freedom, early weight bearing, short-term hospitalisation and early return to work and other activities.

Application. With any form of internal fixation, great importance must always be placed on recognising which cases are best treated in this way. It is equally important to recognise which cases are not suited for treatment by internal fixation and may be better dealt with either surgically or conservatively. It is in the last group that there is often some difficulty, and it is important to remember the risks of surgery, including infection which on occasion can turn a comparatively minor fracture into a disaster. Treatment guidelines are indicated in the regional sections. Note, however, that *in the case of multiple injuries* the prognosis is best when the circumstances allow early rigid fixation of all long bone fractures, particularly those in the lower limbs. (This is mainly due to the fact that many respiratory complications may be avoided by early mobilisation, which rigid internal fixation may permit.)

**Fracture
healing/
complications/
pathological
fractures**

Factors affecting the rate of
    healing of fractures 254
The complications of
    fractures 255
Pathological fractures 264
Recording and
    communicating 266

FACTORS AFFECTING THE RATE OF HEALING OF FRACTURES

- *Type of bone:*
  - *Cancellous bone (spongy bone).* Healing in cancellous bone is generally well advanced at 6 weeks, when protection of the fracture can almost invariably be abandoned: e.g. after 6 weeks, weight-bearing may be permitted after a fracture of the calcaneus, and plaster fixation may be discarded after a Colles' fracture.
  - *Cortical bone (compact bone).* Endosteal callus may take many months to become well established, and many uncomplicated long bone fractures may take 9–18 weeks to unite. In some cases, however, abundant external bridging callus may allow an earlier return of function. For example, conservatively treated tibial fractures take on average 16 weeks to unite, fractures of the humeral shaft can often be left unsupported after 10 weeks, but fractures of the metatarsals, metacarpals and phalanges, where external bridging callus is usually substantial, are usually quite firm in 4–5 weeks.
- *The patient's age.* In children, union of fractures is rapid, the speed decreasing as skeletal maturity approaches. There is then not a great deal of difference in the rate between young adults and the elderly. For example, in a child of 3 years, a fracture of the femoral shaft is usually united after 4 weeks, and a fractured femur in a child of 8 is usually sound after 9 weeks. In contrast, a fracture of the femoral shaft in an adult may take 3–6 months to unite. As well as great rapidity of union it should be noted that children's bones have remarkable powers of remodelling (apart from correction of axial rotation).
- *Mobility at the fracture site.* Excessive mobility at the fracture site may interfere with vascularisation of the fracture haematoma, leading to disruption of early bridging callus and the prevention of endosteal new bone growth. One of the main aims of all forms of internal and external splintage is to reduce mobility at the fracture site and hence encourage union: so it must be adequate.
- *Separation of the bone ends.* Union will be delayed or prevented if the bone ends are separated, for this interferes with the normal mechanisms of healing. Separation may occur under several circumstances:
  - interposition of soft tissue between the bone ends
  - excessive traction
  - following internal fixation, where in some cases a fixation device may hold the bone fragments apart following resorption of bone at the fracture site.
- *Infection.* Infection in the region of a fracture may delay or prevent union.
- *Disturbance of blood supply.*
- *Properties of the bone involved.* Fracture healing is also affected by a number of imperfectly understood factors which lead to variations in the speed of union. The clavicle is a spectacular example; non-union is extremely rare, the time to clinical union is unexcelled by any other part of the skeleton, yet movement at the fracture site cannot be effectively controlled.
- *Joint involvement.* When a fracture involves a joint, union is occasionally delayed. This may be due to dilution of the fracture haematoma by synovial fluid.
- *Bone pathology.* Many of the commonest causes of pathological fracture do not seem to delay union in a material way, although some do.

THE COMPLICATIONS OF FRACTURES

Complications of fracture include the following:

1. *Those associated with any tissue damage:* ● internal and external haemorrhage, oligaemic shock, etc. ● infection ● electrolyte shifts, protein breakdown and other metabolic responses of trauma.
2. *Those due to prolonged recumbency:* ● hypostatic pneumonia ● pressure sores ● deep venous thrombosis ● muscle wasting ● skeletal decalcification and urinary tract calculi ● urinary tract infections, etc.
3. *Those following anaesthesia and surgery:* ● atelectasis and pneumonia ● blood loss leading to anaemia or shock, with their secondary effects ● wound infection.
4. *Those peculiar to fractures:* in summary, these include: ● disorders involving the rate and quality of union ● joint stiffness ● Sudeck's atrophy ● avascular necrosis ● myositis ossificans ● osteitis ● vascular, neurological and tendon complications ● visceral complications and fat embolism ● implant complications.

Slow, delayed and non-union

Slow union. In slow union, the fracture takes longer than usual to unite, but passes through the normal clinical and radiological stages of healing without any departure from normal.

Delayed union. In delayed union, union fails to occur within the expected time. As distinct from slow union, radiographs of the part may show abnormal bone changes. Typically, there is absorption of bone at the level of the fracture, with the production of a gap between the bone ends. External bridging callus may be restricted to a localised area and be of poor quality. There is, however, no sclerosis of the bone ends.

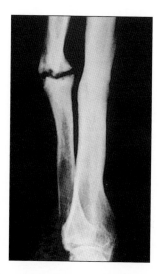

Non-union. In non-union, the fracture has failed to unite, and there are radiological changes which indicate that this situation will be permanent—i.e. the fracture will never unite—unless there is some fundamental alteration in the line of treatment. Two types of non-union are recognised. In *hypertrophic non-union* (see radiograph on left) the bone ends appear sclerotic, and are flared out so that the diameter of the bone fragments at the level of the fracture is increased ('elephant's foot' appearance). The fracture line is clearly visible, the gap being filled with cartilage and fibrous tissue cells. The increase in bone density is somewhat misleading and conceals the fact that the blood supply is in fact good.

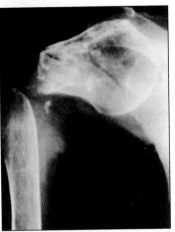

In *atrophic non-union* (see left) there is no evidence of cellular activity at the level of the fracture. The bone ends are narrow, rounded and osteoporotic, and they are frequently avascular.

Treatment

Slow union. Assuming that the fracture is adequately supported, patience should ultimately be rewarded with sound bony union.

Delayed union. The problem is to differentiate between delayed union which is going to proceed with proper encouragement to union, and delayed union which is going to go on to non-union.

The only sure arbiter is time, but the disadvantage of delay is that it tends to encourage irreversible stiffness in those joints which are immobilised with the fracture (besides frequently creating problems from prolonged hospitalisation and absence from work).

If union has not occurred within the time normally required, or if gross mobility is still present at 2 months, there should be a careful appraisal of the radiographs and the methods of fixation. If the radiographs show the changes of slow or delayed union, but none of the changes of non-union, and the fracture is well-supported, immobilisation should be continued and the situation re-assessed, with further radiographs, in 4–6 weeks. Improvement in the radiological appearance will then be an encouraging sign, suggesting that persistence in the established line of treatment will lead to union. If there is no change, or if there is deterioration, this is an indication for more active treatment (e.g. rigid internal fixation).

Hypertrophic non-union. If the fracture can be fixed with absolute rigidity by mechanical means, the cartilaginous and fibrous tissue between the bone ends will mineralise and be converted to bone (by induction). In the femur, this may be accomplished by careful reaming of the medullary canal and the introduction of a stout, large-diameter intramedullary nail. The bone ends are not disturbed. In the tibia and the other long bones, rigid fixation may usually be obtained by compression plating.

There is some evidence that the process of induction which results in the conversion of the tissue at the fracture into bone may also be stimulated by the creation of small electric currents in the gap between the bone ends. This may be achieved by embedding percutaneous electrodes in the fracture gap, or by placing field coils round the limb. Treatment by this method is lengthy (extending over several months) but can often be administered on an out-patient basis and is particularly indicated where it is desirable to avoid surgery (e.g. in the presence of continued infection). Accelerated union has also been reported by the use of ultrasound at the fracture site, and when fractures have been open or surgically exposed, by the local application of a collagen sponge impregnated with recombinant human morphogenic protein-2 (rhBMP-2;dibotermin alfa).

Atrophic non-union. Treatment for atrophic non-union is less easy or reliable, and involves four important aspects: (i) The fracture must be held rigidly: this usually implies internal fixation. (ii) Fibrous tissue should be removed from between the bone ends. (iii) The bone ends should be decorticated from the level of the fracture back to healthy bone. (iv) The area round the fracture is packed with cancellous bone grafts.

Malunion

In practice the term is used in the following circumstances:

- Where a fracture has united with angulation or rotation of a degree that gives a displeasing appearance or affects function.
- Where a fracture has united with a little persistent deformity in a situation where even the slightest displacement or angulation is a potential source of trouble. This applies particularly to fractures involving joints.

Treatment. In treating fractures, one of the main objectives is an adequate reduction and avoidance of malunion. Malunion is sometimes a sign of poor management. If detected before union is complete, angulation may sometimes be corrected by wedging of a plaster or forcible manipulation under anaesthesia. After union, an osteotomy may be considered if the deformity is severe.

Shortening

This is generally a sequel of malunion. In children, bone growth is always accelerated in the injured limb, and any discrepancy in limb lengths is usually quickly made up. In adults, shortening in the lower limb is seen most frequently after fractures of the tibial shaft. Shortening of 1.5 cm is easily tolerated, being compensated for by tilting of the pelvis. Shortening in excess of this may usually be dealt with by alteration of the footwear. A corrective osteotomy may be performed for shortening due to severe, persistent angulation. In the upper limb, shortening seldom causes any problem.

Traumatic epiphyseal arrest

The epiphyseal plate may be damaged as a result of trauma. If the whole width of the plate is affected, then its growth may be arrested, leading to progressive shortening of the limb. The final discrepancy in limb lengths is dependent on the epiphysis affected and the child's age at the time of injury.

More commonly, the epiphyseal plate is incompletely affected so that growth continues more or less normally at one side, while at the other it may be severely retarded or arrested. This leads to some shortening of the limb and to distortion of the associated joint. In all cases of suspected epiphyseal damage, a careful follow-up is necessary. The child should be seen every 6–12 months and any residual deformity carefully assessed by clinical and radiological measurement. In the upper limb, if the deformity is progressive it may produce an unsightly appearance and may be responsible for delayed neurological involvement. In the lower limb, abnormal stresses may be produced in the weight-bearing joints, ultimately giving rise to pain, stiffness, instability and often a rapidly progressive secondary osteoarthritis.

Treatment. It is sometimes possible to treat this problem with an epiphyseolysis. In this procedure the abnormal block of bone bridging the epiphyseal plate is excised, and the defect plugged with fat or bone wax to prevent recurrence. In late cases, a corrective osteotomy may be indicated.

Joint stiffness

This is a common complication which may result from a combination of factors which include pathology within the joint, pathology close to the joint, or problems remote from the joint. In its avoidance, attention should be paid to the following:

- Accurate reduction of the fracture wherever possible.
- Splintage of the minimal number of joints compatible with security.
- Splintage of the fracture for the shortest time compatible with the relief of pain and fracture healing.
- Urgent mobilisation of all unsplinted joints in the limb.
- Elevation of the injured part during the initial stages to decrease joint oedema.
- Where applicable, supporting the joints in such a position that restoration of movement on discarding splintage will be encouraged.
- Where a fracture involves articular surfaces, early movement becomes particularly important if an adequate range is to be regained.
- Where stiffness is present or anticipated, physiotherapy and, where appropriate, occupational therapy should be started as early as possible.
- Anticipate complications, and avoid procrastination, especially with regard to non-union.

When internal fixation is contemplated, there is merit in selecting techniques and devices which will support the fracture to such an extent that the limb may be exercised without external support.

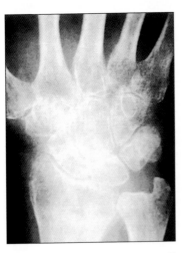

Sudeck's atrophy (post-traumatic osteodystrophy/complex regional pain syndrome)

Aetiology. This condition, which is of uncertain origin, is essentially one where there is chronic post-traumatic pain associated with local autonomic changes. It is seen most frequently after Colles' fractures of the wrist. In most cases it is not recognised until final removal of the plaster. There is swelling of the hand and fingers, and the skin is warm, pink and glazed in appearance. There is striking restriction of movements in the fingers, and diffuse tenderness over the wrist and carpus. This tenderness may at first suggest that the fracture is ununited, but check radiographs will show that this is not the case. Typically, the radiographs demonstrate union of the fracture, with diffuse, osteoporotic mottling of the carpus (see above).

Although seen most often after Colles' fractures, Sudeck's atrophy may follow scaphoid fractures or indeed any injury about the wrist. The condition is also seen in the lower limb, after injuries to the ankle, foot or knee (where its effects may be particularly severe).

Diagnosis. The diagnosis is not often in doubt, but a number of tests are considered to be of value for confirmation, especially if aggressive forms of treatment are being contemplated; these include: • 3-phase radionuclide scintigraphy (which may show asymmetrical blood flow and increased periarticular uptake) • thermography • the measurement of vasomotor and sudomotor response • synovial biopsy.

Relief of symptoms and signs by sympathetic blockade is considered of greatest diagnostic value. Regional sympathetic blockade or a regional perfusion technique may be employed. Relief of pain and an improvement in the clinical signs for 1–4 days after the perfusion is regarded as being diagnostic.

Treatment. The condition is usually self-limiting, with the abnormalities of circulation and decalcification resolving slowly over a period of 4–12 months. There may be some permanent restriction of movements and to minimise this intensive physiotherapy is usually prescribed and continued to resolution. In the more severe cases, additional treatment may be advised. Regional perfusion with guanethidine may be used (although its efficacy has been questioned), with or without the use of oral sympatholytic drugs (such as prazocin or phenoxybenzamine); nifedipine is also sometimes tried, and good results have been claimed following the empirical use of prednisolone. Only rarely are surgical or chemical sympathectomy advised.

In the case of the knee, a particularly aggressive approach which may lead to rapid and complete resolution is advocated. After confirmation of the diagnosis, an epidural blockade is maintained for 4 days, during which time the limb is mobilised vigorously by measures which include continuous passive motion, alternating hot and cold soaks, muscle stimulation and manipulation.

Avascular necrosis
This is death of bone due to interference with its blood supply, and it is seen most often in the femoral head (after some intracapsular fractures of the femoral neck or after dislocation of the hip), in the scaphoid (after certain fractures of the proximal half), in the talus (after fractures or dislocations) and in the lunate (usually after dislocations). The importance of avascular necrosis is that the affected bone becomes soft and distorted in shape, leading to pain, stiffness and secondary osteoarthritis.

Treatment. The natural course of avascular necrosis is for the slow revascularisation of the necrotic bone from the periphery. This process takes 6–18 months, but in spite of it secondary osteoarthritic changes in the affected joints are inevitable. In the lower limb, deformity of the avascular bone may be minimised by the avoidance of weight-bearing, and this is of some value at least in the case of the talus; local bone grafting may speed revascularisation.

Myositis ossificans
In its commonest form, a calcified mass appears in the tissues near a joint, leading generally to considerable restriction of movements. It is seen most often at the elbow after a supracondylar fracture, an elbow dislocation or a fracture of the radial head. It can follow inadvisable passive stretching of joints.

Treatment. Early excision of the mass gives bad results, being almost always followed by a massive recurrence. Late excision (say after 6–12 months), however, is often successful in restoring movement, especially when local radiation therapy is used to discourage recurrence.

Osteitis

Infection in *closed* fractures (due to systemic spread of organisms) is rare and seldom diagnosed until infection is well-established. Infection is a well-known and feared complication of open fractures. It is also seen on occasion after the internal fixation of closed fractures.

Diagnosis. There is usually recurrent pyrexia, a raised sedimentation rate and white count, and unduly prolonged pain, local tenderness and swelling. In addition, there may be a purulent wound discharge with staining of the plaster or dressings which become foul smelling. (Do not be diffident about smelling a cast or wound!) Radiological changes may not be diagnostic and are slow in appearing.

Treatment. (a) The risk of this complication should always be kept in mind in the handling of open fractures or when internal fixation is planned. (b) Once firmly established, bone infections are peculiarly resistant to treatment, and delay must be avoided. (c) If possible, a sample of pus should be obtained so that the bacteriology and antibiotic sensitivity may be firmly established. The appropriate antibiotic must then be administered in adequate dose for an adequate time (usually 4 weeks as a minimum). In patients being treated in plaster casts, access to the wound may be obtained by windowing of the plaster. (d) Unless discovered early, drainage should be established, and regular dressings performed (with a good aseptic technique) to allow healing by granulation. (e) Although discharge from the wound may persist until internal fixation materials are removed, this should be delayed until fracture healing is advanced. (f) When infection is well-established and unresponsive, more radical measures may be called for. These include: • radical excision of all infected bone and open packing of the wound • raising the local concentrate of antibiotics by the use of irrigation tubes or the implantation of beads impregnated with gentamycin or other antibiotics • rarely, amputation may have to be considered.

Acute arterial arrest

The arterial blood flow distal to a fracture is occasionally interrupted, and assessment of the circulation in a fractured limb is an essential part of the examination. Arterial arrest results in loss of the distal pulses, pallor and coldness of the skin, loss of the capillary responses, severe pain in the limb, paraesthesia and eventually muscle paralysis. The commonest cause is kinking of the main arterial trunks by the displacement of a fracture or dislocation. In these cases, the circulation is immediately restored by correction of the deformity, and this should always be carried out as expeditiously as possible. In closed fractures, other arterial disturbances are found, but these are relatively uncommon. (A ragged bone edge may cause arterial rupture, leading to the rapid formation of a large haematoma. A fracture may also give rise to profound arterial spasm, local aneurysm formation or intimal stripping.) In open fractures, where the effects of direct injury may also operate, arterial rupture often declares itself by the nature and the extent of the accompanying haemorrhage.

Diagnosis. If the pulses distal to the injury site cannot be palpated, the patient should be resuscitated and reassessed within an hour. The most reliable guide to the situation is the Doppler pressure. If the limb pressures are not equal, the advice of a vascular surgeon should be sought *immediately*. If no Doppler equipment is available, then advice should be sought, again without delay, should the peripheral pulses on the injured side be reduced or absent.

Treatment. The survival of a useful limb is dependent on restoration of the circulation. Where this is not achieved by reduction of the fracture, exploration of the affected vessel is mandatory. Treatment is then dependent on the findings, and where a vascular procedure such as suture or grafting is required, internal fixation of the fracture is often performed first.

Arterial obstruction leading to muscle death and nerve palsy may also result from swelling within the muscle compartments of a limb, leading to an inexorable rise of pressure beyond the systolic blood pressure. In the leg this will result in muscle necrosis, loss of conduction in the deep peroneal nerve, sensory disturbance in the foot and foot drop. Prompt splitting of the roof of the affected compartment may avert this complication.

Immediate neurological disturbance

Neurological complications occurring immediately after fractures and dislocations are uncommon. In certain situations, a nerve may be stretched over a bone edge in a displaced fracture, or over a bone end in a dislocation. If prolonged this will lead to local ischaemia and interruption of nerve conduction. If stretching is more severe, there may be rupture of axons or of neural tubes: actual nerve division is rare, being seen mainly in association with open injuries. The commoner fractures and dislocations associated with nerve palsies include the following:

Dislocation of the shoulder	Axillary nerve palsy: rarely other brachial plexus lesions
Fracture of the shaft of the humerus	Radial nerve palsy
Dislocation of the elbow	Ulnar nerve palsy; sometimes median nerve affected
Fractures round the elbow	
Dislocation of the hip	Median nerve palsy; less commonly, ulnar nerve, or posterior interosseous nerve
Dislocation of the knee or rupture of lateral ligament of the knee and fracture of medial tibial table	Sciatic nerve palsy
	Common peroneal nerve palsy

Treatment. The majority of nerve lesions are in continuity. Assuming that the fracture or dislocation has been reduced, recovery often begins after 6 weeks, progressing quite rapidly thereafter. The *skin* must be protected during the recovery period against friction, burns and other trauma so long as sensation remains materially impaired. The *joints* should be exercised passively. *Deformity* due to overactivity of unaffected muscles should be prevented, and splintage, fixed or lively may be required.

Where there is a nerve palsy accompanying a fracture which is going to be treated surgically, opportunity may be taken to inspect the affected nerve. Otherwise, when an expected recovery does not occur, electromyography and nerve conduction studies may be of occasional diagnostic value, but exploration is often required. Where there is a nerve division, primary suture should be undertaken if the risks of infection are judged to be slight and facilities are good. Otherwise, elective repair is delayed until sound wound healing has been obtained. If nerve repair is not possible, reconstructive surgery or orthotic support of the paralysed part may be required.

Delayed neurological disturbance
Sometimes a nerve palsy gradually develops long after a fracture has healed.

Tardy ulnar nerve palsy. This is the most striking example. In a typical case the patient gradually develops a progressive ulnar nerve palsy, often after a supracondylar fracture or a Monteggia fracture–dislocation. The striking feature is the interval (often years) between the fracture and the nerve palsy. In a number of these cases there is a cubitus valgus deformity. *Treatment.* This condition is usually treated by early transposition of the ulnar nerve from its position behind the medial epicondyle to the front of the joint.

Median nerve palsy. Signs of median nerve compression may gradually develop a few months after a Colles' fracture. This is generally akin to the partial nerve lesions seen in the carpal tunnel syndrome. Some residual displacement of the fracture may reduce the space available in the carpal tunnel, leading to pressure on the nerve and an incomplete palsy. *Treatment.* Symptoms are usually relieved by carpal tunnel decompression.

Delayed tendon rupture
This uncommon fracture complication is seen most frequently at the wrist, where after a Colles' fracture, a patient loses the ability to extend the terminal joint of the thumb due to rupture of the extensor pollicis longus tendon. The rupture may result from the gradual fraying of the tendon as it rubs against the healing fracture, or it may be caused by traumatic or fibrotic interference with its arterial blood supply, resulting in local sloughing of the tendon.

Treatment. In the case of the thumb, the best results are obtained by transposition and suture of the tendon of extensor indicis.

Visceral complications
(i) Rupture of the urethra or bladder and perforation of the rectal wall may complicate fractures of the pelvis. (ii) Rupture of the spleen, kidney or liver may follow severe local trauma, abdominal compression or crushing. (iii) Rupture of the intestines or tearing of the mesenteric attachments may follow abdominal compression. (iv) Paralytic ileus is occasionally seen following fractures of the pelvis and lumbar spine, the most likely cause being disturbance of the autonomic control of the bowel from retroperitoneal haematoma. It usually resolves promptly with nasogastric suction and intravenous fluids.

The cast syndrome
Abdominal distension, vomiting, shock and prostration sometimes occur in patients being treated in plaster jackets, hip spicas or plaster beds, especially if the spine is hyperextended. It may result from duodenal compression by the superior mesenteric artery.

Treatment. (a) If a plaster jacket has been applied, it should be removed. A patient being nursed in a plaster bed should be transferred to an ordinary bed or a Stryker frame. (b) Insert a large-bore gastric tube and give IV fluids.

Acute respiratory distress syndrome (ARDS)/ Fat embolism syndrome (FES)

Hypoxia and acute respiratory insufficiency are common after trauma, and the causes include upper airway obstruction, chest injury (e.g. due to pneumothorax) and circulatory failure. Most respond to treatment of the underlying cause and the administration of oxygen, but if this fails, other causes, particularly the acute respiratory distress syndrome (ARDS) or the fat embolism syndrome (FES), must be suspected. ARDS is seen most frequently in cases of multiple organ dysfunction occurring after high energy and usually multiple injuries. There is uncertainty about its cause, but it is believed that it may result from an abnormal systemic inflammatory response to trauma, targeting the lungs first and later other organs.

After most fractures, some fat is released into the circulation and causes no problem. In FES, however, the situation is different, and this may be related to the quantity of fat involved. The presence of fat in the pulmonary circulation may result in respiratory problems similar to those found in ARDS. Fat particles may, however, also enter the systemic circulation through pulmonary capillaries and shunts, or through a patent foramen ovale, producing very distinctive features which merit the title 'fat embolus'. This is seen most often after fractures of the femoral shaft and pelvis.

In both ARDS and FES there is no evidence of cardiac failure; chest radiographs show bilateral 'snowstorm' lungs, and there is disturbance of the PaO_2/FiO_2 ratio (arterial oxygen concentration divided by the fractional inspired oxygen concentration). Where there has been a fat embolism the most distinctive features (which may appear two or three days after the injury) are petechial haemorrhages in the skin of the upper trunk and neurological disturbance: the patient may become confused, aggressive or comatose, and focal neurological signs may appear (e.g. epileptiform seizures). There may be evidence of renal insufficiency, and the heart, liver and gastrointestinal tract may also be involved.

Treatment. There is evidence that the risks of these complications developing are reduced by prompt and effective fluid replacement and other resuscitative measures. Many consider that the rigid fixation of femoral fractures in cases of multiple injury is also beneficial. Once established, however, humidified oxygen should be administered, any inadequate fluid replacement corrected, and chest physiotherapy carried out to reduce the risks of secondary pulmonary infection. If oxygenation is inadequate, constant positive airways pressure (CPAP) through a tight fitting mask may be tried, but if this is not enough (as indicated by the blood gas levels), the patient should be transferred to an intensive therapy unit with a view to intubation and ventilation.

Implant complications

Mechanical effects. Plates and intramedullary nails reduce the natural elasticity of the bone in the area where they lie. As a result, the loads to which a bone is subjected are not absorbed evenly throughout its length; stress concentrations tend to occur at the ends of internal fixation devices, and in the femur there is loss of some of the shock distributing elasticity of the bone which may in some cases lead to susceptibility to fracture. For example, after a minor fall on the side which would not normally be expected to cause any problem, someone who has had an intramedullary nailing may sustain a fracture of the femoral neck.

Corrosion. No metal implant is completely inert, and the long-term risks of retention of implants within the body have not been fully evaluated. It is not uncommon for the tissues surrounding a stainless steel implant to become discoloured, with the formation of substantial masses of fibrous tissue. This is especially likely to occur if there has been fretting between components (e.g. between a plate and screw). This may be associated with local aching pain, and is an indication for removal of the device (assuming the fracture is soundly healed).

Treatment. The risks of any long-term effects should be avoided where possible by routine removal of implants once they have served their purpose; this is the general advice in patients under the age of 40. Over that age the indications are less powerful, but as a general rule intramedullary nails should be removed, as should any other device where there is evidence of local tissue reaction.

PATHOLOGICAL FRACTURES

A pathological fracture is one which has occurred in a bone which is abnormal or diseased. In some cases the pathological process leads to progressive weakness of the bone so that fracture may occur spontaneously or after slight injury only. Fracture may occur as an inevitable event in some disease process (e.g. in osteitis), or the disease process may be unknown to the patient and his practitioner, the trivial nature of the trauma giving concern to both.

Where bone strength is not materially impaired, the causal violence producing the fracture may not cause comment; in these circumstances the radiographs taken after the incident may give the first indication to anyone that something else is amiss. It follows that virtually any condition capable of being detected by radiographs of the skeleton may fall into this category—a limitless range of congenital, metabolic and neoplastic disease. As a result, diagnosis may be difficult, but fortunately there is one important point to take into consideration: where a fracture is the presenting feature, the number of conditions commonly responsible is small. These include the following:

Osteoporosis. This is the commonest cause of pathological fracture, being especially important in the spine, the wrist and the femoral neck. It is most frequently due to lowering of hormone levels in association with age or the menopause: less frequently it follows disuse, rheumatoid arthritis or vitamin C deficiency, all of which lead to a failure of osteoid tissue formation and a translucent appearance of bone on the radiographs.

Osteomalacia. This is due to a failure in osteoid mineralisation, and the radiographic appearances may be difficult to differentiate from osteoporosis. It is usually secondary to an inability to utilise vitamin D (adult rickets) but is also seen where calcium is deficient in the diet (or excreted in renal acidosis), where phosphate is excreted in excess (Fanconi syndrome) or where vitamin D is not absorbed (e.g. steatorrhoea). A triradiate pelvis is diagnostic. Stress fractures are common, and areas of bone translucency (Looser's zones) in the pelvis and long bones are characteristic. There are disturbances in the blood chemistry: the serum phosphate is reduced, and the serum calcium normal or reduced.

Paget's disease. This is frequently seen in association with fractures of the tibia and femur. Stress fractures are common, and complete fractures are usually transverse. Sarcomatous change may occur. Note that the bone changes found in hyperparathyroidism and sometimes in metastatic disease may mimic Paget's disease.

Osteitis. Sudden collapse of bone secondary to infection is comparatively uncommon as a presenting feature, but is seen where the destructive processes are comparatively low grade (e.g. in tuberculosis).

Osteogenesis imperfecta. This hereditary disorder (dominant transmission) is characterised by bone fragility leading to bowing of the long bones, deformities of bone modelling, pathological fractures and stunting of growth. Deafness and blue sclerotics are commonly associated. The condition generally declares itself in infancy or childhood, but occasionally may not be diagnosed until skeletal demineralisation is noted later in life. Fracture healing is usually quite rapid, and most fractures may be treated successfully by conservative methods.

Simple bone tumours and cysts. In the metacarpals, metatarsals and phalanges, enchondromata are frequently encountered as a cause of pathological fracture. In children between 5 and 15 years, unicameral bone cyst is one of the most frequent causes of pathological fracture, especially in the proximal humeral shaft. The bone cortex may be thinned, but expansion is rare.

Secondary malignant bone tumours. The commonest malignant bone tumour is the metastatic deposit. Secondaries in bone occur most frequently from primary growths in lung or bronchus, breast, prostate or kidney. Any bone may be affected, but the spine, subtrochanteric region of the femur and the humeral shaft are amongst the commonest sites.

Primary malignant bone tumours. Of these, the commonest include osteogenic sarcoma, chondrosarcoma, fibrosarcoma, Ewing's tumour, and malignant change in an osteoclastoma.

Treatment of malignant bone tumours

Note the following points:

- Without treatment, union of a fracture occurring at the site of a malignant bone tumour seldom occurs.
- If the tumour is responsive to local radiotherapy or to chemotherapy, healing may occur with appropriate splintage, but will be slow.
- In the case of metastatic disease, internal fixation has much to recommend it unless the patient is moribund. Acrylic cement is sometimes used to reinforce a bone defect.
- In the case of primary malignant bone tumours, the occurrence of fracture may in some circumstances be an indication for amputation.

Investigation of pathological fractures

This may require some or all of the following:

- A full personal and family history.
- Full clinical examination, including pelvic examination.
- Radiographs of the chest.
- Radiographs of the pelvis.
- Radiographs of the skull and skeletal survey.
- Estimation of the sedimentation rate.
- A full blood count, including a differential cell count.
- Estimation of the serum calcium, phosphate, alkaline phosphatase and, where appropriate, the acid phosphatase.
- Estimation of the serum proteins.
- Serum electrophoresis.
- Examination of the urine for Bence–Jones proteose.

- A bone scan.
- Marrow biopsy.
- Bone biopsy.
- Occasionally, radiographs of parents or sibs.

RECORDING AND COMMUNICATING
Below are some suggested guidelines.

Records
Careful note-taking is of particular importance, especially in a field of medicine where evidence for insurance claims and litigation is commonly required. There are a number of areas where inadequacy is commonly found:

- Not infrequently, problems arise because entries or letters have been *un-dated*. It is vital that any entry is clearly dated, and in the seriously ill patient whose condition is rapidly changing, the *time* should be stated as well.
- Illegible handwriting is always a problem, but there should be no excuse for numerals and capital letters which are so badly formed that they cannot be read. With contractions, only employ those in common use.
- Paucity of notes (often unfairly) suggests a similarly brief, and, by implication, incomplete examination. In the heat of dealing with a seriously ill patient there is no time for detailed note-taking, but as soon as pressure eases, a full record should be made, and certainly this should be done *on the day of the admission*.
- The interpretation of radiographs should be included in the notes, giving negative as well as positive findings. With the growing tendency to practise a degree of defensive medicine, radiographs should certainly be taken if there is any doubt about the nature or severity of an injury, and if radiographs are not taken, it is perhaps wise to say at the time why this has not been thought to be necessary.

If there is something that you are not sure of, indicate what this is (so that it cannot be claimed later that you had not considered it), and state the course you tend to take (with, if appropriate, the reasons for doing so).

Telephoning
Be clear whether the purpose of your call is to inform, to ask for advice or to seek assistance, and have all the appropriate information at your finger tips. It is necessary to be able to describe a fracture patient in an unequivocal fashion, so that a clear picture of the problem is conveyed. There are undeniably different styles of doing this, but the following method is suggested:

Preamble. After any niceties, including if necessary stating exactly who you are, give the age and sex of the patient along with any special points bearing directly on the call: e.g. 'I have just admitted a 35-year-old man who is a professional ice skater. He has been in a road traffic accident and his main problem is . . .' (Note that it is probably best to avoid contractions such as 'RTA'.)

Precise fracture details. The description of the fracture should always start with whether it is open or closed, and be followed by the bone involved and the level; then the pattern of the fracture, and any displacement or angulation: e.g. '. . . an open fracture of his right tibia in midshaft. It's a transverse fracture, but it's displaced medially and there's some lateral angulation. There's some shortening, and there's no bony contact.'

Particular qualifiers. Where relevant these would include the following:

- Complications of the local injury: this would include a description of the size, nature, location and potential contamination of a wound. It would also include details of any vascular or neurological problem.
- Details of any other injuries such as head injury, chest or abdominal injuries.
- General condition of the patient, with (if appropriate) the time when he would be considered fit enough for anaesthesia and surgery.
- Details of any treatment already carried out.

Reason for call. When this is to *inform only*, the details of the treatment carried out and what is further proposed could with profit be expanded: e.g. 'I am planning to take him to theatre to debride the wound. I think I'll be able to get a good stable reduction under vision and I'll put the limb in plaster afterwards.'

When *advice is sought*, the nature of the problem should be clearly stated: e.g. 'I think this fracture might do best if internally fixed, but I'm wondering whether this should be done right away, or whether I should just reduce it and splint it, and add it to the beginning of tomorrow's list.' (Not generally the best solution!)

When *help is required*, this should be clearly stated, e.g. 'I think this is one you would want to treat by closed intramedullary nailing, and I've laid on theatre for 7:30.'

Clavicular injuries 270
Scapular fractures 275
Dislocation of the shoulder
    276
Fractures of the proximal
    humerus 284
Fractures of the humeral shaft
    292

CLAVICULAR INJURIES

Mechanism of injury. Most (94%) of clavicular injuries result from a direct blow on the point of the shoulder, generally from a fall on the side. Less commonly, force may be transmitted up the arm from a fall on the outstretched hand. *Fracture* is commonest at the junction of the middle and outer thirds, but is also common throughout the middle third and to a lesser extent the outer third. *Subluxations* and *dislocations* may involve the acromioclavicular joint or the sternoclavicular joint.

Common patterns of fracture. *In children*, greenstick fractures commonly occur at the junction between the middle and outer thirds. Fractures may not be particularly obvious in the radiographs and it is often helpful to have both shoulders included for comparison. Healing is rapid, and reduction is not required.

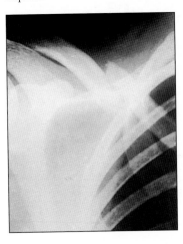

In adults, many fractures are undisplaced and are comparatively stable injuries, with symptoms settling rapidly and minimal treatment being required.

With greater violence, there is displacement of the fracture, often with overlapping of the fragments (e.g. left): sternomastoid elevates the proximal fragment and the shoulder tends to sag downwards and forwards. Nevertheless union is rapid (non-union is a comparative rare event), and remodelling, even in adults, is so effective that strenuous attempts at reduction are unnecessary. Note that pathological fracture may result from radionecrosis (following radiotherapy for breast carcinoma) and may be mistaken for a local recurrence.

Diagnosis. There is tenderness at the fracture site; there may be an obvious deformity with local swelling and later bruising. The patient may support the injured limb with the other hand. Diagnosis is confirmed by radiographs, a single AP projection of the shoulder being adequate.

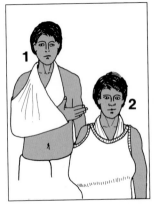

Treatment. The most important aspect of treatment is to provide support for the weight of the arm. As a rule this is best achieved with a broad arm sling (**1**). Additional fixation may be obtained by wearing the sling under the clothes (**2**). No other treatment is needed in greenstick or undisplaced fractures.

Analgesics will generally be required, particularly during the first three days or so.

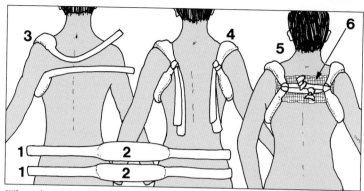

Where there is marked displacement of a clavicular fracture it is common (but not essential) practice to attempt to correct the anterior drift of the scapula round the chest wall. There is no simple way of achieving this. All methods apply pressure to the front of the shoulder and, although they are comparatively ineffective in terms of reduction, are helpful in reducing pain. In the *ring* or *quoit method*, narrow gauge stockingette is cut into two lengths of about a metre each (1). The central portions are stuffed with cotton wool (2). One of the strips is taken and the padded area positioned over the front of the shoulder (3) and tied firmly behind. The second strip is applied in a similar manner to the other shoulder (4). The patient is then asked to brace the shoulders back and the free ends of the ring pads are tied together (5). A pad of gamgee (sandwich of gauze/cotton wool) may be placed as a cushion beneath the knots (6). Alternatively, *figure-of-eight bandages* of wool, applied over pads of cotton wool or gamgee encircling the shoulders may also be tried. Commercially available *clavicle rings*, covered with chamois leather and secured with web straps and buckles may be employed. With all these methods, care must be taken to avoid pressure on the axillary structures and the additional support of a sling is desirable for the first two weeks or so. (Note that elderly patients tolerate clavicular bracing methods poorly, and support with a sling alone may be preferable.)

After-care

- Clavicular braces of all types require careful supervision and, at least initially, may require inspection and possible tightening every 2–4 days.
- Where braces are used in conjunction with a sling, the sling may usually be discarded after 2 weeks.
- All supports may be removed as soon as tenderness disappears from the fracture site.
- Physiotherapy is seldom required except in the elderly patient who has developed shoulder stiffness.
- A child's mother should always be advised that the prominent callous round the fracture is a normal occurrence, and that it will disappear in a few months with remodelling.

Note: If there is evidence of *torticollis* accompanying a clavicular fracture, further investigation of the cervical spine is indicated, as this finding may indicate a coincidental injury at the C1–2 level (locked facet joints). If plain radiographs are insufficient to clarify the situation, a CAT scan should, if possible, be carried out.

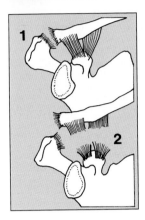

Acromioclavicular joint injuries

Injury to the acromioclavicular joint usually results from a fall in which the patient rolls on the shoulder. Note that in *subluxations and sprains* (1), damage is confined to the acromioclavicular ligaments, and the clavicle preserves some contact with the acromion. In *dislocations* (2) the clavicle loses all connection with the scapula, the conoid and trapezoid ligaments tearing away from the inferior border of the clavicle. The displacement may be severe, and the ensuing haematoma may ossify.

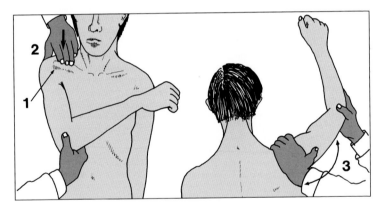

Diagnosis

1. The patient should be standing and the shoulders compared. The outer end of the clavicle will be prominent, and in cases of damage to the conoid and trapezoid ligaments the prominence may be quite striking. Local tenderness is always present.

2. Confirm any subluxation by supporting the elbow with one hand while gently pushing the clavicle down with the other. Improvement in the contour of the outer end of the clavicle will confirm the diagnosis of subluxation or dislocation.

3. Now stand behind the patient and abduct the arm to 90°. Flex and extend the shoulder while gently palpating the acromioclavicular joint. *Failure of the outer end of the clavicle to accompany the acromion indicates rupture of the conoid and trapezoid ligaments.*

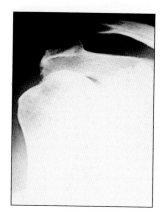

Radiographs. Displacement of the clavicle by a diameter or more relative to the acromion (**left**) suggests rupture of the conoid and trapezoid ligaments. The radiographic appearances may be fallacious as spontaneous reduction tends to occur in recumbency—the position in which AP radiographs are normally taken. *It must be clearly indicated on the radiograph request form that the acromioclavicular joint is suspect.* The films should be taken with the patient standing and preferably holding weights in both hands. It is helpful to obtain views of both shoulders, taken at the same time and on the same film, to allow comparison.

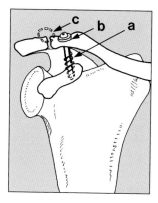

Treatment. (1) If there is no gross instability, treat by the use of a broad arm sling under the clothes for 4–6 weeks. Physiotherapy is seldom required and an excellent result is the rule. (2) In cases of gross instability, good results usually follow conservative management. (3) Although complications are common after surgery, this should be considered in patients who are engaged in work which is heavy or involves prolonged elevation of the arms. The preferred method is to bring the clavicle down into alignment with the acromion, using a lag screw (**a**) run into the coracoid. A washer (**b**) is used to spread local stresses, and some advise reinforcement of the fixation with some absorbable transarticular sutures (**c**). Any tears in the deltoid or trapezius are also repaired. Additional support with a broad arm sling is necessary, and the screw must be removed before the shoulder is fully mobilised. (4) If a dislocation reduces with the arm in abduction, a shoulder spica (**d**) for 6–8 weeks may be used as an alternative to surgery.

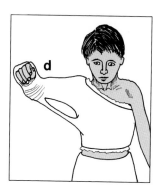

Complications. Symptoms from acromioclavicular osteoarthritis may be relieved by acromionectomy or excision of the outer 2 cm of the clavicle. Fascial reconstruction of the coracoclavicular ligaments can be used for persistent instability.

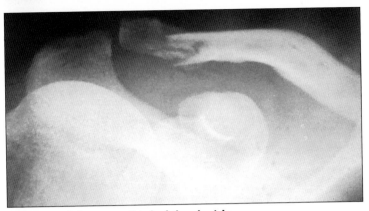

Fractures of the outer third of the clavicle

Displacement is generally minimal (as above) because the coracoclavicular ligaments are not usually torn. When these ligaments are damaged, however, displacement may be marked and give rise (rarely) to non-union. These injuries should be treated along similar lines to acromioclavicular joint injuries: clavicular bracing is valueless and a sling under the clothes for 4–5 weeks is usually quite adequate.

Complications of clavicular fractures. (1) Glenohumeral joint stiffness in the elderly may require physiotherapy. (2) Even after normal remodelling (which continues for may months) a persistent sharp clavicular spike may cause discomfort against the clothes and require excision. (3) Non-union is rare, but if causing symptoms is treated by bone grafting and internal fixation by (a) a reconstruction plate applied superiorly, (b) a dynamic compression plate applied anteriorly, or (c) a T-plate in outer-third fractures. A lag screw between the medial fragment and coracoid may also be used.

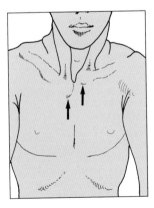

Sternoclavicular dislocation

This is sometimes seen without any history of trauma, but generally the commonest lesion, a minor subluxation, follows a fall or blow on the front of the shoulder or a fall on the outstretched hand. There is asymmetry of the inner ends of the clavicles due to the clavicle on the affected side subluxing downwards and forwards. There is local tenderness. *The diagnosis is essentially a clinical one.*

Radiographs. AP and oblique radiographs are difficult to interpret but are nevertheless usually performed. CAT scans are generally more informative, especially in the uncommon situation when the clavicle passes *behind* the sternum, where it may endanger the great vessels.

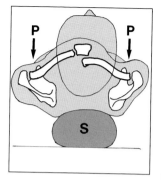

Treatment. *Minor subluxations* should be accepted. Some prominence of the inner end of the clavicle may persist, but a pain-free result is usual. The arm should be rested in a sling for 2–3 weeks until acute pain has settled.

Gross displacements should be reduced under general anaesthesia (but with great caution when the displacement is posterior). A sandbag (**S**) is placed between the shoulders which are firmly pressed backwards (**P**). Apply clavicular braces and a broad arm sling for 4–5 weeks. If the reduction is unstable, surgical repair may have to be considered. The rare irreducible dislocation may require open reduction.

SCAPULAR FRACTURES

Fractures of the blade of the scapula are usually caused by direct violence. Even when comminuted and angled (**left**), healing is usually extremely rapid and an excellent outcome is the rule. Treatment is by use of a broad arm sling and analgesics. Mobilisation is commenced as soon as acute symptoms have settled, and is usually possible after 2 weeks.

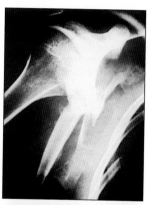

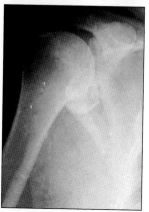

Fractures of the *scapular neck* (**left**) are associated with much bruising and swelling. Comminution is common, sometimes with involvement of the glenohumeral joint. If so, *the position of the humeral head should be checked,* and CAT scans may be required for an accurate assessment.

In spite of frequently daunting radiographs, a good outcome following conservative treatment is the rule, provided mobilisation is commenced as early as possible. However, if damage to the glenoid is extensive with displacement of major fragments, many advocate surgical reconstruction in the younger patient. Fractures of the *scapular spine* or *coracoid* are usually dealt with conservatively.

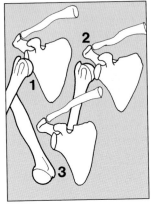

DISLOCATION OF THE SHOULDER

When the shoulder dislocates, the head of the humerus may come to lie *mainly* (1) in front of the glenoid (anterior dislocation of the shoulder), (2) behind the glenoid (posterior dislocation of the shoulder) or (3) beneath the glenoid (luxatio erecta).

Anterior dislocation

Anterior dislocation is *by far* the commonest of these. It most commonly results from a fall leading to external rotation of the shoulder. It is rare in children, common in the 18–25 years age group (from motorcycle and athletic injuries) and comparatively common in the elderly, where the stability of the shoulder may be impaired by muscle degeneration and where falls are common.

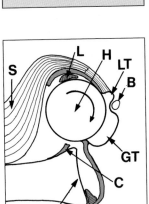

Pathology. The head of the humerus (**H**) externally rotates out of the glenoid (**G**) and comes to lie medially in front of the scapula. This is inevitably associated with damage to the anterior structures. Commonly the capsule is torn away from its attachment to the glenoid (**C**). This is the so-called Bankart lesion, although the frequent simultaneous displacement of the glenoid labrum (**L**) usually attracts this term. (**B** = biceps tendons; **GT** = greater tuberosity; **LT** = lesser tuberosity; S = subscapularis.)

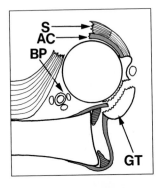

The anterior capsule stretches, but in the older patient especially it often tears (**AC**); there is sometimes associated damage to the shoulder cuff, especially subscapularis (**S**). The greater tuberosity (**GT**) may fracture, and rarely there is damage to the axillary artery. The brachial plexus (**BP**), particularly the axillary nerve, is more commonly affected.

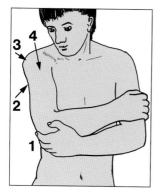

Diagnosis. The shoulder is very painful; the patient resents movement, and to prevent this often holds the injured limb at the elbow with the other hand (**1**). The arm does not always lie into the side, appearing to be in slight abduction. The outer contour of the shoulder may appear to be slightly kinked (**2**) due to the displacement of the humeral head. Palpate under the edge of the acromion (**3**). The usual resistance offered by the humeral head will be absent, and more distally (**4**) the anteriorly displaced humeral head may be palpable. In the doubtful case, palpation in the axilla may be helpful in determining the position of the humeral head.

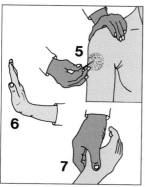

Axillary (circumflex) nerve palsy is the commonest neurological complication. Test for integrity of the nerve by assessing sensation to pin prick (**5**) in its distribution over the 'regimental badge' area over the lateral aspect of the proximal humerus. (Note that the shoulder is usually too painful to assess deltoid activity with certainty.) Exclude other (rare) involvement of the radial portion of the posterior cord (by checking active dorsiflexion of the wrist (**6**) and for involvement of the axillary artery (**7**)).

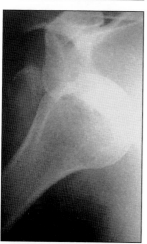

Radiographs. The majority of anterior or posterior dislocations show quite clearly on the standard AP radiograph, unless the humeral head has minimal medial displacement. (This is especially the case in posterior shoulder dislocations.) *A second radiographic projection is essential if the diagnosis is in doubt.* The most useful additional projection is the *axial lateral*, but unfortunately the shoulder may be too painful for this to be taken. *If so, obtain an apical oblique or a translateral projection.* An associated fracture of the greater tuberosity is not uncommon (**left**). This does not influence the initial treatment (by reduction), but it may require subsequent attention. The radiographs may also show evidence of previous episodes of dislocation.

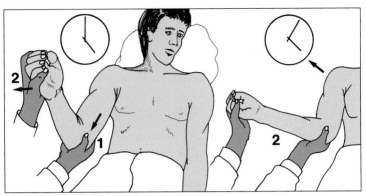

Treatment: reduction by Kocher's method. This may often be carried out in the older patient after the administration of intravenous diazepam, or in the younger patient after a substantial dose of intramuscular pethidine. Severe pain or a muscular patient are indications for general anaesthesia. Apply traction (1) and begin to rotate the arm externally (2). Take plenty of time over external rotation. In the conscious patient, if muscle resistance is felt, stop for a moment while distracting the patient's attention with conversation and then continue. It should be possible to reach 90° of external rotation. (If severe pain and muscle spasm prevent rotation, general anaesthesia will be required.)

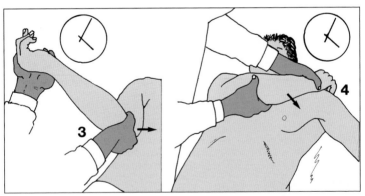

The shoulder frequently reduces with a clear 'clunking' sensation during the external rotation procedure, but if this does not happen adduct the shoulder so that the elbow starts to come across the chest (3). (This and the following movements may be carried out rapidly.) Now internally rotate the shoulder, bringing the patient's hand towards the opposite shoulder (4). If reduction has not occurred, repeat all stages, attempting to get more external rotation in stage 2. If doubt remains, repeat radiographs should be taken. Complete failure is rare under general anaesthesia. In the sedated patient, failure is an indication for general anaesthesia.

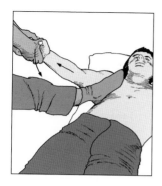

Alternative methods of reduction.
In this common and generally easy to reduce dislocation there is no shortage of alternative procedures.

Hippocratic method. The principle is that traction is applied to the arm and the head of the humerus is levered back into position. The stockinged heel is placed against the chest (without being pressed hard into the axilla) to act as a fulcrum, while the arm is adducted.

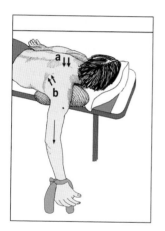

Stimson's method. The patient is given a powerful analgesic (e.g. 200 mg of pethidine in a fit athletic male) with resuscitation facilities available. Alternatively, an injection of 20 ml of 1% Xylocaine, injected over the edge of the acromion into the glenohumeral joint has been found to be effective. The patient should be prone, with the arm dependent, a sandbag under the clavicle and a weight of about 4 kilos tied to the wrist. The joint normally reduces spontaneously within six minutes: if not, with one hand fix the superomedial angle of the scapula (**a**), and with the other push the inferior angle medially (**b**).

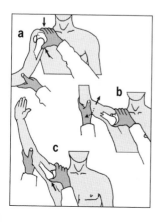

Milch's method. This is based on neutralising the power of the shoulder muscles by abducting the joint. Place the fingers over the shoulder and steady the displaced humeral head with the thumb (**a**). Now gently abduct and externally rotate the arm (**b**). When full abduction is reached, increase thumb pressure to slide the humeral head over the glenoid margin. Variations of this method include the use of traction and an erect posture. Sedation or anaesthesia may or may not be required.

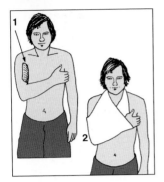

After-care. Check radiographs should be taken. This should be done before any anaesthetic is discontinued if there is doubt about the reduction. The arm should be supported after reduction to lessen the risks of immediate redislocation and to help relieve pain. Begin by placing a gamgee or wool pad in the axilla (for perspiration) (1) and apply a broad arm sling (2).

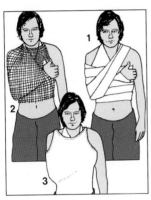

External rotation should be prevented by a body bandage (1), stretchable net (Netelast®) (2) or less securely by the outside clothes (3). The supports may require changing for the sake of hygiene from time to time until they are discarded. If there is some residual pain, an outside sling may be worn for a further week. Mobilisation is usually rapid without physiotherapy being required.

In the younger patient the common practice is to continue supporting the limb for a 4–week period (the rationale being that this gives the torn tissues time to heal), although the efficacy of this is in preventing recurrence (50% incidence in 2 years) is in doubt. If early mobilisation is particularly desirable, or recurrent dislocation certain, curtail the period of support. Thereafter, mobilisation is usually rapid, without physiotherapy being required. *In the elderly patient* the risks of recurrent dislocation are slight, but stiffness is common. Apply a sling under the clothes initially and discard this as soon as pain will permit. Mobilisation of both the shoulder and the elbow may usually be started after 1–2 weeks. Referral for physiotherapy is advisable in nearly all cases. In some elderly patients there may be joint instability problems due to damage to the shoulder cuff. This may be diagnosed and treated arthroscopically.

If there has been an associated fracture of the greater tuberosity which fails to reduce with the dislocation, screw fixation may be required.

Where there has been an axillary nerve palsy with loss of deltoid function, physiotherapy is essential. Although the lesion is usually in continuity and full recovery may occur, this may take several months and is not invariable. Assisted movements will be required—either normally, with the aid of slings and perhaps weights, or by hydrotherapy.

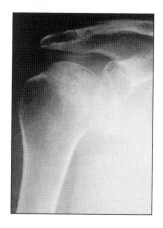

Posterior dislocation of the shoulder

This may result from a fall on the outstretched, internally rotated hand or from a direct blow on the front of the shoulder. The head of the humerus is displaced directly backwards and, because of this, a single AP projection may show little or no abnormality (as illustrated **left**). Nevertheless, clinically there is pain, deformity and local tenderness. *Note:* posterior dislocation may accompany (and be missed) in obstetrical and Erb's palsies. The frequently apparently normal AP projection makes it essential for an *additional lateral view* to be obtained when a posterior dislocation is suspected.

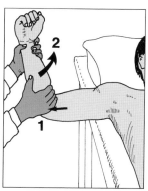

Treatment. Reduction is usually easily accomplished by applying traction to the arm in a position of 90° abduction (1) and then externally rotating the limb (2). If the reduction appears quite stable, the arm should be rested in a sling as described for anterior dislocation of the shoulder. If the reduction is unstable, it is essential that the arm be kept in 60° lateral rotation for 4 weeks to give the torn capsule and labrum a reasonable chance of healing. This can only be reasonably achieved by the application of a shoulder spica, with the shoulder abducted to about 40°, externally rotated by 60° and fully extended.

Luxatio erecta

Diagnosis. In this comparatively rare type of shoulder dislocation, there is obvious deformity, with the arm being held in abduction. The radiographs pose no difficulty in interpretation. The patient should be carefully examined for evidence of neurological or vascular involvement, and reduction carried out without undue delay.

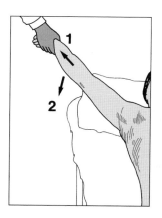

Treatment. Reduction is usually easily obtained by applying traction in abduction (the position in which the limb is lying) (1) and swinging the arm into adduction (2). The shoulder should be supported after reduction as for anterior dislocation.

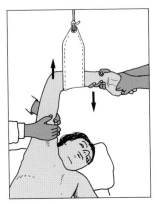

Late diagnosed anterior dislocation

Up until about 6 weeks or so, *closed reduction* (which is often successful) should be attempted. With the patient on his side and under general anaesthesia, the forearm is suspended by a canvas sling or bandage from a ceiling hook. The sling is adjusted so that, by using the arm as a lever, an assistant can exert considerable traction through the patient's body weight. At the time of the actual manipulation a muscle relaxant may be helpful. The humeral head is then manipulated over the glenoid lip. An image intensifier may give considerable assistance. Mobilisation should be commenced at an early stage (say 1 week).

If closed reduction fails, *open reduction* may have to be considered. This is seldom an easy procedure, and a substantial blood replacement may well be required. If the reduction is unstable, temporary pin fixation may be required. If reduction cannot be achieved, resection of the humeral head with or without replacement (excisional arthroplasty, hemi- or total replacement arthroplasty) may have to be considered. In the *elderly patient*, if the dislocation is not discovered until some months after the injury, it should generally be left until the outcome of a prolonged period of physiotherapy has been assessed. (Many become pain-free, albeit with a marked restriction in shoulder movements.) In very late discovered anterior dislocation in the *younger patient*, exploration and open reduction or arthroplasty should be considered.

Late diagnosed posterior dislocation

Manipulative reduction should be attempted as late as a year from the time of the dislocation. The same technique as that described for late diagnosed anterior dislocation may be employed, with in the case of posterior dislocation, pressure being applied from behind the shoulder on the posteriorly displaced head. Failure of reduction should be managed as in anterior dislocation, but using a posterior approach for any operative procedure.

Recurrent anterior dislocation of the shoulder

Even after prompt and adequate early treatment, redislocation may occur. Progressively less trauma is required on each occasion: eventually the patient may be able to reduce the dislocation voluntarily. Pathological features may include: • a Bankart lesion • attrition of the anterior shoulder cuff • a defect with flattening of the posterolateral aspect of the head • rounding of the glenoid margin.

Diagnosis. (1) *History*. This is usually clear, but distinguish between *recurrent dislocation* and *habitual* dislocation. (In the latter the patients are often psychotic or suffer from joint laxity. They can often voluntarily dislocate and reduce the joint without pain. Arthroscopy will reveal a lax capsule and capacious joint, but no other features of recurrent dislocation. This condition has an excellent prognosis in children, and in adults is perhaps best treated by bio-feedback re-education of the shoulder muscles; surgery should be avoided.)

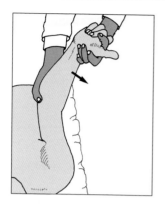

(2) *Clinical examination.* External rotation of the shoulder **(left)** may cause apprehension, and the drawer tests may be positive. (3) *Radiographs.* An axial radiograph may show a defect in the posterolateral aspect of the humeral head (Hill–Sachs lesion); however, this is sometimes seen before or at the time of the first dislocation. (4) *Other investigations.* Arthroscopy or an air contrast CAT scan may show bony defects or Bankart lesions. Look for abnormal excursion of the humeral head by intensifier examination (or taking stress films) with the shoulder in 90° abduction.

Treatment. Two surgical repairs are common: the Bankart and the Putti–Platt. In the former, particular attention is paid to the repair of the Bankart lesion, while in the latter the anterior capsule is also reinforced by dividing subscapularis and sewing it in a double-breasted fashion over the front of the joint. In both anterior and posterior dislocations of the shoulder, where there is a substantial bony defect, the glenoid may be buttressed using blocks of bone screwed to the glenoid (bone-block repair). This may also be used in the rare and generally unrewarding cases where there is a joint laxity syndrome or a paralytic element.

Recurrent posterior dislocation of the shoulder
Surgical repair of the shoulder (using Bankart or Putti–Platt-like procedures through a posterior approach) may be considered, using criteria similar to those for recurrent anterior dislocation. Recurrent dislocation of the shoulder may also be treated by arthroscopic surgery using several techniques including stapling. There is an appreciable failure rate, and the long-term results are not known.

Neurological complications of shoulder dislocations
Any type of brachial plexus lesion may be seen, and most make a good *functional* recovery without surgery. Where there is a diffuse plexus lesion, if joint stiffness is not overcome before neurological resolution occurs, function may be permanently impaired: the lesson is that every effort must be made to mobilise the shoulder as quickly as possible where there is *any* neurological complication. If no recovery has occurred after 3–5 months in major plexus lesions, exploration is indicated.

Shoulder cuff tears
Minor trauma may produce small tears in shoulder cuffs in which degenerative changes have occurred, giving a painful arc of movement from acromial impingement. Physiotherapy and local hydrocortisone infiltrations are usually helpful in relieving symptoms. More extensive tears may give rise to difficulty in initiating shoulder abduction. The diagnosis and the extent of the lesion may be confirmed by arthroscopy or air contrast CAT scans. These injuries are usually treated by prolonged physiotherapy, but if pain remains a problem, open surgical or arthroscopic repair of the tear may be advised. Good results have been obtained as long as 2 years from the onset of symptoms. Repair may be advised at an earlier stage should the problem arise in the younger patient.

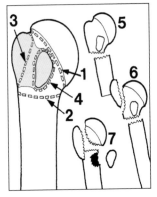

FRACTURES OF THE PROXIMAL HUMERUS

There are many different patterns of fracture which occur in this area. Although some are of considerable rarity, they can be important because of the complications which may follow them. They may involve: (1) the anatomical neck (rare), (2) the surgical neck, (3) the greater tuberosity or (4) the lesser tuberosity. The lesser and greater tuberosities with the bicipital groove between may form a unit, the so-called 'shield' fracture. Combinations of these injuries are common, and it is customary to describe fractures in this region by the number of fragments involved—e.g. two-part (5), three-part (6) and four-part fractures (7).

Classification of proximal humeral fractures

In the commonly used Neer's classification, proximal humeral fractures are divided into 6 groups:

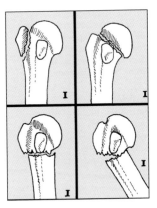

Group I includes *all* fractures in this region (irrespective of the degree of comminution) where there is minimal displacement or angulation. (Minimal displacement is defined as being less than 1 cm; minimal angulation is, surprisingly, defined as being < 45°.)

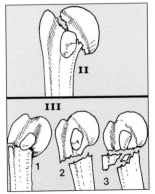

Group II includes all fractures of the anatomical neck displaced by more than 1 cm. These rare injuries may be complicated by avascular necrosis of the humeral head.

Group III includes all appreciably displaced or severely angled fractures of the surgical neck; these generally give no problems with avascular necrosis. They may be (1) impacted, (2) displaced or (3) comminuted. Angulation is often anterior and may give an erroneous impression of abduction or adduction.

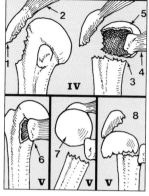

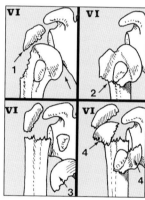

Group IV includes all fractures of the greater tuberosity (1), displaced by the pull of supraspinatus (2). In three-part fractures, a fracture of the surgical neck (3) allows the subscapularis (4) to rotate the head internally, so that its articular surface (5) faces mainly posteriorly.

Group V injuries involve the lesser tuberosity (6). In three-part injuries the humeral head may be abducted and externally rotated so that its articular surface faces anteriorly (7). Four-part injuries (8), identical with four-part injuries of group IV, may render the head avascular.

Group VI comprises the fracture–dislocations. Dislocation of the shoulder with an associated greater tuberosity fracture (1) is included in the two-part injuries in group VI. More serious are the dislocations where the two-part fracture of the proximal humerus is through the surgical neck (2). Most difficult of all are the three- and four-part injuries, especially when the humeral head is completely detached and displaced (3), or worse still, split (4).

The Neer classification has been criticised for poor inter-observer reliability, and it is claimed that a better appreciation of the pathology and more help in performing an open reduction can be obtained from 3-D reconstructions of the proximal humerus using CAT scans. Based on this, five types of fracture have been recognised (Edelson, Kelly et al). These are as follows:

1. *Two-part fractures.* The fracture line involves the surgical neck of the humerus. The fracture may be tilted into varus or valgus and/or impacted. This is by far the commonest of the fractures to be found in this area.
2. *Three-part fractures.* The fracture involves the surgical neck, and the third fragment is the greater tuberosity. The lesser tuberosity remains attached to the humeral head.
3. *Shield-fractures.* These represent a worse form of three-part fractures, where the lesser tuberosity is detached as well as the greater tuberosity, the two having a bony link formed from a portion of the bicipital groove (see p. 284). The shield fracture (named after its shape), has several variations, and itself may be fractured.
4. *Isolated fractures of the greater tuberosity.* A number, if not all of these, may follow momentary anterior glenohumeral dislocation.
5. *Fracture dislocations.* In this group, any of the previous fractures is accompanied by an anterior or posterior dislocation of the glenohumeral joint.

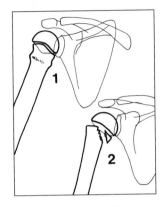

Children's injuries. Note that in children the commonest injury is a greenstick fracture of the surgical neck (**1**); this may be classified as a Neer group I, two-part fracture. Also common is a slight or moderately displaced proximal humeral epiphyseal injury with an associated juxta-epiphyseal fracture (**2**) (Salter & Harris type 2 injury.) This would fit into Neer group I or II, depending on the displacement and angulation.

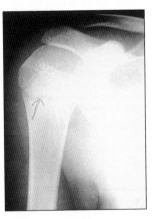

Diagnosis

The patient tends to support the arm with the other hand, there is tenderness over the proximal humerus and, in severely angled or displaced fractures, there may be obvious deformity. Later, gross bruising gravitating down the arm is an outstanding feature. *The diagnosis is established by the radiographs.* Note that a *second projection* of the shoulder is essential for a clear assessment of these injuries—either by means of an apical oblique or a good translateral. Note that in children that part of the epiphyseal line (see arrow in the normal shoulder on the **left**) is frequently mistaken for a fracture.

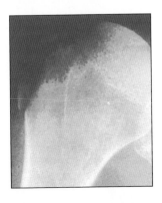

Treatment guidelines

The following examples are arranged in order of severity.

Group I injuries (undisplaced fracture of the greater tuberosity).

(1) This type of injury may occur in isolation or be seen in association with a dislocation of the shoulder which has reduced—either spontaneously or after manipulation. The arm should be supported in a collar and cuff sling until the acute symptoms have resolved (1–2 weeks), when mobilisation may be carefully commenced. Watch carefully in case of late displacement.

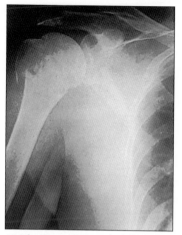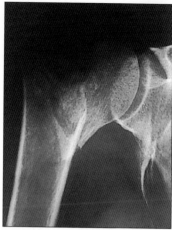

(2) The illustration on the **left** is of a three-part impacted fracture involving the greater tuberosity as well as the surgical neck. There is minimal displacement and angulation showing in this single projection, and confirmed in a lateral.

(3) Illustrated on the **right** is a two-part fracture of the surgical neck. In spite of not being impacted, there is an appreciable area of cancellous bone in contact, which will generally assure rapid healing. Secondary displacement is unlikely provided the limb has some initial protection (required anyway to relieve the severe pain, aggravated by movement, which often accompanies these injuries).

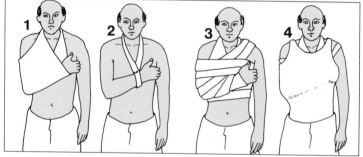

Slightly displaced and moderately angled humeral neck fractures may be treated satisfactorily by external support alone. Firstly, the arm should be placed in a sling. Where disimpaction is undesirable (e.g. 2 above) a *broad arm* sling (1) is preferable. Where the fracture is disimpacted (e.g. 3 at the top of the page), then a *collar and cuff* sling (2) may allow gravitational correction of any angulation. Placing the arm under the clothes gives some protection from rotational stresses; this may be improved with a body bandage (3) (e.g. of crepe bandages) under the clothes (4), or by using an expanding net support (e.g. Netelast®). Pain is often severe and analgesics will be required.

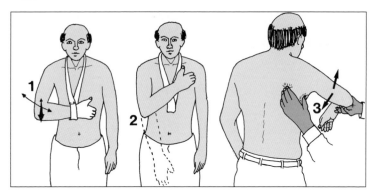

After-care. *After 2 weeks*, the body bandage may be discarded unless pain is commanding. The sling should be worn under the outer clothes. The patient is advised to commence rocking movements of the shoulder (abduction, flexion (1)) and to remove the arm from the sling three or four times per day to flex and extend the elbow (2).

At 4 weeks the sling can be placed outside the clothes. Gentle active movements should be practised throughout the day. Over the next 2 weeks the patient should be encouraged to discard the use of the sling in gradual stages.

At 6 weeks the patient should be referred for physiotherapy if, as is usual, there is considerable restriction of movement. The range of movements (particularly glenohumeral, 3) should be recorded at fortnightly intervals, and physiotherapy discontinued when gains cease. Some permanent restriction of glenohumeral movement is common, but seldom incapacitating.

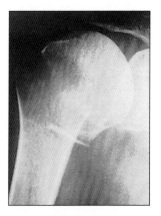

Group II injuries (displaced fractures of the anatomical neck).

These uncommon fractures are often complicated by avascular necrosis of the humeral head. Unless the displacement is very severe (e.g. with off-ending) or there is some complication (such as vascular obstruction in the arm), avoid manipulation or open reduction and treat conservatively with a sling as described on the previous page, and with measures to prevent rotational stresses. If manipulative reduction is required, the method described on the following page may be employed. If avascular necrosis ensues, joint replacement may have to be considered.

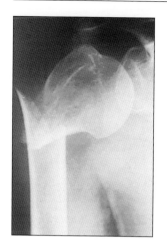

Group III injuries (severely displaced or angled fractures of the surgical neck). In the elderly patient a good result can be expected in injuries of this pattern, where the deformity is accepted and conservative management is pursued along previously indicated lines. Nevertheless, there will be some restriction of abduction, so where the deformity is particularly severe or the patient very active, open reduction and internal fixations should be considered. (Methods include using an intramedullary nail (with screws into the humeral head and locking screws into the humeral shaft), Rush pins, or a T-plate and screws. An external fixator may also be effective.)

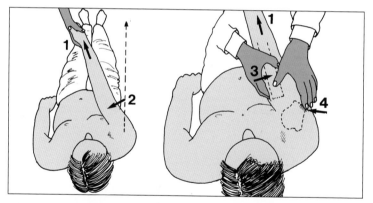

Alternatively, *manipulative reduction* may be attempted if the circumstances are against internal fixation. The patient is anaesthetised; if an image intensifier is available it should be employed and positioned in such a way that the surgeon has adequate access to the shoulder. Apply traction in the line of the limb (1) and swing the arm into *adduction* (2). An assistant maintains traction in adduction (1). Now apply pressure on the humeral shaft, pushing it laterally (3). At the same time, attempt to control the proximal fragment with the other hand, applying firm pressure beneath the acromion (4). If the medial edges of the fracture can be opposed, reduction may be completed by the assistant abducting the arm, and then gently and gradually releasing the traction. After reduction of the fracture, the limb should be supported in a broad arm sling and body bandage.

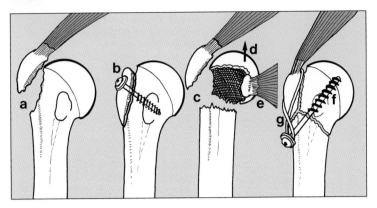

Group IV injuries (displaced fracture of the greater tuberosity).

Two-part injuries (**a**) may be reduced by closed methods, but are liable to displace as the result of the unopposed action of the supraspinatus. It is probably best to internally fix these fractures, and this may be done with a single cancellous screw with a washer under the head (**b**). This is also indicated in group I injuries where there is late displacement.

In *three-part injuries* (**c**) the articular surface of the humeral head (**d**) is directed posteriorly by the pull of subscapularis (**e**). The viability of the head is usually preserved. In the unfit elderly patient, these injuries are best treated conservatively, but if the patient's condition will allow, joint replacement should be considered. In the young and active, consider open reduction and internal fixation. This is usually technically difficult, but it may be possible to reduce the three parts of the fracture using a cancellous screw (**f**) to oppose the head and shaft, and a tension band (**g**), anchored to the screw head, for the tuberosity.

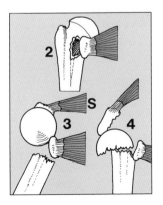

Group V injuries (displaced fractures of the lesser tuberosity).

Two-part injuries (**2**) are rare and should be treated conservatively. In *three part injuries* (**3**), supraspinatus (**S**) is unopposed and the humeral head points forwards. Treat as three-part group IV injuries. Group V *four-part injuries* (**4**) are identical with four-part injuries in group IV; there is a high incidence of avascular necrosis of the detached head. These injuries may also be managed conservatively, and complications dealt with as they arise.

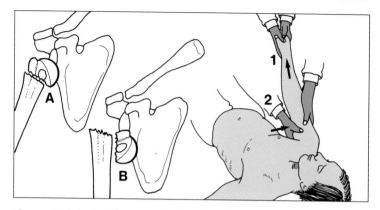

Group VI injuries (fracture–dislocations). Two-part injuries in which there is a dislocation of the shoulder and a fracture of the greater tuberosity are dealt with as though they were uncomplicated dislocations, i.e. by manipulative reduction. The greater tuberosity usually returns to its normal location, but if it remains severely displaced, reduction should be undertaken.

When a two-part injury involves a fracture of the surgical neck of the humerus, the degree of separation of the fragments affects the chances of a satisfactory closed reduction. Where there is little separation (**A**), an intact periosteal sleeve will generally permit manipulative reduction. Where there is wide separation of the elements (**B**), closed reduction is difficult. The risks of failure are high, and an open procedure may become necessary.

Closed reduction technique. Apply strong traction in the neutral position or slight abduction (**1**) and manual pressure to the head via the axilla and front of the shoulder (**2**). Avoid hyperabduction.

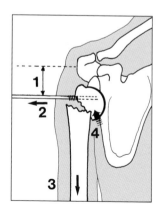

If the previous technique fails, pass a threaded pin into the humeral head (under intensifier control); introduce the pin on the lateral aspect of the arm 3 cm below the acromial arch (**1**). Apply lateral traction to the pin (**2**), with slight traction to the arm (**3**) and manual pressure over the humeral head (**4**). *After care* is as for group III injuries.

Where closed methods fail, open reduction should be considered unless there are serious contraindications. In *three-* and *four-part injuries,* especially where there is splitting of the head fragment, the risks of avascular necrosis with persistent pain and stiffness are high; excisional arthroplasty, hemiarthroplasty or total joint replacement should be considered.

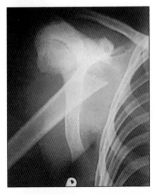

Treatment of children's fractures of the proximal humerus. Unimpacted fractures of the proximal humerus may be of adult pattern (as illustrated), or they may be group 2 (Salter and Harris) epiphyseal injuries. *Open reduction should be avoided in all cases.* Manipulate as described, but if the deformity recurs on bringing the arm to the side apply a shoulder spica in abduction. Bony apposition should be obtained, but persisting angulation in excess of 30° should not induce pessimism as rapid recovery of function through remodelling is the rule. Note that pathological fracture from simple bone cyst is common in the proximal humeral shaft in children, and should be treated as an uncomplicated fracture.

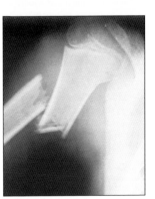

FRACTURES OF THE HUMERAL SHAFT

Fractures of the humeral shaft may result from both direct and indirect violence. In the upper third, as illustrated, the proximal fragment tends to be pulled into adduction by the unopposed action of pectoralis major, while in fractures involving the mid-third, the proximal fragment tends to be abducted by deltoid. Radial nerve palsy, non-union and open fractures are commonest in those involving the *middle third*.

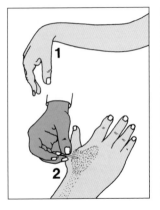

Diagnosis. The arm is flail and the patient usually supports it with the other hand. Obvious mobility at the fracture site leaves little doubt regarding the diagnosis. Confirmation is obtained by radiographs which seldom give difficulty in interpretation. In all cases, look for evidence of radial nerve palsy—drop wrist (1)—and sensory impairment on the dorsum of hand (2). This is, in fact, an uncommon complication, as a slip of brachialis lies beneath the nerve; this generally prevents it from coming in contact with the musculospiral groove or the fractured bone ends. If, however, radial nerve palsy accompanies an open fracture, exploration is mandatory.

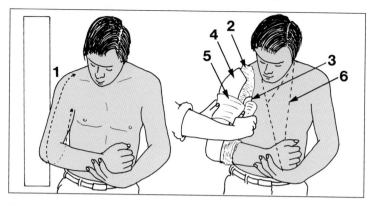

Treatment

U-slab method. Closed fractures may be treated by the application of a U-plaster. If angulation is slight, no anaesthetic is required. The patient should be seated and a plaster slab prepared of about eight thicknesses of 15 cm (6″) plaster bandage (1). The length should be such as to allow it to stretch from the inside of the arm round the elbow and over the point of the shoulder. Wool roll is then applied to the arm (2) from the shoulder to a third of the way down the forearm. The slab is wetted and applied to the arm, starting on the medial side at the axillary fold (3) and then bringing it round the elbow up to the shoulder (4). The slab should be carefully smoothed down. The plaster is secured with wet open weave cotton bandages (5). During the setting of the slab, the fracture may be gently moulded and any slight angulation corrected. Thereafter, the arm should be supported in a sling (6), which should be worn under the clothes. If the fracture is badly displaced, heavy sedation or general anaesthesia is desirable. An assistant should apply light traction to the arm, and a U-slab applied as before. The cast is carefully moulded in the regions of the fracture as the plaster sets. Again, a sling should be worn under the clothes.

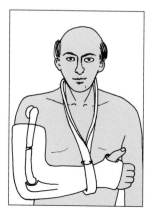

Hanging cast method. This is only suitable for ambulant patients, as the principle is that the weight of the limb and the cast reduce the fracture and maintain reduction. A long arm plaster is applied along with a *collar and cuff sling*. With either method of fixation, and after the initial pain has settled (say 2–3 weeks), a polythene sleeve or other form of functional bracing may be substituted, but many prefer to continue using a cast until union. Check for this clinically and with X-rays at 9 weeks. If judged sound, a sling may be worn as an additional precaution for 2 weeks, but mobilisation of the shoulder and elbow should be commenced. Physiotherapy may be required.

Internal fixation. This should be considered if:
- there are two or more fractures in the one limb
- both arms are fractured
- there are multiple injuries
- a prolonged period of recumbency is likely
- there is a radial nerve palsy in an open and otherwise suitable fracture
- a radial nerve palsy occurs after manipulation.

Methods include dynamic compression plates applied to the posterior aspect of the humerus; crossed Rush pins or Nancy nails inserted through small incisions made on either side of the elbow; intramedullary nails introduced from below, just proximal to the olecranon fossa, or from above, from the region of the greater tuberosity.

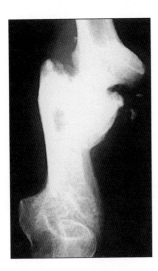

Complications of humeral shaft fractures

Non-union. (A *hypertrophic non-union* is shown left). Non-union is seen most frequently in middle-third fractures, especially in the obese patient where support of the fracture may be difficult, or where gravitational distraction has occurred. Rigid internal fixation (e.g. with a well-fitting Küntscher, AO or Seidel nail, or by compression plating), complemented with bone grafting, are usually advised. Visualisation of the radial nerve is recommended to avoid damaging it, and a posterior approach is frequently used. *Atrophic non-union* is found in association with radionecrosis, often secondary to radiotherapy for carcinoma of the breast.

Radial nerve palsy. This is generally a lesion in continuity, and recovery often commences 6–8 weeks after the initial injury. If there is no indication for initial exploration (e.g. where a radial nerve palsy is found to be present in a closed fracture of the humerus), the patient should be treated expectantly. He should be provided with a drop-wrist splint, preferably of the lively type, as soon as possible, and he should attend the physiotherapy department so that he can be encouraged in active and passive movements of the fingers, thumb and wrist.

If there is no evidence of recovery in 8 weeks, an electromyographic examination should be performed. If this shows no sign of recovery, exploration of the radial nerve should be undertaken.

Fractures in children 296
Adult fractures 306
Dislocation of the elbow
  308
Fractures of the olecranon
  311
Fractures of the radial head
  312
Fractures of the radial neck
  314

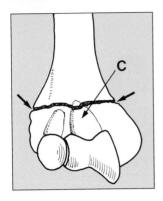

FRACTURES IN CHILDREN
Supracondylar fracture
The term is applied to fractures of the humerus in the distal third lying just proximal to the bone masses of the trochlea and capitulum (capitellum). The fracture line often runs through the apices of the coronoid (**C**) and olecranon fossae, and is generally transverse. It is a common fracture of childhood; its incidence reaches a peak about the age of 8 years. It generally results from a fall on the outstretched hand, and should always be suspected when a child complains of pain in the elbow after such an incident.

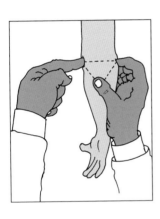

Diagnosis. The olecranon and medial and lateral epicondyles preserve their normal equilateral triangular relationship (unlike dislocation of the elbow, also common in children). There is tenderness over the distal humerus, there may be marked swelling and deformity, and the child generally resists examination.

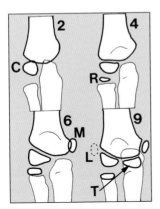

Radiographs. The interpretation of radiographs is made difficult by the changing complexities of the epiphyses. Typical appearances at ages **2**, **4**, **6** and **9** years are shown on the left.

Note:

C = capitulum (present usually within the first year of life).
R = radial head (appears 3–5 years).
M = medial epicondyle (present by 6).
T = trochlea (appears 7–9).
L = lateral epicondyle (11–14).
   (Olecranon—8–11 years.)

Variations in these appearances occur, and if there is any difficulty in interpreting the radiographs, comparison films of the other side should be taken.

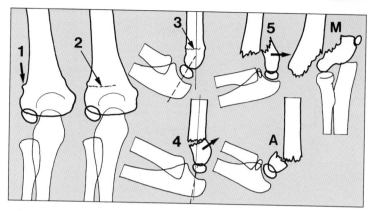

When there is minimal violence (in a child), the only sign may be of slight cortical irregularity (1). With progressively greater violence the following may occur:

- There may be a hairline crack (2), visible in the AP view only.
- Next, the fracture line will be detectable in the lateral as well as the AP projection (3).
- Then the distal fragment is tilted (4) in a backward direction.
- With still greater violence there is backward displacement (5) of the distal humeral complex, often leading to loss of bony contact.

In the AP view there is often medial (M) or lateral shift of the epiphyseal complex. The complex may also be rotated (generally lateral (external) rotation). Rarely (as a result of other mechanisms of injury), the distal fragment is displaced and tilted *anteriorly* (A)—the anterior or reversed supracondylar fracture.

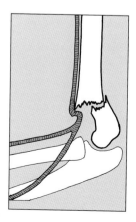

Vascular complications. Where the fracture is appreciably displaced, the brachial artery may be affected by the proximal fragment with the risk of Volkmann's ischaemic contracture. In the majority of cases this is no more than a kinking of the vessel, but occasionally there may be structural damage to the wall. In every case, the circulation should be assessed and recorded *prior* to any manipulation. If the radial pulse is absent, seek other evidence of arterial obstruction (pallor and coldness of the limb, pain and paraesthesia in the forearm, and progressive muscle paralysis). Look for excessive swelling and bruising.

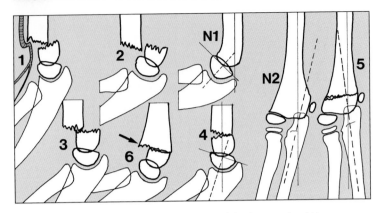

Indications for reduction. Manipulation of the fracture should be undertaken (other things being equal) under the following circumstances: **(1)** If there is evidence of arterial obstruction and the fracture is displaced and/or angulated. **(2)** If there is off-ending of the fracture. **(3)** Ideally, if there is less than 50% of bony contact.
Reduction should also be considered if there is:

(4) Backward tilting (anterior angulation) of the distal fragment of 15° or more. Note that in the normal elbow the articular surfaces of the distal humerus lie at 45° to the axis of the humerus (**N1**).
(5) Medial or lateral tilting of 10° or more. Note that the normal 'carrying angle' of the elbow is about 10° (**N2**); cubitus varus and cubitus valgus do not remodel well and may ultimately be associated with tardy ulnar nerve palsy.
(6) Severe torsional deformity (axial rotation).

   Assuming that no vascular complications are present, pure posterior displacement, lateral displacement or medial displacement of 50% or less *may be accepted as remodelling is generally rapid and effective.*

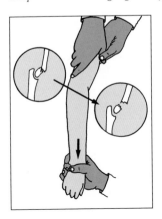

Manipulation techniques. The arm should be manipulated under general anaesthesia. Gentle/moderate traction is applied at about 20° of flexion while an assistant applies countertraction to the arm. This should lead to rapid disimpaction of the fracture. Some surgeons advise that this and the following stages should be carried out with the arm in supination.

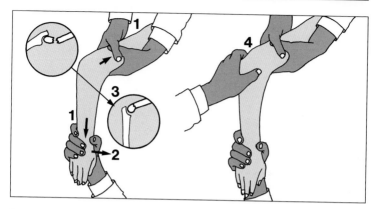

Now, maintaining traction and countertraction (**1**), flex the elbow to 80° (**2**). This lifts the distal fragment forwards, thereby reducing any posterior displacement and correcting any backward tilting (**3**). During this manoeuvre, the epiphyseal complex may be further coaxed into position by grasping it in the free hand (**4**). (The thumb can be used to steady the proximal humeral shaft.) Lateral displacement and torsional deformity (axial rotation) may also be corrected in this way.

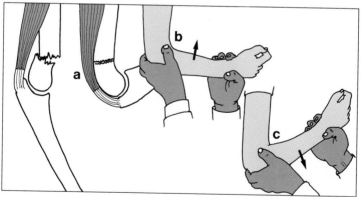

Fixation. Flexion of the elbow stretches the triceps over the fracture, often splinting it most efficiently (**a**). *The aim should be to flex the elbow as far as the state of the circulation will permit.* Assuming that at 80° a pulse is present (if present before the manipulation it should still be there, and if absent it will have hopefully been restored), continue flexion of the elbow (**b**) until the pulse disappears (due to the elbow flexure crease along with the swelling compressing the brachial artery). Now extend the elbow slowly (**c**) till the pulse just returns. *This is the position in which the arm should be maintained.* If 110–120° or more of flexion can be preserved, a sling and body bandage, well secured with adhesive strapping, may suffice for fixation.

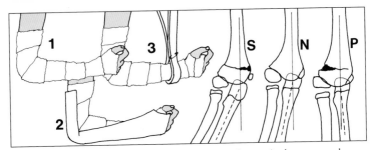

Unfortunately, further extension of the elbow may be required to restore the circulation. In such cases, apply a generous layer of wool (1), followed by a long arm plaster slab (2) secured with bandages and a sling (3). *Many surgeons favour this in every case.* Warning: never apply a *complete* plaster because of the risks of swelling. While the slab is being applied, the risks of recurrence of valgus or varus deformity may be reduced by careful positioning of the forearm: viz. if there has been valgus deformity (lateral tilting, medial angulation), place the arm in supination (S). With varus place the arm in pronation (P). With insignificant angulation, the neutral position (N) may be employed.

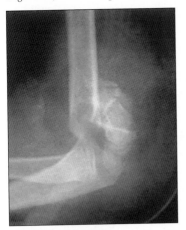
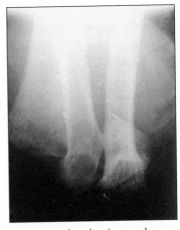

Check radiographs. Check radiographs must now be taken in two planes. The lateral projection (**left**) shows an unsatisfactory reduction, with the distal fragment completely off-ended and displaced proximally. AP views, which must be taken with the elbow flexed, are hard to interpret. The view on the **right** shows an unsatisfactory medial displacement of the epiphyseal complex. If a good reduction has been achieved, the anaesthetic can be discontinued. The child should be admitted for overnight observation. The arm should be elevated in a roller towel or similar device which allows good access for observation of the pulse and circulation in the fingers. *If the radiographs show a poor reduction, then two further attempts at manipulation may be permitted under the same anaesthetic.*

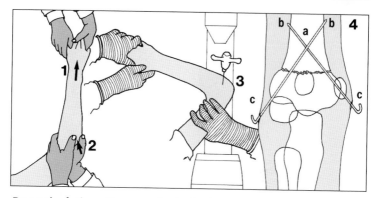

Remanipulation. If a poor reduction has been obtained, the preceding technique may be repeated; alternatively, while an assistant applies light traction to the forearm (1), the distal fragment is pushed forwards with the thumbs (2) while the fingers control the proximal fragment. *In most cases, the problem is actually one of excessive instability of the fracture.* Image intensification (which is highly desirable) may confirm this, and allow a good reduction to be obtained and stabilised (3). For the latter, two crossed Kirschner wires (4) (a) may be inserted. They should engage the opposite supracondylar ridge (b), remain proud of the skin and be further supported with a plaster back slab. It is unwise to repeat manipulation beyond the third attempt, owing to the risks of increasing swelling. In these circumstances, marked displacement (but not angulation) may be accepted, relying on later remodelling. If the fracture cannot be reduced and the position is very poor, open reduction is not recommended. Instead, continuous traction may be used (e.g. Dunlop (skin) traction, or by a screw in the olecranon).

Management of vascular complications

Absent pulse after manipulation. If immediately after manipulation, the pulse is *not* palpable, the elbow should be flexed to *not more than 100°* and maintained in that position with a sling and a back slab. The anaesthetic should be continued while check radiographs are taken.

Absent pulse, adequate circulation. If a good reduction has been obtained and the pulse remains absent, the circulation should be checked more critically. The use of a pulse oximeter is often helpful. Clinically, if the hand is warm and pink, with good capillary return in the nail beds, there is no immediate indication for further intervention. *Admission, elevation and close observation for 24 hours* are essential. (Generally the pulse returns spontaneously over 2–3 days.)

Absent pulse, ischaemia. If there are incontrovertible signs of gross ischaemia, either in the face of a good reduction or a failed reduction, *exploration of the brachial artery* must be undertaken. This should be performed by an experienced vascular surgeon in case a specialised procedure is required.

Late development of ischaemia. If while under observation the pulse disappears, and especially if there are other signs of ischaemia, all encircling bandages should be cut, and all wool in front of the elbow teased out. If this does not lead to improvement, the elbow should be placed in a more extended position (e.g. by cracking the slab and slackening the sling).

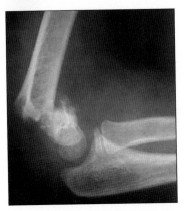
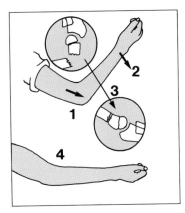

The anterior (reversed) supracondylar fracture. Uncommonly, the distal fragment is displaced anteriorly. *This deformity is aggravated by flexion of the elbow.* Traumatic separation of the epiphyseal complex (Salter & Harris type 1 or 2) with a similar displacement is a related injury. To reduce either of these, traction is applied to the elbow in the flexed position to disimpact the fracture. Continuing the traction (**1**) the elbow is slowly extended (**2**), reducing the angulation (**3**). The arm is put in a plaster back slab in a position of 10° flexion (**4**). *This position should not be maintained for more than 3 weeks.* At that stage the elbow should be gently flexed (usually about 70–80° can be achieved) and supported either with a sling or further plaster slab till union occurs.

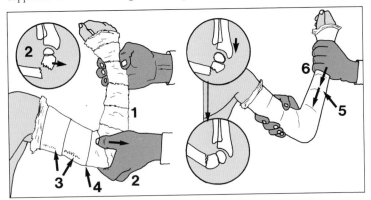

An alternative technique is to apply wool to the limb (**1**) and disimpact the distal fragment by direct traction on the epiphyseal complex (**2**). A plaster cuff (**3**) is then applied by an assistant and allowed to set. Care must be taken to avoid ridging at the distal end (**4**). The rest of the plaster is quickly applied (**5**), and while it is still soft, flex to 110° or less and exert pressure on the distal fragment through the forearm (**6**). The position is held till the plaster has set. Check radiographs are taken and fixation continued as for a normal supracondylar fracture.

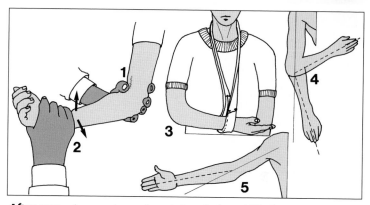

After-care. Assess union at about 3–4 weeks for a child of 4 years, and about 4–5 weeks for a child of 8, by means of radiographs and the assessment of fracture site tenderness. A further useful test is to place your thumb over the biceps tendon (**1**), and then flex and extend the elbow (**2**) through a total range of 20°. Spasm of the biceps indicates that the elbow is not yet ready for mobilisation. Mobilisation itself may be commenced from a sling (**3**) (i.e. the arm is removed from the sling for 10 minutes' active exercises, 3–4 times per day). The sling is discarded as soon as any discomfort has settled. This procedure may also be used where there is a little residual fracture tenderness. Physiotherapy is indicated if after 2 weeks' mobilisation there is still gross restriction. The range should be recorded at every clinic attendance; physiotherapy can be safely stopped when 25–120° (**4**) is reached (normal 0–145°). On no account should passive movements be allowed, and *the parents should be warned against this*. If any cubitus varus or valgus (**5**) is present it should be recorded and the child assessed yearly regarding deterioration and the need for a corrective osteotomy.

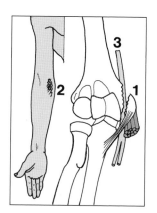

Medial epicondylar injuries

The medial epicondyle may be injured by direct violence. It may also be avulsed by the ulnar collateral ligament if the elbow is forcibly abducted, or by sudden contraction of the forearm flexors which are attached to it (**1**). Suspect this injury if there is bruising on the medial side of the joint (**2**), and always test the integrity of the ulnar nerve (**3**). The degree of displacement varies with the severity and direction of the forces applied: separation may be slight or marked. Comparison films may be helpful in the doubtful case. Injuries of these types may be treated by immobilisation in a long arm padded plaster for 2–3 weeks. In some cases tardy ulnar nerve palsy may occur.

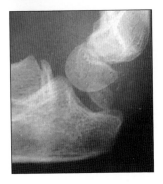

The potentially most serious injury is when the medial epicondyle is trapped in the elbow joint. This is often missed. It may follow the manipulative or the spontaneous reduction of a dislocated elbow.

Radiographs. *Note:* in the normal *lateral projection*, the medial epicondyle cannot be seen; if it can (as it is left), it is lying in the joint. If the child is over 6 years and the medial epicondylar epiphysis cannot be seen in the *AP view*, it is probably in the joint. So note the child's age, examine both views carefully, and if in doubt obtain comparison films.

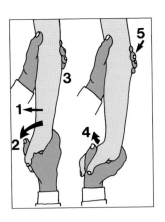

Treatment. Removal by manipulation is often successful. Under general anaesthesia, increase valgus (1), supinate (2), extend the elbow (3) and jerk the wrist into dorsiflexion (4). A finger placed over the medial side of the elbow (5) may detect the medial epicondyle slipping out of the joint. If the previous method fails, (a) electrical stimulation of the flexor muscle mass under general anaesthesia may be tried, or (b) carry out an open reduction through a small anteromedial incision, with fixation either with a Kirschner wire (retained for 3 weeks) or a soft-tissue suture.

Complications. The majority of ulnar nerve palsies found in association with medial epicondylar injuries are lesions in continuity; commencement of recovery can be expected in 3–6 weeks.

Lateral epicondylar injuries

The epiphysis for the lateral epicondyle is inconstant, but usually appears at about 11 years, fusing with the main epiphysis 2–3 years later (1). It may, however, ossify by direct extension from the capitellum (2). It may be detached as a result of an adduction stress. Only very rarely does it become trapped in the joint after a dislocation.

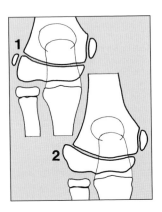

Treatment. These injuries may be treated along the lines suggested for medial epicondylar injuries.

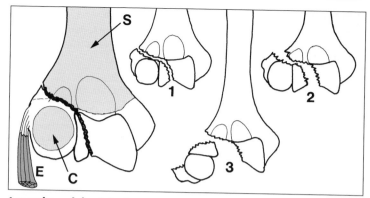

Lateral condylar injuries

The common pattern of injury involves the *whole of the capitellum and nearly half the trochlea.* This large fragment may be displaced by the forearm extensors (**E**) or the lateral ligament. As the capitellar epiphysis (**C**) and the shaft (**S**) may be the only structures visible on the radiographs, *their relationship may be the only clue to injury.* Fractures of the lateral condyle may be (**1**) undisplaced, (**2**) laterally displaced, (**3**) rotated.

Treatment. *Undisplaced fractures* should be treated conservatively by a long arm padded back shell and sling for 3–4 weeks. Radiographs should be taken at weekly intervals in case of late slip. Where there is *slight to moderate lateral shift* of the complex, closed reduction may be attempted by applying local pressure. If this is successful, a long arm padded back shell should be applied and retained with a sling for 3–4 weeks. Again, it is vital to detect any slipping by weekly radiographs. Where there is *lateral displacement which is unstable,* or late slipping occurs, Kirschner wire fixation (under image intensifier control) is indicated, with the additional support of a cast. The wires may be removed after 2–3 weeks and mobilisation commenced at 4 weeks.

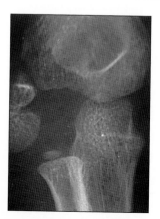

In injuries where there is rotation of the complex (e.g. **left**), closed methods are unlikely to give a satisfactory reduction, so that there is risk of non-union, growth disturbance and progressive cubitus valgus. Open reduction and Kirschner wire fixation are therefore indicated. (Note that if there is some uncertainty over the position or extent of the epiphyseal fragments, films taken after the injection of a radio-opaque dye into the fracture haematoma or an MRI scan may be helpful.)

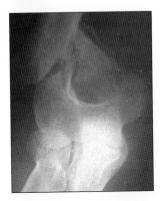

ADULT FRACTURES
Supracondylar fractures

In adults, the fracture line tends to lie a little more proximal than in children: comminution, spiralling and angulation are common. Nevertheless, many may be treated successfully as in children by manipulation and plaster fixation; 6–8 weeks' immobilisation is usually required. If instability is a problem, it may be possible to control the fracture with percutaneous wires. If this fails, or if there are other factors favouring primary internal fixation (e.g. multiple injuries), then AO plating or other techniques may be used. In all cases, early mobilisation is essential to minimise stiffness.

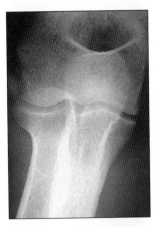

Medial and lateral epicondylar fractures

Displacement of these fractures is seldom severe and, although potential instability of the joint may be present, symptomatic treatment only is usually required. A crepe bandage applied over wool to limit swelling and a sling for 3–4 weeks is usually adequate. A short period in a long arm plaster is indicated if pain is severe.

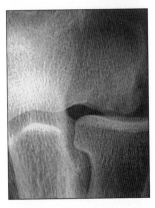

Fractures of the capitellum (capitulum)

(1) The cartilaginous and bony surfaces of the capitellum may be damaged by force transmitted up the radius from a fall on the outstretched hand. This is often seen in association with radial head injuries. Late complications include osteochondritis dissecans and osteoarthritis. *Treatment:* initially this should be symptomatic, with a collar and cuff sling and analgesics. Later, any loose bodies should be excised and the capitellum drilled to encourage revascularisation.

(2) A small flake may be detached from the capitellum as a result of force transmitted up the radius; it may come to lie in the front of the joint. It should be treated as a loose body and excised.

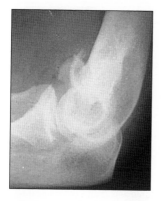

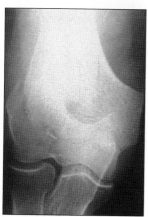

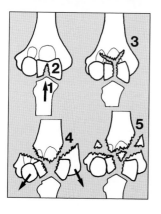

(3) A more serious fracture involves the major portion of the anterior half of the articular surface of the capitellum. Generally the corresponding part of the trochlea is involved. Severe disability will result if this is not accurately reduced, and generally exposure through an anterior approach will be necessary. Smillie pins or a Herbert screw may be used for fixation. (Occasionally reduction may be achieved by pressure over the fragment while traction is applied to the arm, but an imperfect reduction should not be accepted. After reduction, a long arm padded plaster should be retained for approximately 5 weeks before mobilisation.)

Fracture of a single condyle

Fracture of the lateral or medial condyle may be caused by the mechanisms responsible for the more severe Y-fractures. *Treatment:* if displacement is minimal, as illustrated, or the patient elderly and frail, apply a long arm plaster (over wool) and a sling. The plaster may usually be discarded safely after 4–5 weeks, and mobilisation commenced from the sling. Where there is appreciable displacement and the patient fit, the best results are obtained by open reduction and internal fixation: this can usually be achieved using one or two cancellous screws.

Intercondylar Y- or T-fracture

This injury is caused by the coronoid (1) being driven into the trochlea (2), often by a blow on the elbow. The vertical split bifurcates (3), and the two main fragments may separate (4). Comminution may occur (5). *Treatment.* (a) If undisplaced, treat conservatively. (b) If there is separation of the fragments, but open reduction is thought inadvisable (e.g. because of the patient's age, or great comminution), apply a long-arm plaster over wool; before this sets, apply traction, and side-to-side pressure. Remove the plaster and mobilise from a sling at an early date (e.g. 4–5 weeks). (c) In displaced fractures in the younger patient, open reduction and internal fixation is the treatment of choice.

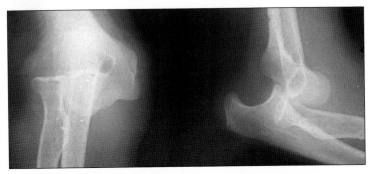

DISLOCATION OF THE ELBOW

Dislocation of the elbow is common in both children and adults, often resulting from a fall on the outstretched hand. It is sometimes confused with a supracondylar fracture (where however there is distortion of the equilateral triangle formed by the olecranon and epicondyles). *Radiographs:* These radiographs show a typical posterolateral dislocation of the elbow. Accompanying fractures are comparatively uncommon, but the coronoid and radial head should be carefully examined. In children, fracture of the epicondyles or the lateral condyle may occur, and these should be excluded as a routine.

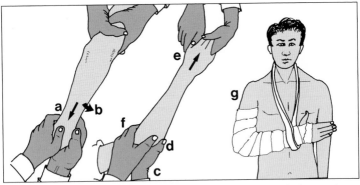

Complications: Damage to the ulnar nerve, median nerve or brachial artery is uncommon, but should always be sought. *Treatment:* Apply strong traction in the line of the limb (a) under general anaesthesia, and if necessary slightly flex the joint (b). A fair amount of force is often required, although the use of a muscle relaxant will reduce this. Success is usually accompanied with a characteristic reduction 'clunk'. If this is not successful, clasp the humerus from behind (c) and push the olecranon forwards and medially (d) while an assistant applies traction in moderate flexion (e). (The fingers apply countertraction (f).) Always take check radiographs. Support with a padded crepe bandage and sling (g) for 2 but not more than 3 weeks. Too early or too vigorous mobilisation runs the risk of myositis ossificans, and passive movements must be avoided.

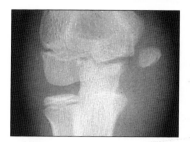
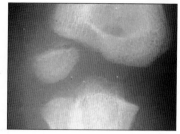

Associated injuries

(1) In children, the medial epicondylar epiphysis may be detached. *On reduction of the elbow*, it will generally be restored to an acceptable position (as above **left**). A plaster slab and a sling are advised for 4 weeks. (2) *The medial epicondyle may be retained in the joint:* this pattern of injury must always be excluded, and dealt with as already described. (3) The capitellar epiphysis (along with half the cartilaginous trochlea, as above **right**) may be displaced. If it is found to be in a displaced position after reduction of the dislocation, it must be appropriately treated as previously described.

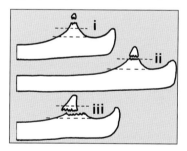
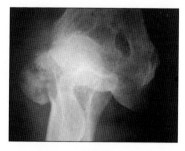

(4) The coronoid may fracture: three common patterns are found: **(i)** simple avulsions; **(ii)** fractures involving half or less of the coronoid; **(iii)** fractures involving more than half. Groups (i) and (ii) may be treated conservatively, commencing mobilisation before 3 weeks. Group (iii) injuries may be internally fixed to reduce the risk of recurrent dislocation. *Established recurrent dislocation* may be treated by bone block reconstruction of the coronoid and/or repair of the capsule and medial ligament. (5) The radial head may fracture, and if highly comminuted (above **right**), reduce the elbow dislocation and *delay excision of the radial head for at least 4–8 weeks* to lessen the risks of myositis ossificans. Minor fractures of the radial head need no special care. (6) If the radial neck is fractured, reduce the elbow and proceed as for this injury.

Treatment of late diagnosed posterior dislocation in children.

Between 3 weeks and 2 months, open reduction carries an unacceptable risk of myositis; if the dislocation is discovered within that period, treat conservatively by mobilisation alone. A quarter do well and need no further treatment; in the remainder (and in cases discovered later than 2 months), operative reduction should be attempted.

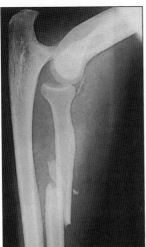

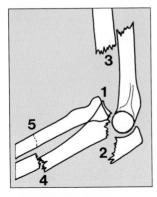

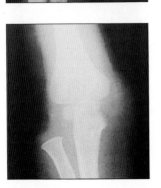

Anterior dislocation of the elbow.

This may accompany a fracture of the olecranon (see Hume fracture and Monteggia fracture–dislocation). A more complex form is seen in the side swipe injury (**left**). This occurs when a driver rests his elbow on the window ledge, and he is struck by a passing vehicle. Typically this injury includes anterior dislocation of the elbow (**1**), with fractures of the olecranon (**2**), the humerus (**3**), the ulna (**4**) and sometimes the radius (**5**). It is vital to reduce the dislocation immediately, fixing it internally or by a cast (in extension for 2–3 weeks) prior to delayed internal fixation of the olecranon. The other injuries may be treated with less urgency conservatively or surgically. It is not often wise to attempt immediate fixation of all the elements of this severe injury.

'Isolated' dislocation of the ulna.

Dislocation of the ulna may occur in association with a fracture of the radial shaft. As the fracture in the radius may be quite distal, it is important that adequate radiographs of the forearm are taken. This double injury may be treated by manipulative reduction of the elbow followed by a long arm plaster until the fracture of the radius unites (assuming a satisfactory reduction has been obtained). Alternatively, internal fixation of the radius may permit earlier mobilisation, and this is always desirable.

Isolated dislocation of the radius.

Lateral, anterior or posterior dislocation of the proximal end of the radius is almost invariably part of a Monteggia lesion which may not at first be obvious if the ulnar fracture is of greenstick pattern as illustrated. Great care must be taken in the assessment and treatment of these injuries which is dealt with separately (see Ch. 21, Monteggia fracture–dislocation, p. 323).

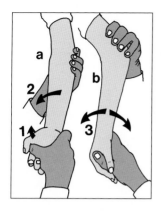

Pulled elbow. This is due to the radial head slipping out from under cover of the orbicular ligament. It occurs in the 2–6 age group and is normally caused by a parent suddenly pulling on a child's arm. *Diagnosis:* The child is usually fretful and has tenderness over the lateral aspect of the joint. *Supination is limited* and the radiographs are usually normal. *Treatment:* Reduction can usually be achieved by (a) placing the wrist in full radial deviation (1) and forcibly supinating the arm (2); or (b) by rapidly pronating and supinating the forearm (3). If these fail, rest the arm in a sling, when spontaneous reduction usually occurs within 48 hours.

FRACTURES OF THE OLECRANON

The olecranon may be fractured as a result of a fall on the point of the elbow or by sudden triceps contraction. In either case, displacement may occur as a result of muscle pull.

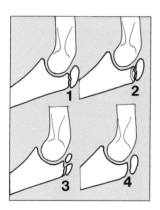

Diagnosis. This is usually straightforward, but beware of the following fallacies: (1) the normal epiphyseal line; (2) duplication of the normal line due to obliquity of the projection; (3) a normal bifid olecranon epiphysis (the epiphyses appear between the ages of 8 and 11 and fuse at 14 years); (4) patella cubiti due to ossification in the triceps tendon (note rounded edges).

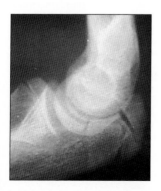

Treatment. If the fracture is hairline and undisplaced, it may be treated by immobilisation in a long arm plaster (3–4 weeks in a child, 6–8 weeks in an adult). Note in the radiographs shown on the left the three lines running through the olecranon: the most distal is a fracture, the middle the epiphyseal line, and the most proximal either a bifid epiphysis or a fracture of the epiphysis. Which of these it is would be determined by localising tenderness.

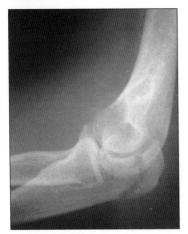
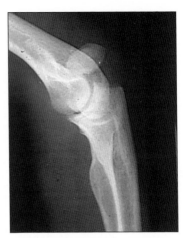

If the fracture line is *pronounced but still undisplaced* (**left**), it may be treated in the same way, but radiographs should be taken at weekly intervals during the first 3 weeks in case of (unlikely) late displacement. Minor epiphyseal separations may also be treated conservatively in a similar manner. Slight to moderate displacement may be accepted in the frail elderly.

In the young adult, where the *olecranon fragment is small (a third or less of the articular surface) and significantly displaced by triceps pull* (**right**), surgical excision with repair of the tear in the triceps insertion gives excellent results. (The stability of the elbow must be tested on the table, and if the joint can be in any way subluxed, the olecranon must be retained). The elbow may be mobilised after 2 weeks.

If the olecranon fragment is substantial it must be reduced and held by some form of internal fixation. The methods available include tension band wiring, lag screws and plating. The security of fixation dictates the need for additional external fixation and when mobilisation may be safely commenced.

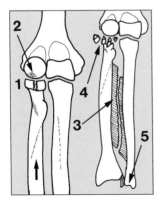

FRACTURES OF THE RADIAL HEAD

The radial head is most frequently fractured by direct violence, such as a fall or blow on the side of the elbow, but may often follow a fall on the outstretched hand where force is transmitted up the radius; the radial head strikes the capitellum (capitulum) and fractures (**1**). The articular surface of the capitellum may also be damaged (**2**), prolonging recovery. In some cases, where violence is severe, the interosseous membrane tears (**3**), severe comminution of the head occurs (**4**) and there is *subluxation of the distal end of the ulna* (**5**) due to proximal migration of the radial shaft. (Essex–Lopresti fracture–dislocation.)

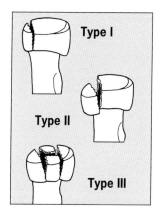

Type I

Type II

Type III

Classification of radial head fractures.
Mason's classification recognises three types:

Type I fractures are small and marginal, with displacements of less than 2 mm: they do not compromise stability or affect rotation.

Type II includes large two-part fractures displaced by 2 mm or more; any fracture that restricts rotation; and comminuted fractures amenable to operative fixation.

Type III fractures are highly comminuted ones where operative fixation is not possible.

Diagnosis. There is complaint of pain in the elbow and there may be local bruising and swelling. In *minor fractures*, tenderness may not be apparent until the damaged portion of the head is rotated under the examining thumb (placed over the radial head) while gently pronating and supinating the limb. The range of pronation and supination is often full, but elbow *extension* is usually restricted.

Radiographs. Most radial head fractures will show in the standard lateral and (supination) AP projections, but if there is clinical evidence of fracture and negative radiographs, *additional* AP projections should be taken in the midprone and full pronation position, so that all portions of the radial head will be visualised in profile.

Assessment. Assess the type and severity of the fracture from the radiographs, and always examine the forearm and wrist to exclude an Essex–Lopresti fracture–dislocation.

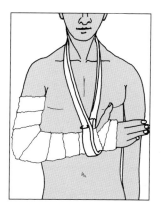

Treatment. Non-displaced fractures (Mason I above) should be treated with a light compression bandage and a sling before mobilisation from the sling is commenced after 2–3 weeks. The sling alone may be worn for a further 2 weeks. If pain is initially very severe, a plaster back slab may be used. An excellent outcome is usual, but note that many months may elapse before full *extension* is regained.

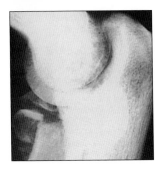

Severely comminuted fractures (Mason III and **left**) should be treated by immediate excision of the radial head. The arm is then rested in a sling for 2–3 weeks before mobilisation. A prosthetic replacement is carried out if there is valgus instability or proximal radial drift, and mobilisation started earlier. Displaced marginal and segmental fractures (Mason II) may be treated conservatively and reassessed after 2–3 months. If movements are severely restricted, *late excision* of the radial head should be considered.

Note: In any case of fracture, excision of the radial head should be performed *either* within the first 48 hours *or* after union (between carries the risk of myositis ossificans). A painful late Essex–Lopresti lesion may be treated by excision of the distal end of the ulna, albeit with some weakening of the grip.

The 'terrible triad'. This is used to describe a fracture of the radial head along with a coronoid fracture and dislocation of the elbow. Immediate surgery is advised for this complex injury. The elbow is reduced and the coronoid internally fixed. Then the radial head is fixed or replaced and the lateral ligament repaired. If the joint remains unstable, the medial ligament is also tackled. If the joint is still unstable, a hinged external fixator is then used to allow early movements.

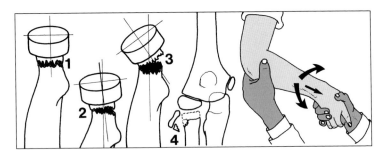

FRACTURES OF THE RADIAL NECK

The mechanisms of injury and the diagnosis are similar to fractures of the head. They may be hairline and undisplaced (1) or result in slight (2) or gross tilting (3). In children, the epiphysis of the head may be completely separated and widely displaced (4). *Treatment:* With slight or no tilting (1 and 2) and up to 30° in children, treat conservatively. With marked tilting (3) (20° or more in adults) manipulate (**above right**). To do so, apply traction and gently pronate and supinate, feeling for the prominent part of the radial head to present; then apply pressure when the head is at its zenith. Where there is gross epiphyseal displacement, *operative reduction* is indicated. If locking does not occur on reduction, a Kirschner wire may be used to achieve stability. In some cases, insertion of a temporary percutaneous wire into the radial head may allow it to be levered back into position under intensifier control without opening the joint.

CHAPTER

21

Regional injuries: the forearm bones

Patterns of injury 316
Treatment of forearm
    fractures 319
Isolated fracture of the ulna
    322
Monteggia
    fracture–dislocation 323
The Galeazzi
    fracture–dislocation 325
Isolated fractures of the
    radius 325

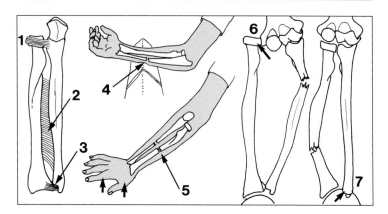

PATTERNS OF INJURY

The radius and ulna are bound together by (1) the annular (orbicular) ligament, (2) the interosseous membrane, (3) the (inferior) radioulnar ligaments and the triangular fibrocartilage. With direct violence it is possible for either of the forearm bones to be fractured in isolation (4). More commonly, the forearm is injured as the result of indirect violence, such as a fall on the back or the front of the outstretched hand, when both bones fracture (5). If *one* forearm bone is seen to be fractured and angled, it has inevitably become relatively shorter, leading to dislocation of the other. The commonest fracture–dislocation of this type is a fracture of the ulna with a dislocation of the radial head (Monteggia injury) (6). The same pattern of injury occurs in the Galeazzi fracture–dislocation, when a dislocation of the distal ulna accompanies a shaft fracture of the radius (7). *Never accept a single forearm bone fracture as an entity until a Monteggia or Galeazzi injury has been eliminated.*

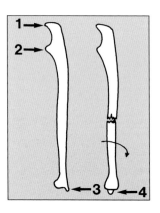

Axial rotation of the ulna. In any forearm injury, when the ulna fractures it may angulate or displace like any other bone. Axial rotation is rare, but always check to see that this is not present. To do so, note that in the lateral projection, the olecranon (1), the coronoid (2) and the styloid process (3) should be clearly visible. This relationship is lost in the presence of axial rotation (4).

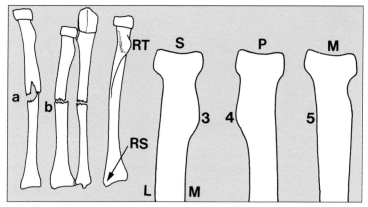

Axial rotation of the radius. This is much commoner than in the case of the ulna. It may be suspected by the shape of the mating parts of the fracture (**a**), by a discrepancy in the widths of the fragments at the fracture level (**b**) and by the relationship (**c**) between the radial tubercle (**RT**) and the styloid process (**RS**). In *full supination* (**S**) the radial tubercle lies *medially* and is prominent (**3**). In *pronation* (**P**) it lies *laterally* (**4**). In the *mid position* (**M**) it is concealed (**5**). The positions of the radial styloid and the radial tubercle should always correspond.

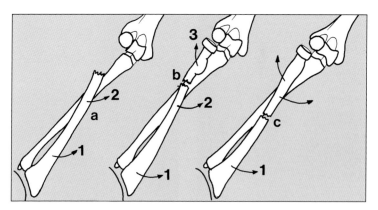

Forces responsible for axial rotation
(**a**) In all radial shaft fractures, pronator quadratus tends to pronate the distal fragment (**1**). In all upper (proximal) third fractures, pronator quadratus is assisted in this movement by pronator teres (**2**).
(**b**) In upper third fractures, the *proximal* fragment is fully supinated by biceps (**3**) while the *distal* fragment is fully pronated by pronator teres and quadratus (**1, 2**), (i.e. there is a maximal tendency to axial rotation).
(**c**) In fractures distal to the proximal third, biceps is opposed, so the proximal fragment tends to lie in the mid-position.

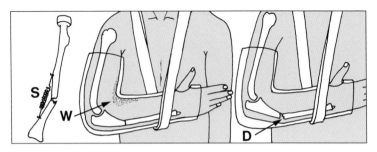

Factors responsible for increasing angulation. In children's greenstick fractures, any intact periosteum on the original concave surface of the fracture exerts a constant, springy force (**S**) which may cause recurrence of angulation if the plaster slackens, impairing three-point fixation. *Frequent check films may be essential in any conservatively treated fracture*. Another contributory cause of fracture slipping is when muscle wasting (**W**) occurs in a patient in a full arm plaster wearing a collar and cuff sling. Loss of brachialis and brachioradialis bulk leads to plaster slackening and angulatory deformity (**D**). *Patients with conservatively treated fractures should be given broad arm slings.*

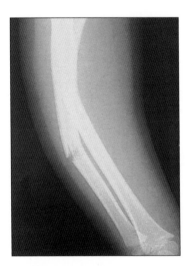
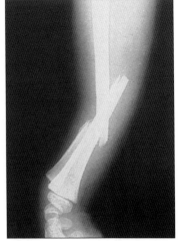

Patterns of fracture of both bones of the forearm in children.
Most forearm fractures in children are greenstick in pattern (**left**), with angulation but minimal displacement. An extensive, intact periosteal hinge can be assumed and reduction of such a fracture involves correction of the angulation only. When there is off-ending (**right**) there is potential instability. Shortening, angulation and axial rotation are more likely, and reduction may therefore be more difficult.

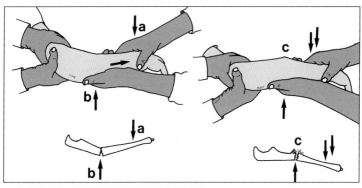

TREATMENT OF FOREARM FRACTURES
Children
Undisplaced fractures. In the undisplaced angulated greenstick fracture, the child should be given a general anaesthetic and the angulation corrected. One hand applies a little traction and the corrective force (**a**), while the other acts as a fulcrum under the fracture (**b**). If the fracture is overcorrected (**c**), the periosteum on the initially concave side of the fracture will be felt to snap. This will immediately give the fracture more mobility. While this has the advantage of reducing the risks of late angulation, it has the disadvantage of requiring greater care during the initial positioning of the arm in the plaster.

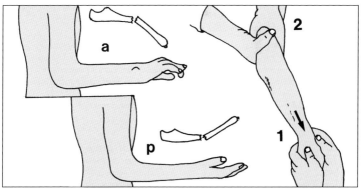

In the *undisplaced greenstick fracture* (i.e. with no axial rotation), the position of the forearm is important in preventing re-angulation while in plaster. Fractures with *posterior tilting* (anterior angulation) (**a**) should be placed in full pronation. The commonest fractures with *anterior tilting* (posterior angulation) (**p**) should be placed in full supination.

Displaced fractures. Axial rotation of the fragments should be looked for and the appropriate position in the pronation/supination range evaluated. The forearm is then placed in that position. Strong traction (**1**) is applied for a quarter of a minute or so, with the patient well relaxed under a general anaesthetic. The elbow is flexed at a right angle for countertraction (**2**).

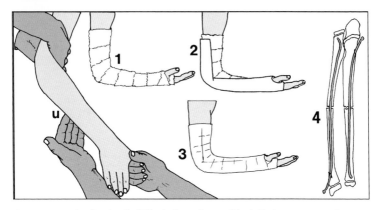

Assessment of reduction is difficult, but often residual displacement may be detected by feeling the subcutaneous surface of the ulna (**u**) in the region of the fracture. In the difficult case it is sometimes possible to gain bony apposition by applying traction and *increasing* the deformity before finally correcting it. Only rarely is open reduction and internal fixation indicated.

Fixation. To lessen the risks of ischaemia, apply a back shell only while maintaining traction. Wool (**1**) is followed by the shell (**2**), held by cotton bandages (**3**). Just before the plaster sets, give a final moulding. Review the check radiographs before withdrawing the anaesthetic. (Note that some proximal third fractures in children are only stable with the elbow in extension, and this position can be maintained for 5 weeks with relative safety.)

Internal fixation. This should be reserved for the rare (4%) unstable fractures. While plating of both bones is the commonest procedure, the use of elastic stable intramedullary nails (ESIN or Nancy nails) using an image intensifier is less invasive (**4**). Failure to obtain a reduction while introducing these nails can be dealt with by making a small incision over the fracture. Good results have been claimed when only one bone is fixed, with the arm subsequently held in a cast.

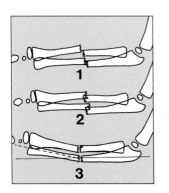

Assessment of radiographs. (1) Persistent displacement without angulation may be readily accepted. (2) Complete off-ending without angulation: remanipulate, and if no improvement can be gained either accept (when careful surveillance to detect early angulation is essential) or internally fix. (3) Slight angulation (10° or less) while undesirable *will* correct with remodelling in the younger child, and should be accepted. Marked angulation requires remanipulation.

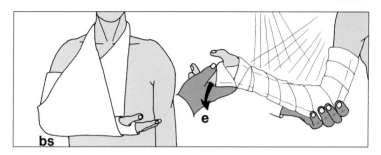

After-care. Apply a broad arm sling **(bs)**, keeping the arm well elevated and the fingers exposed. If there is much swelling, or the reduction has been difficult, then admit for elevation of the arm and circulatory observation: otherwise the child must be seen within 24 hours of the application of the plaster and the parents given the usual warnings regarding the possibility of circulatory impairment.

On review, the fingers should be checked for swelling, colour and active movements. If there is some doubt, slowly and gently extend the fingers **(e)**—if this produces excessive pain, it is suggestive of ischaemia. If ischaemia is present, the encircling bandages must be split and the situation carefully re-assessed after a short interval. If the circulation is perfect, the plaster may be completed.

In a conservatively treated unstable injury, check the plaster and the position of the fracture at weekly intervals for 3–4 weeks; if satisfactory, the sling may then be discarded. The plaster is maintained till union (usually after a further 1–2 weeks in a child of 4, and a further 3–4 weeks in a child of 10 years). In stable injuries, fortnightly checks will usually suffice. Mobilisation may be commenced from a sling.

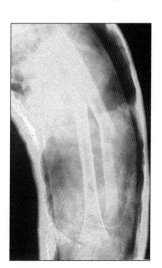

Management of late angulation.
Slight angulation of up to 10° may be accepted, especially under the age of 10, but a slack plaster must be changed to prevent *further* angulation. Where angulation is more severe and has been detected before callus has appeared **(left)**, the plaster should be changed under general anaesthesia and the angulation corrected by manipulation.

In a young child, if callus has appeared, accept any angulation unless gross (20° or more). *In the older child*, say 10 years or over, if angulation is marked remanipulation should be considered even in the presence of callus, as the powers of remodelling are less good. Union after remanipulation is usually rapid.

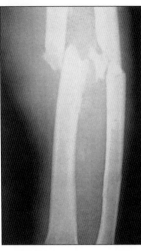

Adult fractures

In the adult, displacement is often quite marked **(left)**, and rotational deformities frequent. Closed reduction is often difficult and hard to maintain. In consequence, the best treatment for displaced fractures of the forearm bones in the fit adult is *open reduction and internal fixation. If the internal fixation is rigid, no external support may be necessary and the arm can be fully mobilised from the start*. Where the fixation is less good, a cast may be used until there is reasonable callus formation round both fractures. When rigid fixation has been obtained by the use of AO dynamic compression plates, these should be retained for not less than 21 months.

It is, however, reasonable to treat fractures of the forearm bones in the adult conservatively, if the fractures are undisplaced; in the elderly; or in patients where the duration of anaesthesia required for open reduction and internal fixation is considered hazardous. The following precautions must be taken:
• the arm must be carefully positioned in order to minimise any tendency to axial rotation • the plaster should be checked weekly for slackness, and changed if necessary (a complete plaster, applied over wool, should be used in an adult) • only a broad arm sling should be used • weekly X-rays should be taken to detect and allow correction of early slipping.

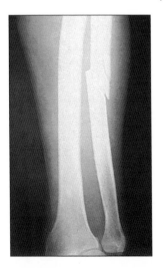

ISOLATED FRACTURE OF THE ULNA

This injury **(left)** may result from direct violence (e.g. in warding off a blow from a stick or falling object, or by striking the arm against the sharp edge of, for example, a machine or a step). In all cases, however, the whole of the radial shaft should be visualised to exclude in particular an associated dislocation of the radial head.

Treatment. Displacement is generally slight, and if this is the case a long arm plaster should be applied with the hand in mid-pronation. Beware of late slipping. The plaster is retained until union is advancing (usually about 8 weeks). If angulation is marked, then open reduction and internal fixation will have to be considered.

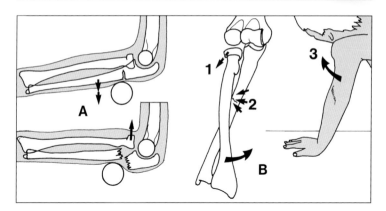

MONTEGGIA FRACTURE–DISLOCATION

Here a fracture of the ulna is accompanied by a dislocation of the head of the radius. *Mechanisms of injury:* (**A**) The most easily understood mechanism is when a violent fall or blow on the arm fractures the ulna and displaces the radial head anteriorly. (**B**) More commonly, the injury results from forced *pronation*. The radius is forced against the ulna, levering the radial head away from the capitellum (**1**) and fracturing the ulna (**2**). A fall on the outstretched arm accompanied by rotation of the trunk above (**3**) is often responsible. Rarely, the radial head may dislocate without damage to the ulna. *Supination of the arm is needed for reduction.*

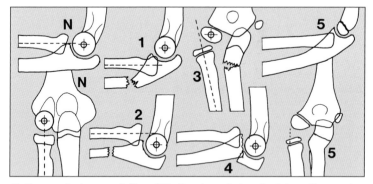

Patterns. In the normal elbow (**N**) a line through the axis of the radius cuts the centre of the capitellum. The radial head may dislocate backwards, with posterior angulation of the ulna (posterior Monteggia) (**1**); the radial head may dislocate anteriorly, with anterior angulation of the ulna (anterior Monteggia) (**2**); the radial head may dislocate laterally, with lateral angulation of the ulna (lateral Monteggia) (**3**); the radial head may dislocate anteriorly and be associated with a fracture of the olecranon (Hume fracture) (**4**); a greenstick fracture of the ulna (**5**), often difficult to detect, partly accounts for the fact that Monteggia lesions are frequently overlooked in children. *Always* check the position or the radial head in both views, and *always* look for distortion and kinking of the ulna.

Treatment. The key to successful management of this potentially difficult injury is accurate reduction. In the adult (and in children with displaced fractures), this is best achieved by open reduction and internal fixation of the ulnar fracture (commonly using a plate and screws, but in children an elastic intramedullary Nancy nail may be used). Thereafter, the elbow should be placed in right-angled flexion. *The position of the radial head should be checked by palpation and by radiographs.* Full supination *may* be required to maintain reduction, but generally once the ulna has been fixed, the neutral position will be satisfactory in maintaining stability. If the radial head will not reduce in full supination, it should be exposed, any loose cartilage fragments removed and any tear in the orbicular ligament sutured.

After-care. The plaster is changed at 3 weeks and the stitches removed. The cast may be finally discarded when you assess that there is adequate stability. Your opinion will be based on the type of fixation, its technical adequacy, callus formation, etc. In practice, mobilisation from a sling may often be started about 6 weeks. Physiotherapy is often required.

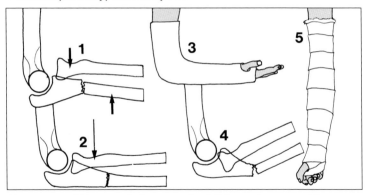

Treatment of Monteggia fractures in children. Any greenstick angulation of the ulna should be manipulated (1) to obtain correction (2). Put up an *anterior* Monteggia fracture in a position of 90° flexion at the elbow and in supination (3). *Posterior* Monteggia fractures (4) are often stable in full extension and may be fixed for not more than 3 weeks in this position (5); the elbow should be brought into a more flexed position for the remainder of the time in plaster. The position of the radial head must be confirmed by weekly radiographs; if there is any evidence of incongruity, exploration may have to be considered.

Late diagnosed Monteggia lesions. In *the adult*, some restriction of elbow movements may be the only complaint. Excision of the radial head may give temporary relief, but is often followed by subluxation of the ulna at the wrist. Tardy ulnar nerve palsy may be the first complaint; transposition of the ulnar nerve may arrest its progress. In *children*, excision of the radial head is contraindicated (it would lead to growth disturbance). In some cases, manipulative correction may be possible depending on the delay. In exceptional circumstances, the condition may be very late in being brought to light. In children under 10, good results have been claimed for surgery performed as late as 4 years.

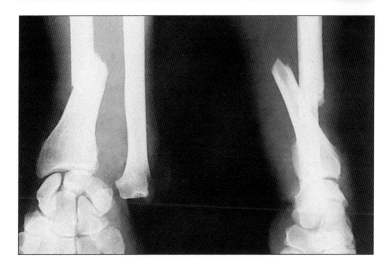

THE GALEAZZI FRACTURE–DISLOCATION

This is a fracture of the radius associated with a dislocation of the inferior radioulnar joint (as above).

Treatment. *Children:* these should be manipulated and put up in plaster in supination. Open reduction is seldom required. *Adults:* open reduction and plating of the radius through an anterior incision eliminate the risks of late slipping. Reduction of the radius is usually followed by spontaneous reduction of the ulnar subluxation, and only in exceptional circumstances does the inferior radioulnar joint require opening. With stable internal fixation and an intact ulna, there is less need for additional external fixation. *Late diagnosed Galeazzi lesions:* prominence of the ulna with pain in the wrist is the commonest complaint and excision of the distal ulna may give relief.

ISOLATED FRACTURES OF THE RADIUS

These usually result from direct violence. Although the inferior radioulnar joint may initially appear to be intact, late subluxation may occur if the radial fracture angulates. The rule is that if the radius is fractured, you should *always* look for subluxation of the ulna, and if it is not present to begin with, be on guard for it developing later. When assessing the radiographs note that in the normal wrist the distal end of the ulna (excluding the styloid process) lies just proximal to the articular surface of the radius, the space between being occupied by the triangular fibrocartilage.

Treatment. *Adults:* if there is no significant angulation or rotational deformity these may be treated in plaster, generally with the arm in supination. (Slight axial rotation may be controlled by careful positioning of the forearm.) In all cases, careful surveillance is vital to detect early slipping, an indication for operative intervention. *Children:* in children, isolated fractures of the radius should also be treated conservatively.

22

Regional injuries: the wrist and hand

Colles' fracture 328
Fracture of the scaphoid 343
Dislocations of the carpus 347
Injuries to the metacarpals and phalanges 352

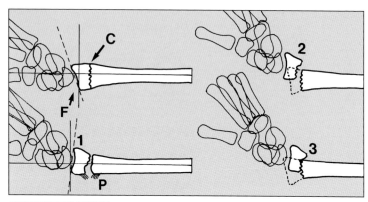

COLLES' FRACTURE

A Colles' fracture (**C**) is a fracture of the radius within 2.5 cm of the wrist, with a characteristic deformity if displaced. It is the commonest of all fractures and is seen mainly in middle-aged and elderly women. Osteoporosis is a frequent contributory factor. It often results from a fall on the outstretched hand.

Deformities. The position of the radial fragment has no less than six characteristic features which the radiographs elucidate. The force of impact (**F**) fractures the radius through the cancellous bone of the metaphysis. With greater violence the anterior periosteum tears (**P**), and the distal fragment tilts into *anterior angulation* (**1**) with loss of the normal 5° forward tilt of the joint surface. With still greater force there is *dorsal displacement of the distal fragment* (**2**). The shaft of the radius is driven into the distal fragment leading to impaction (**3**). (The dotted lines indicate the position of the distal fragment prior to any displacement.)

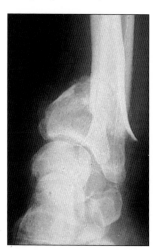

The altered contour of the wrist in a badly displaced Colles' fracture is striking, and is referred to as a 'dinner fork' deformity. (When viewed from the side, the wrist has the same curvature as a fork, with the fingers resembling the tines.)

The radiograph shows a typical displaced Colles' fracture. The anterior angulation, dorsal displacement and impaction are obvious (deformities 1,2,3). In the radiograph the *posterior surface* of the radiograph lies on the *left*.

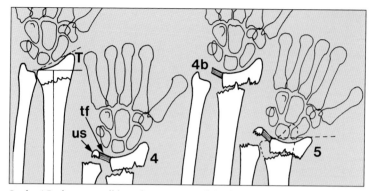

In the AP plane, a small lateral component of the force of impact causes *lateral* (radial) *displacement of the distal fragment* (**4**). (Note that in the AP projection of the normal wrist that the joint surface has a tilt of 22° (**T**).) The distal fragment is attached to the ulnar styloid by the triangular fibrocartilage (**tf**), which generally avulses the ulnar styloid (**us**). Sometimes the triangular fibrocartilage is torn (**4b**). In either case there is disruption of the inferior radioulnar joint. The distal fragment tilts laterally into *ulnar angulation* (**5**) (reducing the tilt to less than 22°) and impacts. The sixth feature is a rotational or torsional deformity which is not obvious in either AP or lateral projections.

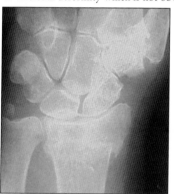

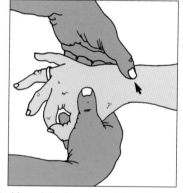

The AP projection on the **left** shows typical lateral displacement of the radial fragment, with ulnar angulation and impaction. There is avulsion of the ulnar styloid process.

Diagnosis

If there is *pain in the wrist* and *tenderness over the distal end of the radius* (**right**) after a fall, radiographs must always be taken. The site of maximum tenderness will help to exclude a fracture of the scaphoid (unless there is a double injury). Where there is *marked displacement* the characteristic appearance leaves little diagnostic doubt. Note that in the normal wrist the radial styloid lies 1 cm distal to the ulnar styloid.

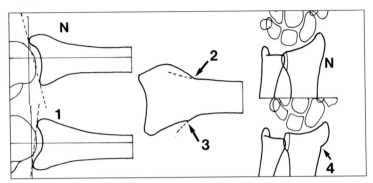

Radiographs. In most cases the fracture is easily identified, but sometimes impaction may render the fracture line inconspicuous. If in doubt, look at the angle between the distal end of the radius and the shaft in the lateral (**1**). Decrease to less than 0° is suggestive of fracture (but enquire about previous injury). The minimally displaced fracture may also reveal itself by an increase in the posterior radial concavity, often with local kinking (**2**), or by separate or accompanying breaks in the smooth curves of the anterior (**3**) or lateral surfaces (**4**). If there is any doubt, return to the patient *and confirm whether there is any localised tenderness over the suspect area.* (**N**=Normal.)

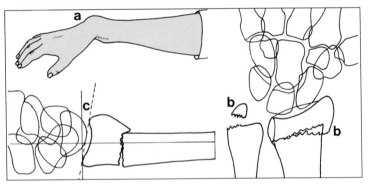

Treatment
Does the fracture require manipulation? If the fracture is grossly displaced, it is obvious that it should be reduced. If undisplaced, no manipulation is needed. Between these extremes, the following are indications for manipulation: (**a**) if there is a readily appreciated naked-eye deformity (deformity, not swelling). (**b**) If there is displacement of the ulnar styloid or marked ulnar angulation of the distal fragment. (These indicate serious disruption of the inferior radioulnar joint, and an attempt at correction should be made *irrespective of other appearances*.) (**c**) If the joint line in the lateral projection is tilted 10° or more posteriorly rather than anteriorly, the fracture should be manipulated; but in the very old, frail patient somewhat greater degrees of deformity may be accepted.

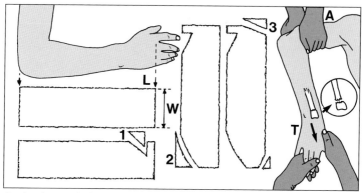

Reduction technique. *Anaesthesia* is necessary, either general or regional (Bier block). Both require the ready availability of good resuscitation facilities. Where there is a preference for general anaesthesia, but the patient attends late at night with a history of recent intake of food or drink, it is permissible and often safer to apply a temporary plaster back shell and an arm sling, and delay reduction till morning. Before any manipulation, prepare a suitable plaster back slab. The length (**L**) should equal the distance from the olecranon to the metacarpal heads. The width (**W**) in an adult should be 15 cm (6″), and it should be about eight layers thick. The slab should be trimmed with a tongue (**1**) for the first web space, a large radial curve to allow elbow flexion (**2**), and a cut for ulnar deviation (**3**). The essential next stage is to disimpact the distal radial fragment. The elbow is flexed to a right angle and the arm held by the interlocked fingers of an assistant (**A**). Traction is applied in the line of the forearm (**T**). Traction need only be applied for a few seconds, and disimpaction may be confirmed by holding the distal fragment between the thumb and index; it should be easy to move anteriorly and posteriorly.

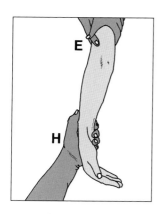

The elbow is now extended (**E**). The heel of one hand (**H**) should be placed over the dorsal surface of the distal radial fragment, and the fingers curled round the patient's wrist and palm. This grip allows traction to be re-applied to the disimpacted fracture.

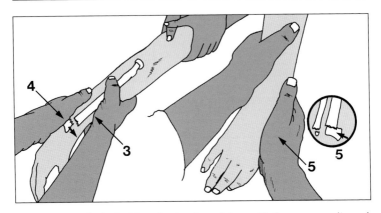

Now, by using the heel of the other hand as a fulcrum (3), firm pressure directed anteriorly (4) will correct all the remaining deformities normally visible in the *lateral* radiographs of the wrist (posterior displacement, anterior angulation).

Still maintaining traction, alter the position of the grip so that the heel (here of the right hand) is able to push the distal fragment ulnar-wards and correct the radial displacement (5). Ulnar angulation, the other deformity seen in the AP radiograph, is corrected by placing the hand in full ulnar deviation at the wrist.

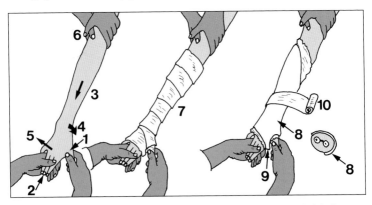

Change the grip to allow free application of the plaster. One hand holds the thumb fully extended (1) while the other holds three fingers (2) to avoid 'cupping'. Maintain slight traction (3). The wrist should be in *full pronation* (4), *full ulnar deviation* (5) and *slight palmar flexion*. The elbow must be *extended* (either by an assistant (6), or by resting the upper arm against the edge of the table). The skin should be protected with wool roll (7), but if stockingette is preferred this must be applied *prior* to reduction. Fit the wet slab over the anterior, lateral and posterior aspects of the radius (8), tucking the tongue into the palm (9). Secure it with two wetted 10 cm (4″) open weave bandages (cotton, gauze or Kling® (10). The end can be secured with a scrap of plaster bandage.

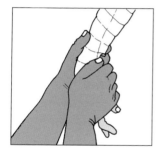

Before the plaster sets, many surgeons like to apply further pressure over the posterolateral aspect of the distal fragment, and maintain this until setting occurs ('final moulding'). This precaution ensures maintenance of the reduction, but care should be taken not to dent the plaster.

A collar and cuff sling should be applied, making sure that there is no constriction at the elbow or at the wrist. Try to flex the elbow beyond a right angle so that the forearm is not dependent.

Alternative techniques. It is not unexpected that in this common fracture, methods of reduction are legion. As it is generally an easy fracture to reduce, it follows that success can rightly be claimed for many techniques. The method given is logical in so far as it correlates with the pathology as seen on the radiographs. Note, however, the following: (1) a direct, simple and extremely effective procedure is to disimpact the fracture, apply a plaster slab, and correct the deformity before the plaster sets by applying pressure on the posterolateral aspect of the distal fragment (as in the 'final moulding' described above). (2) In the elderly patient unfit for general anaesthesia (but preferably after intravenous diazepam), a *marked* dorsal displacement may be corrected by quick application of pressure (without previous disimpaction) over a dorsal slab.

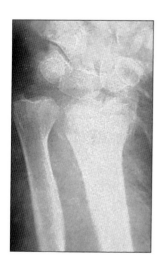

Check radiographs. These should be taken and studied preferably before the anaesthetic is discontinued or wears off. Severe persisting deformity, *especially in the AP projection* (as illustrated **left**), should not be accepted, and remanipulation should be undertaken.

If the position is acceptable, the patient is shown finger exercises and advised regarding normal plaster care.

If the fracture is very unstable and difficult to control, the use of an external fixator should be considered, particularly in a young adult.

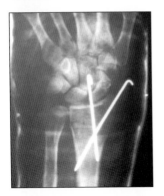

Alternative fixation methods

If during manipulation, instability is found to be very marked (often due to comminution and marked local osteoporosis) or if the check radiographs taken after manipulation confirm that the reduction is poorly controlled by plaster fixation alone, then the position may be held with two or more Kirschner wires (as shown **left**). Additional cast support will be required. The wires may be removed after 3–4 weeks.

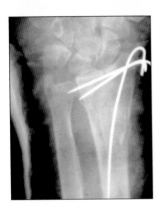

In this further example of Kirschner wiring, there has been some comminution of the distal fragment, and this has been secured with two transversely placed wires. The reconstructed distal fragment has then been aligned with the shaft using a longitudinal wire. An additional plaster cast has been required. The positioning of the K-wires may be managed using an image intensifier or by direct vision using an arthroscope.

A T-plate screwed to the radial shaft, either on its anterior or posterior surface, may also be considered.

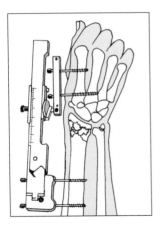

An external fixator may also be used. Commonly two pins are inserted into the distal third of the radial shaft and two into the lateral aspect of the metacarpal shaft of the index finger. The two half-pin sets are then secured by a suitable linking device; this is then adjusted to obtain a good correction in all planes. In the Agee–Wristjack™ illustrated, traction and palmar flexion are readily controlled.

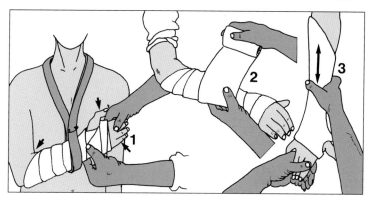

After-care

The patient is seen *the next day*. The circulation is checked and swelling assessed (1). Examine the palm, fingers, thumb and elbow for constriction caused by bandaging or elbow flexion, and make any adjustments.

In 2–5 days (usually at a fracture clinic), the plaster is completed if finger swelling is slight. (If it is marked, delay completion.) *Superficial* layers of cotton bandage are removed, the slab retained and encircling plaster bandages applied (2). The patient is instructed in elbow and shoulder exercises, and unless there is still a fair amount of swelling the sling may be discarded. *At 2 weeks* the plaster is checked for marked slackening (3) (replace), softening (reinforce) and technical faults. Movements in the fingers, elbow and shoulder are examined and appropriate advice given or physiotherapy started. In some centres, radiographs are taken at this stage; slight slipping is inevitable, but marked slipping may be an indication for remanipulation (not usually a profitable procedure). At this stage the plaster may be replaced by a resin cast should this be thought desirable.

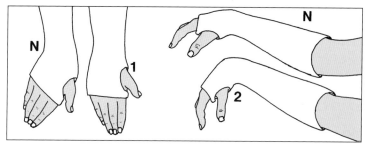

Checking for positional errors. The commonest fault is lack of ulnar deviation (1). This should be sadly accepted if discovered at 2 weeks (but replaster if found earlier). Lack of ulnar deviation increases the risks of non-union of the ulnar styloid or other problems arising from the inferior radioulnar joint. Excessive wrist flexion (2) is liable to lead to difficulty in recovering dorsiflexion and a useful grip, and if present, the plaster should be re-applied with the wrist in a more extended position. (**N**=Normal, i.e. correct position.)

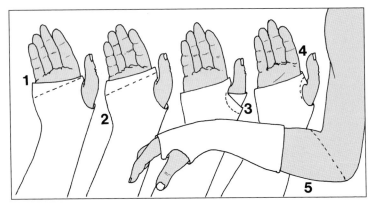

Checking for plaster faults. The following faults are common. The distal edge of the plaster may not follow the normal oblique line of the MP joints, and movements of the little (1) and sometimes the other fingers (2) are restricted. The thumb may be restricted by a few turns of plaster bandage (3), or the plaster may dig into the skin of the first web (4). In all these cases, the plaster should be trimmed to the dotted line to permit free movement. The plaster may be too short (5), impairing support of the fracture: it should be extended posteriorly to the olecranon and anteriorly as far as will still permit elbow flexion.

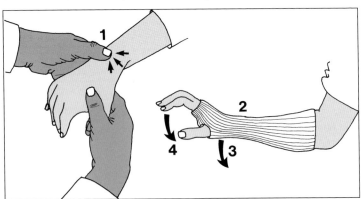

Assessment of union. The plaster should be removed at 5 weeks (or 6 weeks in badly displaced fractures in the elderly), and the fracture assessed for union. (Radiographs are of limited value.) *If there is marked persisting tenderness* (1), a fresh plaster should be applied and union re-assessed in a further 2 weeks. *If tenderness is minimal or absent*, a circular woven support (e.g. Tubigrip (2)) or a crepe bandage may be applied (to limit oedema and to some extent increase the patient's confidence). The patient is instructed in wrist (3) and finger exercises (4) and encouraged to practise these frequently and with vigour. Elbow and shoulder movements should be continued. Arrange review in a further 2 weeks.

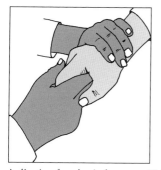

Assessing the need for rehabilitation. At about 7 weeks post-injury, you must decide whether to discharge the patient or refer her for rehabilitation. Base your decision on:
• *Finger movements* lack of 'tuck-in' (i.e. the last few degrees of flexion) is an indication for physiotherapy. • G*rip strength*—assess by first asking her to squeeze two of your fingers as tightly as possible while you try to withdraw them. Compare one hand with the other. Repeat with a single finger. Marked weakness is an indication for physiotherapy. • *Wrist movements*—initially, material restriction of *palmar flexion* is normal and by itself is of little importance. If, however, the total range of *pronation* and *supination* is less than half normal, physiotherapy is advisable. • *Functional requirements*—where there is only slight restriction of movements and power, rehabilitation may still be indicated because of the patient's occupation or domestic needs.

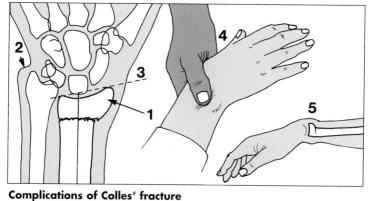

Complications of Colles' fracture
Persistent deformity or malunion. Radial drift of the distal fragment results in prominence of the distal radius (**1**). Radial tilting and bony absorption at the fracture site lead to relative prominence of the distal ulna (**2**) and tilting of the plane of the wrist as seen in the AP radiographs (**3**). These deformities may be symptom-free, and surgery on purely cosmetic grounds is seldom indicated. In some cases there is quite marked pain in the region of the distal radioulnar joint, owing to its severe disorganisation. There is generally quite marked *local tenderness* (**4**) and supination in particular is reduced. Physiotherapy in the form of grip strengthening and pronation/supination exercises is indicated. If symptoms remain severe, excision of the distal end of the ulna may be considered. Uncomplicated persistence of dinner-fork deformity (**5**), with persistent deformity in the lateral but not necessarily in the AP radiographs, is accompanied by some loss of palmar flexion, but significant functional disturbance is unusual. This type of residual deformity is generally accepted.

Sudeck's atrophy/complex regional pain syndrome. This is often detected about the time the patient comes out of plaster. The fingers are swollen and finger flexion is restricted. The hand and wrist are warm, tender and painful. Radiographs show diffuse osteoporosis. *Treatment:* the mainstay of treatment is intensive and prolonged physiotherapy and occupational therapy, but if pain is very severe a further 2–3 weeks rest of the wrist in plaster may give sufficient relief to allow commencement of effective finger movements. If the MP joints are stiff in extension and making no headway, manipulation under general anaesthesia followed by fixation in plaster (MP joints flexed, IP joints extended) for 3 weeks only may be effective in initiating recovery. In severe cases, a chemical sympathetic blockade may be attempted.

Delayed rupture of extensor pollicis longus. This may follow a Colles' fracture, and be due to attrition of the tendon by roughness at the fracture site or by sloughing from interference with its blood supply. Disability is often slight, and spontaneous recovery may occur. There is no urgency regarding treatment, and in the elderly this complaint may be accepted or treated expectantly. In the young, an extensor indicis proprius tendon transfer is advocated.

Carpal tunnel (median nerve compression) syndrome. Paraesthesia in the median distribution is the main presenting symptom, but look for sensory and motor involvement. *If detected before reduction:* (a) Complete lesion: reduce, plaster and re-assess. If no improvement, explore and divide not only the roof of the carpal tunnel but the antebrachial fascia. (b) Partial lesion: reduce and apply a cast; if motor symptoms remain or if symptoms persist for a week, decompress. *If detected after reduction:* release the splints, put the wrist in the neutral position and use Kirschner wires or an external fixator to hold the reduction; if symptoms persist, explore. *If detected after union:* exploration is generally advised, as symptoms otherwise tend to persist.

Persisting stiffness. Restriction of movements, even after prolonged physiotherapy, is not uncommon but is seldom severe enough to impair limb function to a material extent. This is due to compensatory (trick) movements developed by the elbow, shoulder and trunk (e.g. in the case of loss of supination.)

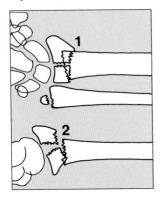

Comminution of the radial fragment. This may show as a vertical crack in the AP view (1), while in other cases the fracture may run horizontally. The scaphoid may separate the fragments (2). In the latter case, in the young adult, internal fixation is indicated. Some permanent joint stiffness is the rule, and prolonged physiotherapy will be required.

Associated scaphoid fracture. The scaphoid fracture may be internally fixed, the Colles' fracture manipulated and fixation discontinued as soon as the latter has united. Alternatively, manipulate the Colles' fracture and apply a scaphoid plaster. After the Colles' fracture has united, a further period of immobilisation may be required for the scaphoid fracture.

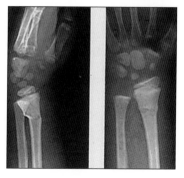

Related fractures

A number of fractures of the distal radius have similarities with the classical Colles' fracture.

Greenstick fracture of the radius. *Undisplaced:* this is common and may be overlooked, as the only sign may be slight local buckling of the bone **(left)**. It may be treated by a plaster slab which can usually be completed after 1–2 days. Fixation for about 3 weeks only is required. *Angulated:* in this type of injury there is both clinical and radiological deformity. Manipulation is required as for a Colles' fracture, with fixation for 3 or 4 weeks, depending on the age of the child.

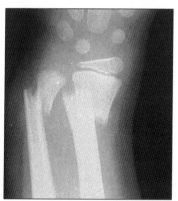
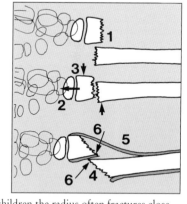

Overlapping radial fracture. In children the radius often fractures close to the wrist, with off-ending of the fragments. *On the ulnar side* there may be:
• detachment of the triangular fibrocartilage • separation of the ulnar epiphysis • fracture and angulation of the distal ulna • fracture and displacement of the distal ulna **(left)**, in effect a fracture of both bones of the forearm • dislocation of the ulna (Galeazzi fracture–dislocation). *Treatment:* if the fracture line is transverse **(1)**, reduction is straightforward by traction **(2)** and local pressure **(3)**. When, however, there is an oblique fracture running from front to back **(4)**, reduction by traction is often impossible owing to the integrity of the periosteum on the dorsal surface **(5)** and the overlapping bony spikes **(6)**.

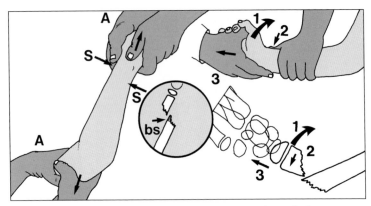

In those circumstances, two closed techniques may be tried. For the first, two assistants (**A, A**) are essential to apply *maximal* traction to the limb. While this is being strongly maintained, the surgeon should press forcibly with the heel of one hand on the distal fragment and use the other to apply counter-pressure (**S, S**). Reduction is achieved by shearing off one of the bone spikes (**bs**). Alternatively, by *increasing* the deformity (**1**) and applying pressure directly over the distal radial fragment (**2**), whilst maintaining traction (**3**), reduction may be achieved. After the fragments have unlocked, the angulation is corrected. Thereafter, plaster fixation is carried out as in other fractures in this region. If shortening is marked and closed methods fail, open reduction may be considered. This may be performed through a small dorsal incision under a tourniquet; internal fixation is not required, although a Kirschner wire may be used to hold the fracture temporarily—being withdrawn as soon as the plaster has been applied. Nevertheless, if persisting overlap is reluctantly accepted, a good result from remodelling is the usual outcome *provided* any angulation is corrected.

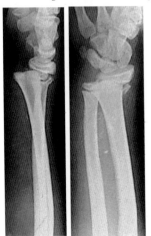

Slipped radial epiphysis. This injury is common in adolescence, and the displaced distal radial epiphysis is usually associated with a small fracture of the metaphysis (Salter–Harris type 2 injury, as shown on the AP radiographs on the left). Unless displacement is minimal, manipulation followed by plaster fixation (as for a Colles' fracture) is indicated. Growth disturbance is rare, but reduction should be carried out promptly as this injury is often difficult to reduce after 2 days.

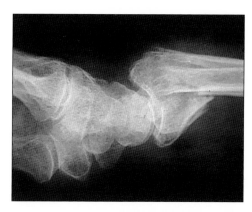
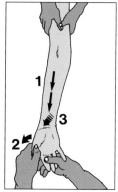

Smith's fracture. The distal radial fragment is tilted into posterior angulation and may be displaced anteriorly. It is often referred to as a reversed Colles' fracture, as when viewed from the side the deformities are in the opposite direction. (In the AP, however, the two may be identical.) Comminuted Smith's fractures may also involve the articular surface of the radius (**left**). Greenstick fractures of Smith's pattern are common. *Treatment:* to reduce, apply traction (**1**) in supination (**2**) until disimpaction is achieved. Pressure may be applied with the heels of the hands to force the distal fragment dorsally (**3**).

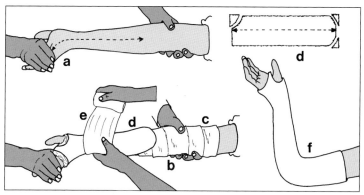

The reduction, although difficult to hold, may be maintained in supination and dorsiflexion (**a**). A long arm, complete plaster applied in two stages is best. First extend the elbow (**b**) and apply wool roll (**c**), an anterior slab (trimmed as shown, **d**), and encircling plaster bandages (**e**). The fracture may be moulded during setting of the cast. Now flex the elbow and extend the plaster above the elbow (**f**). *After-care:* split the plaster if necessary. Radiographs should be taken weekly for the first 3 weeks to detect any significant slipping (treat by remanipulation or moulding). A slack plaster should be carefully changed. Six weeks' fixation is usually required, followed by physiotherapy.

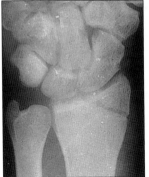

Fracture of the radial styloid. This fracture is sometimes caused by an engine starting-handle kickback or by a fall on the outstretched hand. Displacement is usually slight, and manipulation seldom of value. *Treatment.* If displacement is minimal, fixation in a Colles' type plaster usually gives good results. Physiotherapy may be required to deal with wrist stiffness. Where the distal articular surface of the radius is disturbed because of displacement, internal fixation is advisable, and some advocate its use in all cases. Sudeck's atrophy (complex regional pain syndrome) is a common complication of this fracture.

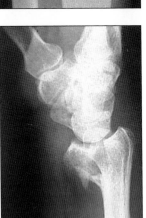

Barton's fracture. This is a form of Smith's fracture in which the anterior portion only of the radius is involved. Closed reduction may be attempted along the lines indicated for Smith's fracture, but this may fail, with the carpus wedging the fragments apart. If this occurs, open reduction and internal fixation (e.g. by means of a cancellous screw or an anterior-placed buttress plate) are indicated, particularly in the younger patient.

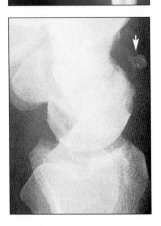

Avulsion fractures of the carpus. Forcible palmar flexion may result in a minor avulsion fracture of the carpus (**left**) at a ligament insertion.

Impingement fracture of the radius. If the wrist is forcibly palmar flexed or dorsiflexed, the carpus impinging on the distal end of the radius may produce a marginal chip fracture of the radius. *Treatment:* only symptomatic treatment (e.g. 2–3 weeks in a plaster back slab) is required for these last two injuries.

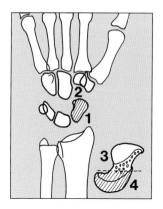

FRACTURE OF THE SCAPHOID

Features. The scaphoid plays a key role in wrist and carpal function, taking part in the radiocarpal joint (**1**) and in the joint between the proximal and distal rows of the carpus (**2**). In some cases this dual role may contribute to displacement of the fracture, difficulty in fixation, non-union and carpal instability. If the fracture disrupts the blood supply to the bone (much of which enters in the region of the waist) (**3**), avascular necrosis of the proximal pole (**4**) may ensue.

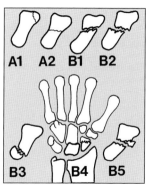

Fracture patterns (Herbert classification). **A1** = fractures of the tubercle; **A2** = hairline fracture of the waist. The prognosis is good in these *stable* injuries. The prognosis is poorer in *unstable* injuries, which include oblique fractures of the distal third (**B1**), displaced fractures of the waist (**B2**), proximal pole fractures (**B3**), fractures associated with carpal dislocations (**B4**) and comminuted fractures (**B5**). The commonest site for fracture is the waist (50%); 38% of fractures occur in the proximal half and 12% in the distal half.

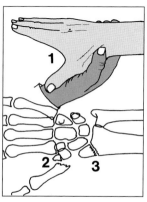

Mechanisms of injury. Scaphoid fractures often result from 'kickback' when using engine starter handles or from falls on the outstretched hand.

Diagnosis

Suspect when there is pain on the lateral aspect of the wrist following any injury (or frequently repeated stress). In some cases there may be marked swelling of the hand and wrist. Tenderness in the snuff box (**1**) is suggestive, but is also a feature of many wrist sprains. In a true scaphoid fracture, tenderness will also be found over the *dorsal* and *palmar* aspects of the scaphoid. Beware too of tenderness which may be a sign of a Bennett's fracture of the thumb metacarpal (**2**) or of a fracture of the radial styloid (**3**).

Radiographs. Note the following important points: Request cards should be clearly marked 'scaphoid' and not 'wrist', to ensure that *at least* three views of the scaphoid are obtained. 'Carpal box' views helpfully show the scaphoid elongated and magnified. The fracture is often hairline and hard to see, so that in all suspected but unconfirmed cases, radiographs should be repeated at 10–14 days, when local decalcification may reveal a previously hidden fracture. If doubt remains, a bone scan may be helpful.

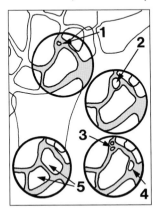

Note that there is a 20% rate of false positive reporting of scaphoid radiographs, and *clinical confirmation of the diagnosis is mandatory*.

Again, a number of abnormalities in ossification may be confused with fractures. The *os centrale* may be small (**1**), large (**2**) or double (**3**). The *os radiale externum* (**4**) lies in the region of the tubercle and in some cases may represent an old, un-united fracture; certainly the so called 'bipartite scaphoid' (**5**) is now generally regarded as being due to this. (Rounded edges differentiate these from fresh fractures.) Note that MRI scans may help in diagnosis and giving a prognosis.

Treatment of suspected fracture

When there is local tenderness and normal radiographs, apply a scaphoid plaster and sling. Remove the plaster and re-X-ray at 2 weeks. Absorption of bone at the site of any hairline fracture is by then likely to have revealed it. If a fracture is confirmed, apply a fresh cast and treat as for a frank fracture. If the radiographs are negative, the patient is presumed to have suffered a sprain and is treated accordingly: but if symptoms persist, re-examine and X-ray after another 2 weeks.

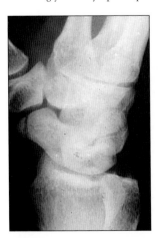

Treatment of fractures of the tuberosity of the scaphoid

Avascular necrosis never occurs in fractures of this type (**left**), and non-union here does not give rise to significant symptoms. Symptomatic treatment only is needed (e.g. a crepe bandage or plaster, depending on pain). Some extend this line of treatment to include all distal pole fractures, but generally plaster fixation is the mainstay of treatment of all fractures through the body of the scaphoid.

Treatment of undisplaced fractures of the body of the scaphoid

For fractures of the waist undisplaced by more than 1mm, some advocate the semi-closed insertion of a Herbert or cannulated screw, claiming good results without the necessity of plaster fixation. Conservative treatment in plaster appears to give equally good results and avoids operative complications: it remains the mainstay of treatment for this class of fracture.

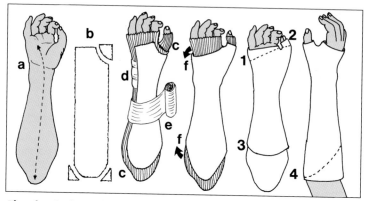

The classical scaphoid plaster.

The *position of the hand* is of importance and this should be made clear to the patient prior to the application of the plaster. The wrist should be fully pronated, radially deviated and moderately dorsiflexed. The thumb should be in mid-abduction and able to form a circle with the index (**a**).

An anterior plaster slab is frequently used, being made from 6–8 layers of 10 cm (4″) plaster bandage or taken from a slab dispenser. The corners should be trimmed and a cut-out made to accommodate the swell of the thenar muscles (**b**).

Stockingette, which is later turned down, is applied to the arm and thumb (**c**). A turn of wool is used to protect the bony prominences of the wrist (**d**). If there is a lot of early swelling (suggesting perhaps more to come), more generous wool padding is applied round the wrist and hand.

The plaster slab may then be wetted and applied to the forearm, taking care not to extend it beyond the proximal palmar crease. Encircling plaster bandages are then applied, using 15 cm (6″) bandages for the forearm, 10 cm (4″) for the wrist and 7.5 cm (3″) for the thumb. The edges of the stockingette are turned down before completion (**f**).

Check that there are none of the common faults, such as (**1**) the plaster including the MP joints of fingers or (**2**) the terminal phalanx of the thumb, restricting flexion. Check that the cast is not too short (**3**), impairing fixation, or too long (**4**), restricting elbow flexion. (Note that to give the best support to a scaphoid fracture there is some questioning of the position of the wrist and the need to include the thumb. Some use a Colles' plaster in neutral, 20° extension, or slight flexion, without radial deviation.)

A sling should be worn for the first few days until swelling subsides. Analgesics are usually required initially.

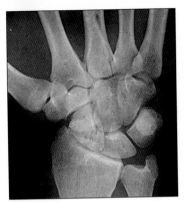 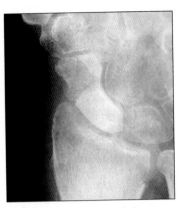

After-care. The patient is reviewed at *2 weeks* (assuming the initial plaster check has been satisfactory). If the plaster is unduly slack, it should be changed. Any softening in the palm should be reinforced.

At *6 weeks* the plaster should be removed and the scaphoid assessed clinically and with radiographs. There are several possibilities: (i) If there is no tenderness over the dorsal surface and in the snuff-box, and the fracture appears united on the radiographs, the wrist should be left free and reviewed in 2 weeks (usually for discharge, or further radiographs if pain recurs). (ii) The fracture line may still show clearly on the radiographs **(left)**. (iii) The radiographs may suggest union, but there is marked local tenderness. (iv) There is some uncertainty on either score. These all suggest delayed union, and a further 6 weeks' fixation is desirable.

At *12 weeks*, there may be: (a) evidence of *avascular necrosis* (**right:** note density of proximal half), (b) clear evidence, clinically and radiologically of *union*. In these circumstances, there is no advantage in continuing with plaster fixation.

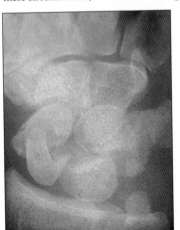

At *12 weeks* there may be: (c) no evidence of union, (d) evidence of established non-union: internal fixation should be considered. In (d), local bone grafting will also be required. If surgery is not entertained in (d), the cast should be discarded, while in (c), a further period in plaster may be considered if there is marked persistent pain and local tenderness.

Treatment of displaced fractures of the scaphoid

Where there is marked displacement **(left)**, make a careful analysis of the radiographs to exclude a carpal dislocation. Where the displacement or angulation exceeds 1 mm or 15° respectively, open reduction and internal fixation are indicated.

Complications of scaphoid fracture

Avascular necrosis. This is of immediate onset, but 1–2 months may elapse before increased density betrays its presence on the radiographs. There is usually slow but progressive bony collapse and radiocarpal osteoarthritis, leading to worsening pain and stiffness in the wrist. It occurs in about 30% of fractures of the proximal pole of the scaphoid. Surgery should be carried out before secondary changes occur in the wrist. Procedures include excision of the scaphoid with or without the insertion of a prosthetic replacement.

Non-union. Cystic changes at the fracture site are followed by marginal sclerosis. The edges may round off and form a symptomless pseudarthrosis, or osteoarthritis may supervene. (Note that non-union can occur without avascular necrosis, and that most fractures with avascular necrosis are united.) Late diagnosed non-union, seen 3–6 months after injury, may still be effectively treated by plaster fixation and pulsed magnetic fields, *provided* that there is no displacement, carpal collapse or osteoarthritic change. If there is displacement, or if seen later than 6 months and symptoms are present, internal fixation and bone grafting may be attempted. If an early impingement osteoarthritis threatens, satisfactory results may be obtained from excision of the radial styloid, even although the midcarpal joint is unaffected by this. Symptomless non-union of the scaphoid, sometimes discovered by accident, should have the risks of secondary osteoarthritis assessed; if the appearances indicate that these are insignificant, then no treatment is indicated.

Advanced osteoarthritis. This generally occurs as a sequel to avascular necrosis or non-union. It may be treated by radiocarpal fusion (where pronation and supination movements are retained, but all other wrist movements are lost); or by excision of the proximal row of the carpus (where although some movements remain, the results are somewhat unpredictable); or the use of an orthotic support.

Sudeck's atrophy. Treat as described under Colles' fracture.

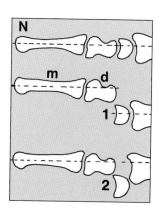

DISLOCATIONS OF THE CARPUS

These are comparatively uncommon injuries. There are *two main groups*: in the first, the metacarpals (**m**), the distal row of the carpus (**d**) and *part* of the proximal row dislocate dorsally. In classifying injuries within this group, the prefix 'peri' is used to describe the undisplaced structures in the proximal row (e.g. 'perilunar dislocation of the carpus' (**1**)). Occasionally, one of the carpal bones fractures, part remaining in alignment and part displacing with the distal row of the carpus. In the second main group of injuries, the distal row of the carpus re-aligns with the radius and part of the proximal row is extruded (e.g. dislocation of the lunate (**2**), the most common of the carpal dislocations). (**N** = normal wrist alignments.)

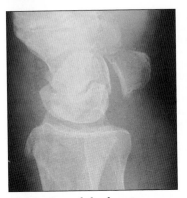
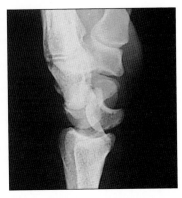

Dislocation of the lunate

This is the most common of all the carpal dislocations. Note in the *normal* radiograph of the carpus **(left)** that the pisiform bone stands out to a varying degree from the rest of the volar surface. The *shape* of the dislocated lunate is quite different. The *concave surface* in which the capitate usually sits is *rotated* anteriorly, and the crescent moon shape of the bone (and hence its name) is rendered obvious **(right)**. It is *displaced* anteriorly. (In the AP projection, the lunate is sector shaped.) *Diagnosis:* this is established on the basis of a history of injury, local tenderness and the radiographs. Look also for evidence of median nerve involvement resulting from the direct pressure of the displaced bone.

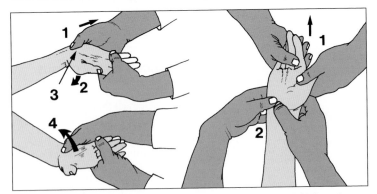

Treatment. Reduction can generally be achieved by closed methods under general anaesthesia. **(1)** Apply traction to the supinated wrist. **(2)** Extend the wrist, maintaining traction. **(3)** Apply pressure with the thumb over the lunate. **(4)** Flex the wrist as soon as you feel the lunate slip into position. Alternatively, an assistant applies traction in supination and extension as before **(1)** while you use both thumbs to push the lunate posteriorly and distally **(2)**. When it is felt to reduce, the wrist is flexed. The reduction should be checked with radiographs before the anaesthetic is discontinued. (Failure is an indication for open reduction.)

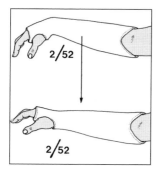

The wrist is encased in plaster in a position of moderate flexion. Check X-rays should be taken to ensure that the reduction has been maintained. After 1–2 weeks, the plaster is changed for one with the wrist in the neutral position for a further 2 weeks.

Physiotherapy may then be required, depending on the degree of residual stiffness. Swelling may be a problem initially, and the usual precautions should be taken (e.g. generous padding, elevation, a sling, vigorous finger movements, etc.).

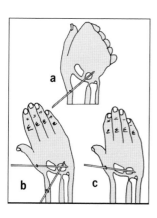

Many prefer Kirschner wire fixation in all cases. To do this the wrist is put in flexion and full ulnar deviation, and the lunate fixed to the radius with a K-wire (a). The wrist is then positioned in dorsiflexion, and radial deviation and a second wire passed through the scaphoid into the lunate (b). The wrist is then placed in a more neutral position and the first wire removed (c). A light cast is applied and the remaining wire removed at 4 weeks. The cast is retained for a further 2 weeks before mobilisation is commenced.

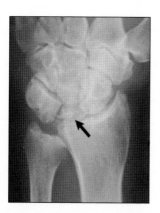

Complications
Avascular necrosis. This leads to collapse of the lunate and a secondary osteoarthritis, which advances with great rapidity. *All cases of dislocated lunate should have monthly radiographs for 6 months* to allow early detection of this complication. If detected early, excision with or without prosthetic replacement may prevent progressive osteoarthritis. In many cases, and certainly at the later stages, arthrodesis of the wrist is preferable.

Note that repeated trauma to the wrist, without frank dislocation of the lunate, may lead to similar X-ray appearances (Kienbock's disease); this condition is found particularly in manual workers such as carpenters, cobblers and pneumatic drill operators, etc.

Late diagnosis. If there is delay in making the diagnosis, manipulative reduction becomes increasingly difficult, and after a week may not be possible. Open reduction is then necessary, and carries with it the greatly increased risk of avascular necrosis. Surgery should be performed through an anterior incision, and every effort made to reduce the bone without disturbing any of its remaining intact ligamentous attachments (particularly those lying on the posterior surface) or further damaging the median nerve if it has been involved.

Median nerve palsy. Prompt reduction of the dislocation is usually followed by complete recovery soon afterwards. After late reduction, recovery may be incomplete but seldom requires separate treatment.

Sudeck's atrophy/complex regional pain syndrome. This is a common complication and is treated along previously described lines.

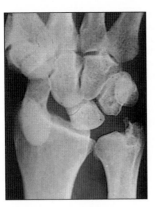

Dislocation of the scaphoid
Treatment. If the displacement is anterior and complete **(left)**, manipulate as for dislocation of the lunate. In many cases, dislocation is incomplete, with the proximal pole being tilted posteriorly and the distal pole anteriorly. Such injuries have often a toggle-like instability within the dorsiflexion/palmar flexion range (and the stable position within this phase must be found by trial and error during reduction). Reduction may be achieved by pressure over the proximal pole. If possible, an image intensifier should be used to check the reduction and stability.

If a stable position is found, the wrist should be put up in plaster in that position, with some added radial deviation; the plaster should be retained for 6 weeks, with frequent radiographs to check the position. If instability is not easily controlled, then the scaphoid should be fixed with Kirschner wires.

Other carpal injuries
Dislocation of the lunate and half the scaphoid. This may be treated by closed reduction in the same way as an uncomplicated dislocation of the lunate. Thereafter, however, the scaphoid fracture dominates the picture, and the treatment should follow the lines described for that injury. If after reduction there is gross carpal instability, internal fixation of the scaphoid is advised.

Trans-scapho perilunar dislocation of the carpus. This corresponds to dislocation of the lunate and half the scaphoid. It is the commonest of the first group of carpal dislocations. In some cases there may be associated fractures of the styloid process of the radius and the ulna. Reduction by traction is usually easy. Thereafter, the management is that of fracture of the scaphoid. If there is instability, or the scaphoid reduction is poor, internal fixation is advised.

Perilunar dislocation of the carpus. This corresponds to isolated dislocation of the lunate and may be reduced by traction. A cast with the wrist in flexion should be applied and retained for 1–2 weeks before changing to one with the wrist in the neutral position. This should be retained for a further 2 weeks.

Dislocation of both the lunate and scaphoid. Treat as for dislocation of the lunate.

Periscapholunar dislocation of the carpus. Treat as for perilunar dislocation of the carpus.

Dislocation of the trapezium, trapezoid or hamate. These are rare. Closed reduction should always be attempted, but open reduction is frequently required. In the face of instability, transfixion by Kirschner wires may be helpful.

Fractures through the bodies of any of the carpal bones other than the scaphoid. These are also rare and should be treated symptomatically by 6 weeks' fixation in a Colles' or scaphoid plaster. Fractures of the hamate and pisiform may be complicated by ulnar nerve palsy, which should be treated expectantly.

Small chip fractures of the carpus. These common injuries generally result from hyperflexion or hyperextension injuries of the wrist. The bone of origin is often in doubt. Rest of the wrist in plaster for 3 weeks is all that is required.

Fracture of the hook of the hamate. This is seen most often as a result of a heavy golf or tennis swing, but may follow a fall or a direct blow in the palm. There is local pain and tenderness. The fracture is best shown by a CAT scan of both wrists taken in the praying position, or by carpal tunnel films. The best treatment is to excise the hamate fragment.

Carpal instabilities. In these rare conditions there is a loss of normal carpal alignment, which develops early or late after a wrist injury. In *static carpal instabilities* there is an abnormal carpal alignment which can be seen by careful studies of straight films of the wrist. There are a number of clinical patterns. In *dynamic carpal instabilities*, routine films are normal, but the patient is usually able to toggle his carpal alignment from normal to abnormal and back. Manipulation of the scaphoid by the examiner may reproduce the sensation of pain and instability of which the patient complains. To help establish the diagnosis, lead markers may be placed on the skin over points of local tenderness and radiographs taken in both stable and unstable positions. A number of other investigations are available, including intensifier visualisation of carpal movements. *Scapholunate dissociation* is the commonest of the carpal instabilities and may be diagnosed by AP X-ray projections of the wrist in both radial and ulnar deviation. The most striking feature is the widening of the space between the scaphoid and lunate. If untreated it may be followed by osteoarthritis. In the acute case, manipulative reduction using the image intensifier should be undertaken (followed by closed pinning), or open repair of the torn ligaments. In chronic cases, reattachment of the avulsed scapholunate ligament may be carried out, but where there are arthritic changes and subluxation, prosthetic replacement of the scaphoid and a midcarpal arthrodesis may have to be considered. There is continuing controversy over the pathomechanics and management of these injuries, which is now highly specialised.

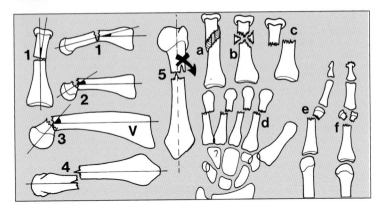

INJURIES TO THE METACARPALS AND PHALANGES

Assessment

Begin by making sure there is no significant soft-tissue involvement, such as nerve or tendon injury, or substantial skin loss.

Now, from the radiographs, assess whether the *bony alignment* is acceptable. Generally speaking, the position of a metacarpal or phalangeal fracture can be considered acceptable if: • angulation does not exceed 10° in either the lateral or AP projections (1), but in the lateral, 20° may be accepted in the metaphysis (2) and 45° in the neck of the fifth metacarpal (3) • there is at least 50% bony contact (4) • there is no rotational deformity (5). Rotational deformity may not always be obvious on the radiographs, or clinically when a finger is in the extended position. *Note, however, that when the fingers are individually flexed that they all strike the palm close to the scaphoid.* Check that this is the case. (The same precaution should be taken when the quality of a reduction is being assessed or when splintage is being applied.)

Now assess the stability of the fracture. Undisplaced transverse and longitudinal fractures are generally *stable*, but the following are usually *unstable:* **(a)** rotated spiral and some oblique fractures; **(b)** multifragmentary fractures; **(c)** severely displaced fractures; **(d)** multiple fractures; **(e)** fractures through the neck of a proximal phalanx; **(f)** displaced articular fractures. If there is some remaining doubt, assess the *functional stability* of the fracture. This is done by asking the patient to flex the injured finger (without assistance) and assessing the range of movements in the joints on either side of the fracture. If the fracture is functionally stable, the range obtained should reach 30% of the normal range, i.e. MP = 27° (N = 90°); PIP = 30° (N =100°); DIP =24° (N = 80°).

Treatment: general principles

If there is no significant soft-tissue injury, if the fracture is in an acceptable position and if it is clinically and radiologically stable, treatment should be directed at controlling the initial pain and swelling. Elevation of the arm in a sling may be helpful, *provided the sling is applied in such a way that the hand is not dependent.* Any pressure dressing should be applied in such a way that it avoids any local constriction and the fingers and hand should be mobilised early.

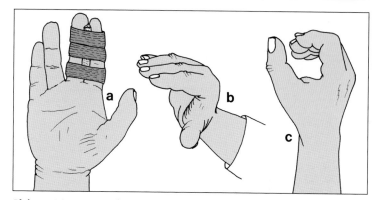

If the *position is unsatisfactory,* the fracture should be manipulated. If a good stable position can be obtained, treat as described on the previous page.

If the *position is acceptable,* or an acceptable position has been obtained by manipulation but the fracture is unstable, splintage will be required. For the less severe injuries, garter ('buddy') strapping to an adjacent finger with interdigital felt padding provides the ideal combination of stability while retaining movement (a).

If the *injury is more severe,* and a more restricting cast or bandaging is necessary, close attention must be paid to the position of the fingers. The MP joints should *never* be splinted in extension. When recovery of movements is hoped for, the MP joints should be flexed to 90°, the IP joints extended and the thumb abducted (b). MP joint extension should be studiously avoided. This position reduces the effects of fibrosis in the collateral ligaments, and places the finger joints in a favourable position for mobilisation. It must be carefully differentiated from the position of *fixation* (c), where no return of function is anticipated (e.g. the position a joint is placed in for fusion). In the latter case, the MP and IP joints are put up in mid-flexion.

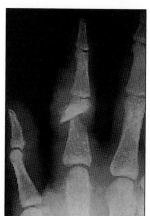

If the *fracture cannot be reduced* (e.g. as on the **left** where the radiographs shows an open unstable fracture of proximal phalanx in an unacceptable position) or *if it cannot be held with simple splintage in acceptable position,* then open reduction and/or surgical stabilisation should be considered.

Other indications for internal fixation include: • the presence of a significant soft tissue injury • the presence of multiple fractures • fractures involving or disrupting joint surfaces.

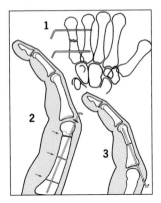

Internal fixation methods

Kirschner wires remain the single most useful method of stabilising a fracture. They may be inserted percutaneously, using an image intensifier as an aid to correct positioning, but if the reduction cannot be obtained by closed methods, the fracture may have to be exposed through a small incision. A shaft or neck fracture may be supported using 2–4 wires placed transversely (**1**). Intramedullary wires may be used to help maintain the alignment of metacarpal fractures at any level (**2**), or phalangeal fractures (**3**). Resistance to torsional stresses may have to be reinforced with additional support (e.g. 'buddy' strapping or a cast).

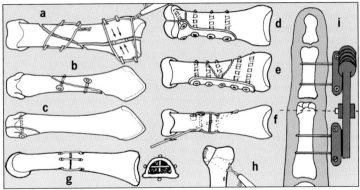

Kirschner wires may also be used in open procedures and can be cut off before the skin closure. They may be used for tension band wiring (**a**) in conjunction with malleable stainless steel wire which when twisted can draw the bone fragments together. Small screws may be used in pairs to hold oblique and spiral fractures (**b**), or singly for articular fragments (**c**). T- and Y-fractures may require the use of a T-plate and screws (**d**). Transverse and comminuted diaphyseal fractures may be held with a small plate and screws (**e**). Transverse fractures which have to be opened for reduction may also be held by a number of wiring techniques. In *Type A interosseous wiring*, the fracture is first reduced and held with a K-wire. A single malleable wire is then used to draw the fragments together, and its twisted ends are buried in a small hole drilled in one of the bone fragments (**f**). In *Type B interosseous wiring*, two wires are used at right angles to one another; additional K-wire support is not required (**g**). Interarticular fragments may also be wired (**h**). External fixators may be used, and these come in many patterns. The Compass PIP joint hinge™ (**i**) permits a degree of distraction to aid the alignment of interarticular fragments. Its axis is centred on the joint, and its hinge fixed or adjusted to permit active movement or stretching.

Soft-tissue management. Where there is necrotic or foreign material, a thorough debridement should be performed under a tourniquet to minimise the risks of infection. There is little tissue to spare in the hand, and wide excision of wounds is to be avoided. Every attempt should be made to ensure that healing will be achieved as quickly as possible to permit early mobilisation. The exposure of fractures, joints and bones should be avoided, and if the situation permits, a primary skin grafting procedure or plastic repair should be carried out.

If there is division of both neurovascular bundles to a finger, amputation should be advised unless facilities for microsurgery are available and the particular circumstances (e.g. employment, hobbies, etc.) make an attempt at preservation particularly desirable. In all cases, the maximum length of thumb must be preserved.

If there is appreciable risk of infection (e.g. a ragged wound or a dirty causal instrument), primary suture of nerves and also of tendons in the 'no man's area' of the tendon sheaths should not be undertaken. Where, however, the circumstances are ideal, the experienced surgeon may achieve the best results by primary repair.

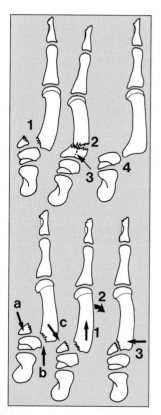

Injuries to the base of the thumb

The commonest injuries involving the base of the thumb are: (1) Bennett's fracture (or Bennett's fracture–dislocation as it may be more aptly called); (2) fracture of the base of the thumb metacarpal. When there is a vertical extension into the joint, converting it into a T- or Y-fracture (3), the prognosis is less good (Rolando fracture); (4) carpometacarpal dislocation of the thumb.

Diagnosis. The cause is usually force applied along the long axis of the thumb or forced abduction. Unlike scaphoid fractures, the tenderness is maximal distal to the snuff box and deformity may be obvious.

Bennett's fracture. Note the distinctive features of this fracture: (a) a small medial fragment of bone which may tilt but maintains its relationship with the trapezium; (b) the (vertical) fracture line involves the joint between the thumb metacarpal and the trapezium (trapezometacarpal joint); (c) the proximal and lateral subluxation of the thumb metacarpal.

Treatment. Reduction is achieved by applying traction to the thumb (1), and abducting it (2) while applying pressure to the lateral aspect of the base (3). Maintaining reduction can be troublesome, and careful attention must be paid to the details of plaster fixation.

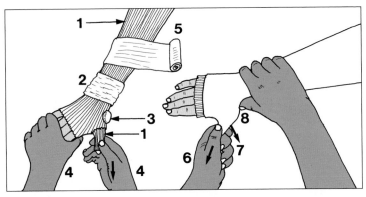

Apply stockingette to the arm and thumb (**1**). Bony prominences should be protected as required with wool roll (**2**). A small felt pad (**3**) is placed over the base of the thumb metacarpal, *on top* of the stockingette to avoid skin problems. An assistant applies traction to the thumb and steadies the lateral three fingers (**4**). Two to three 15 cm (6″) POP bandages (with or without an anterior slab) are applied to the forearm (**5**). Two 10 cm (4″) POP bandages are then quickly applied to the wrist and up to the IP joint of the thumb. The surgeon now takes the thumb (the plaster being set on the forearm while the distal part remains soft). He must apply traction (**6**), abduct the thumb (**7**), maintain pressure over the base of the first metacarpal (**8**) and mould the plaster well into the MP joint on its flexor aspect. *After-care:* Check radiographs are taken to confirm the reduction, and the arm is elevated in a sling. The patient should be seen at weekly intervals for the first 2–3 weeks and the thumb X-rayed. If the plaster is slack or if there is evidence of slipping, it should be changed; during the setting of the plaster, light traction should be applied to the thumb while the plaster is well moulded, with light pressure round the base. Plaster fixation is maintained for 6 weeks.

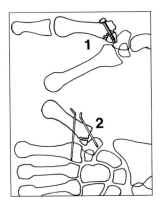

Alternative methods of treatment. A good result is the rule following reduction and plaster fixation. While a perfect reduction is desirable, it is not essential. So long as the metacarpal is aligned with the trapezium, a step of 2 mm or less can be accepted, as this degree of displacement is not followed by secondary osteoarthritis. A number of alternative methods of holding this fracture are practised. These include: (**1**) screw fixation (e.g. using the AO small fragment set); (**2**) the use of two Kirschner wires to stabilise the thumb metacarpal.

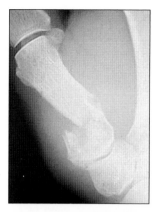

Fractures near the base of the thumb metacarpal.
Greenstick fractures of this type are common in children. Angulation is usually slight or moderate (**left**) and should be accepted; gross angulations should be manipulated, using the technique described for Bennett's fracture. Plaster fixation for about 5 weeks is desirable. Rolando fractures require careful reduction, and good results are claimed for stabilisation with an external fixator, the pins being placed in the metacarpal and the trapezium.

Carpometacarpal dislocation of the thumb.
The thumb may dislocate at the joint between the metacarpal base and the trapezium, or the whole of the first ray may be involved, the trapezium remaining with the thumb metacarpal, with the dislocation taking place between the trapezium and the scaphoid (**left**). Both these injuries result from forcible abduction of the thumb. *Treatment:* reduce by applying traction to thumb and local pressure over the base. Thereafter, apply a well-padded plaster of scaphoid type for 3 weeks. Elevation of the limb for the first few days is desirable. Physiotherapy is seldom required.

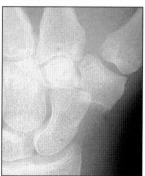

Injuries at the MP joint of the thumb.
Posterior dislocation. This injury generally results from forcible hyperextension. It is common in children. In a number of cases there is 'button-holing' of the capsule by the metacarpal head, and closed methods of reduction will fail. Nevertheless, manipulation should be tried first in all cases. Manipulative reduction may often be attempted without anaesthesia (by the quick confident application of traction to the thumb with simultaneous pressure over the anterior aspect of the metacarpal head). When open reduction is required this should be performed through a lateral incision under a tourniquet. In all cases a light plaster splint should be worn for 2–3 weeks after reduction.

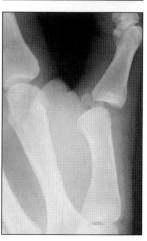

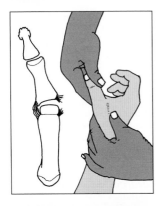

Rupture of the ulnar collateral ligament (Gamekeeper's thumb).
This injury is caused by forcible abduction. If unrecognised and untreated, there may be progressive MP joint subluxation. This may lead to interference with grasp and cause a significant permanent disability.

Diagnosis. Suspect this injury when there is complaint of pain in this region. Look for tenderness on the medial side of the MP joint. Test for abnormal 'give' on stressing the ulnar collateral ligament **(left)**. Compare the sides, and if necessary take stress radiographs.

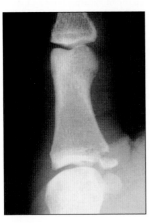

An avulsion fracture **(left)** may betray this type of injury, and if present, note the position of the fragment. (Marked displacement or rotation are indications for surgery.)

Treatment. (a) Slight laxity (incomplete tear) or minimally displaced avulsion fracture: scaphoid cast for 6 weeks; (b) rotated fragment: reduction and internal fixation, e.g. by wiring; (c) gross laxity (complete tear): conservative treatment may give a good result, but many prefer primary surgical repair; (d) late diagnosed complete tear: repair of the capsuloligamentous complex with a palmaris longus free tendon graft; or as a salvage procedure, MP joint fusion.

Other injuries to the thumb
Fracture of the proximal phalanx.
The severely angled fracture **(1)** should be reduced by traction and local pressure. Hold with a dorsal (or volar) slab **(2)** to which is added a girdered extension **(3)**, held on with bandages. If the position cannot be readily held, internal fixation is indicated. The minimally angled fracture **(4)** or the splinter fracture **(5)** may be protected by a local slab (similar to 3) bandaged in position. Elevation may be required.

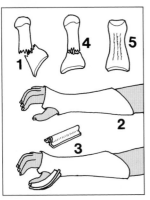

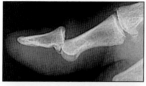

IP joint dislocation of the thumb.
Reduce by traction as described for MP joint dislocations. Only occasionally is anaesthesia required (ring or Bier block). Thereafter, splint for 2-3 weeks with a local plaster slab.

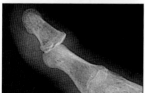

Fractures of the terminal phalanx.
Crushing accidents are the usual cause, and any soft-tissue damage takes priority in management. A light local splint (e.g. of plaster) will prevent pain from stubbing.

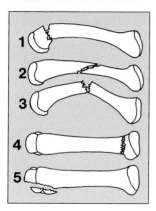

Injuries to the fifth metacarpal
The commonest fractures involving the metacarpal of the little finger are: (1) fractures of the neck; (2) spiral fractures of the shaft, usually undisplaced; (3) transverse fractures of the shaft, often angulated; (4) fractures of the base; (5) fractures of the head.

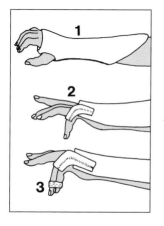

Fractures of the neck of the fifth metacarpal.
These are nearly always caused by the clenched fist meeting resistance—for example, as a result of a fight. Angulation and impaction are common.

Treatment. When *angulation is slight* or moderate, the position should be accepted and the fracture supported for 3–4 weeks until local pain settles. A simple dorsal slab (1), completed after a few days, may be quite satisfactory. Better fixation is achieved by the addition of a finger extension (2) to the basic slab. Still more support is provided by the use of garter strapping (3) and the inclusion of the ring and little fingers in the extension. (In 2 & 3 the left hand is illustrated, and the securing bandages have been omitted for clarity.)

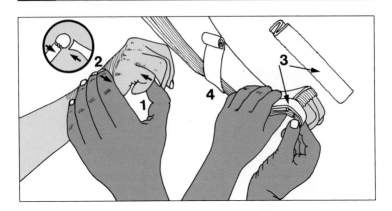

If *angulation is gross* (more than 45°), an attempt should be made to correct it. The MP joint is flexed; pressure is then applied to the displaced head via the proximal phalanx, using the thumb (1); the fingers apply counter-pressure to the shaft (2). Reduction is generally easy. The position may be maintained using a Kirschner wire or with a plaster cast.

In the latter case, stockingette is applied to the arm and to the little finger, over the dorsal surface of which is fixed a thin strip of felt. A substantial dorsal slab is applied. The finger should be flexed into the palm and the striking point checked. A finger slab, made from a thrice-folded slab formed from three layers or so of 10 cm (4″) plaster bandage (3) is applied from the wrist to the finger tip. Pressure is maintained while the slab is setting following the principles already described. Meanwhile an assistant can be securing the slabs with a wet gauze bandage (4). The plaster should be completed in 2–3 days and retained for 4–5 weeks only.

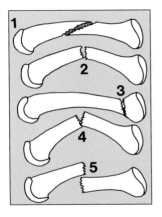

Fractures of the shaft and base of the fifth metacarpal. Spiral fractures of the shaft (1), transverse fractures of the shaft with slight or moderate angulation or displacement (2) and fractures of the base (3) may be treated quite adequately by the application of a Colles' plaster for 3–4 weeks.

Where there is marked angulation of a shaft fracture (4), apply traction and local pressure prior to plaster fixation. Displaced fractures (5) may be similarly reduced, but soft tissue between the bone ends may necessitate an open procedure. Reduction may be maintained by percutaneous Kirschner wiring or other methods.

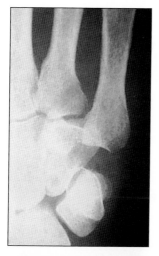

Dislocation of the base of the fifth metacarpal (left). Injuries of this pattern are usually easily reduced with traction, but they sometimes require stabilisation with percutaneous Kirschner wires.

Fractures of the head of the fifth metacarpal. Fractures of the head of the fifth metacarpal may be treated by garter strapping and early mobilisation; if symptoms are marked, a dorsal slab may also be used for the first 1–2 weeks. If the fragment is substantial and displaced, internal fixation may be considered.

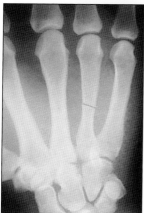

Fractures of the index, middle and ring metacarpals

The commonest fracture is a spiral fracture of the shaft (especially of the ring metacarpal), but fractures involving the base and neck are frequent, as are transverse fractures (**left**) of the shaft.

Treatment. Undisplaced fractures may be supported by a Colles' type slab, but be on guard for swelling which can be severe, especially in multiple fractures.

Severely displaced fractures of the index metacarpal should be managed along the lines described for fractures of the fifth metacarpal, with reduction and, if necessary, some form of internal fixation. If Kirschner wires are used they should be retained for 3 weeks; plaster fixation may be needed for a further 2 weeks.

When the AP radiographs show the presence of an isolated off-ended fracture of the middle or ring metacarpal, or moderate angulation or shortening, the position can generally be accepted. The striking point of the finger should be checked, a dorsal slab applied and the limb elevated to counteract swelling. If off-ending or angulation is conspicuous in the *lateral projection*, reduction should be carried out, either by manipulation or by an open procedure, and if unstable, Kirschner wire fixation employed.

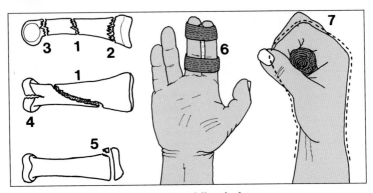

Fractures of the proximal and middle phalanges

Undisplaced, simple, stable fractures—e.g. of the shaft (**1**), base (**2**), neck (**3**), intercondylar region (**4**) or epiphyseal injuries (**5**)—seldom present any problem. Garter ('buddy') strapping (**6**) for 3–4 weeks may give adequate support, but if symptoms are marked this may be supplemented by the use of a volar or dorsal slab, with finger extension.

There is a tendency for angulation to occur due to intrinsic muscle pull; if more than 10°, this should be corrected under general anaesthesia by gentle traction, using the thumb as a fulcrum. Generally, these fractures are stable in flexion, and to maintain this several methods are available. A rolled bandage can be held in the palm; this may be used as a fulcrum, the injured finger being flexed over it (**7**) and secured with adhesive tape. Additional encircling bandaging is required for security, but even so dislodgement may occur. Some surgeons use a (wetted) POP bandage in the palm. Alternatively, a volar plaster slab with a substantial finger extension may be used, moulding the fracture while this is setting; thereafter, the plaster is secured with wet open-weave bandages. If this arrangement appears too flimsy, it may be reinforced with a dorsal slab and dorsal finger extension. Where the fracture is unstable in any position, some form of internal fixation is advisable.

After-care. In all cases: • uninjured fingers should be left free and exercised • rigid fixation should be discarded as soon as possible. In many situations, garter strapping may be substituted after 2 weeks, and often all support after 4. *In no instance should the MP joints be fixed in extension.*

Complications

Finger stiffness is the commonest and most disabling complication and is due to joint adhesions, fibrosis in the adjacent flexor tendon sheaths and collateral ligament shortening. Infection in open fractures may be a major contributory factor. Stiffness may be minimised by the procedures described (e.g. elevation, correct splinting, early mobilisation) and by intensive physiotherapy and occupational therapy. Physiotherapy and occupational therapy should be continued with vigour until the range of movements and finger power become static. This implies careful recording at frequent intervals of these parameters. In this respect it is helpful to note the *total active range of motion* (TAM) in each digit. This overall movement can be assessed by a single goniometer measurement; it is a little less than the sum of the normal maxima of flexion of the individual joints, the normal value of TAM being taken to be 250°.

Early return to work should be encouraged to foster re-adaptation. Inability to work and a static response to physiotherapy require most careful assessment of the following: • the possibility of redeployment • the possibility of improvement from further surgery (e.g. tenolysis) • amputation. This as primary treatment must be raised in open phalangeal fractures when they are associated with flexor tendon division. Division of one or both neurovascular bundles, skin loss or severe crushing are additional factors weighing in favour of this procedure (in contrast to attempted repair where treatment is likely to be prolonged and the final result uncertain). With these factors must be considered the patient's age, sex and occupation.

Malunion. Problems may arise from: • recurrence of deformity • failure to correct the initial deformity • torsional deformity. In some cases, epiphyseal displacement may have escaped attention. In the latter, remodelling may lead to correction, and in the others, trick movements and postural adaptations may remove the patient's initial strong desire for corrective surgery. It is wise not to offer surgical correction until at least 6 months have passed since the injury.

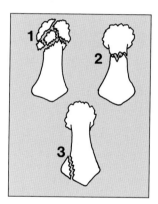

Fractures of the terminal phalanx

Fractures of the terminal tuft (often comminuted) (1), of the neck (2), and the base (3) are painful but relatively unimportant injuries. Treatment of any associated soft tissue injury takes precedence (e.g. debridement and suture of pulp lacerations).

Nevertheless, strapping the finger to a spatula or the use of a plastic finger splint may relieve pain and prevent any painful stubbing incidents.

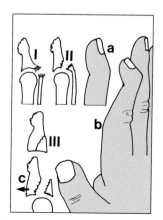

Mallet finger

This is caused by forcible flexion of an extended finger. The distal extensor tendon slip is torn at its attachment to bone (type I injury) or avulses a fragment of bone (Type II). The patient is unable to extend the DIP joint fully (a); drooping of the finger tip may be slight or severe. In late cases there may be hyperextension of the PIP joint (b). In Type III injuries, more than 20% of the articular surface of the distal phalanx is involved, sometimes with anterior subluxation of the phalanx (c).

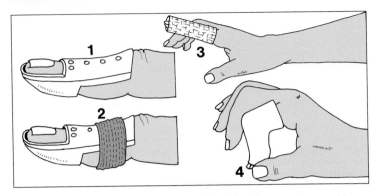

Treatment. All cases, excepting Type IIIs with subluxation, may be treated by splinting the distal joint in extension. A Stack or Abuna splint (1) may be used, choosing the size with care to lessen the risks of skin ulceration. It is strapped to the finger (2), worn for 6 weeks constantly, and then for a further two at night only. It may be removed for skin hygiene so long as extension is preserved.

Alternatively, support the distal joint with a short length of padded spatula strapped to the volar surface. Where the patient's cooperation is in doubt, a Smillie plaster for 6–8 weeks may be used. Form a 4-layer tube of 7.5 cm (3") dry POP bandage round the finger (3). Dip the hand momentarily in water, asking the patient to flex the PIP joint and extend the DIP joint against the thumb (4) while the plaster is smoothed.

If there is *subluxation*, see if reduction can be achieved in either flexion or extension, and splint accordingly. If not, consider operative repair. Where mallet finger is diagnosed *late*, extension splintage may be successful even up to 6 months. If there is a *swan-neck deformity*, some advise an oblique retinacular ligament reconstruction.

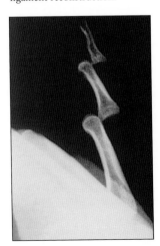

MP and interphalangeal joint dislocations

These may be simple or multiple (left), and as they result from hyperextension they are almost always posterior dislocations. Reduce as already described for the thumb. Thereafter, garter strapping should be applied for 2 weeks unless there is any evidence of instability—when plaster of Paris splintage may be required for a slightly longer period.

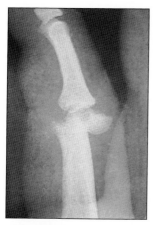

Fracture–dislocation

It is essential that the joint surface is correctly relocated, and important that mobilisation is commenced as soon as possible. Open reduction is usually required, and fixation may be achieved with intraosseous wiring, small fragment set screws, T-plating or a motion-permitting external fixator. Any additional external support should be removed after 2–3 weeks and mobilisation commenced using garter strapping for the first week or so until the fracture becomes more stable.

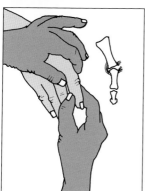

'Sprains' and lateral subluxations

These are usually caused by falls in which the side of a finger strikes some resistant object. There is avulsion or tearing of a collateral ligament. Spontaneous reduction is the rule.

Diagnosis. The injury should be suspected on the basis of the history, the presence of local tenderness and the demonstration of laxity on testing the collateral ligament (**left**).

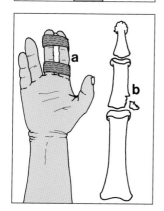

Radiographs may show a tell-tale avulsion fracture. If doubt remains, stress films may be taken.

Treatment. (**a**) Garter strapping for 5 weeks should be adequate. (**b**) If an avulsion fracture is present and has rotated, it should be replaced.

Complications. Fusiform swellings of the finger may persist for many months, even in the treated injury.

Regional injuries: the spine

General principles 368
Cervical spine injuries 370
The upper two cervical
    vertebrae: atlanto-
    occipital subluxations
    and dislocations 381
Soft tissue injuries of the
    neck (whiplash injuries)
    386
Fractures of the thoracic and
    lumbar spine 388
Other injuries of the spine
    394
Neurological assessment of
    spinal injuries 395
Treatment of spinal paralysis
    397

GENERAL PRINCIPLES

- The main concern in any spinal injury is not with the spine itself, but with the closely related neurological elements (the spinal cord, issuing nerve roots and cauda equina).
- If there is no neurological complication, risks of later neurological involvement must be assessed; if there is some risk of this, *precautions must be taken to see that this is avoided at all stages.*
- If there is an incomplete paraplegia complicating the injury, *great care must be taken to see that no deterioration is allowed to occur.*
- If paraplegia is present and complete, the prognosis regarding potential recovery must be firmly established as early as possible. Only if the paraplegia is pronounced *total* and *permanent* can vigilance in the handling of the spinal injury be relaxed.

Assessment of spinal injuries

In managing any case of spinal injury it is important to determine which structures have been involved and the extent of the damage they have suffered; with this information an assessment may be made of the risks of complications. *Note:* • the history may direct you to the type of injury to suspect • the clinical examination may be a valuable guide to the extent of bony and ligamentous injury, and any neurological complication • investigation by X-ray and CAT scan is likely to provide the most information.

It is important to make an early assessment of the stability of the spine—i.e. to assess whether it is able to withstand any stress without progressive deformity or further neurological damage. *Instability may be purely mechanical* (e.g. in some compression fractures where further kyphotic deformity may occur). *Instability may be neurological* (e.g. where shifting or further extrusion of bone fragments within the spinal canal may lead to neurological deterioration). *Combined mechanical and neurological instability* may be present.

In assessing instability it may be helpful to regard the spine as having three main elements or columns.

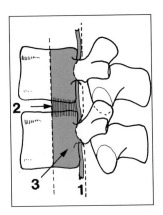

1. The middle column. This consists of the posterior longitudinal ligament (1), the posterior part of the annular ligament (2) and the posterior wall of the vertebral column (3). Unstable injuries occur when damage to the middle column is combined with damage to either the anterior column or damage to the posterior column.

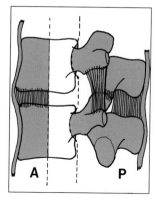

2. *The posterior column (P).* This comprises the neural arch, the pedicles, the spinous process and the posterior ligament complex.

3. *The anterior column (A).* This is formed by the anterior longitudinal ligament, the anterior part of the annular ligament and the anterior part of the vertebral body. Note that the concern is the integrity of these columns, and that failure in their role as supports can be due to either bone or ligamentous involvement (or a combination).

Classification of spinal injuries
There are four common types of spinal injury:

1. compression fractures
2. burst fractures
3. seat-belt type injuries
4. fracture–dislocations.

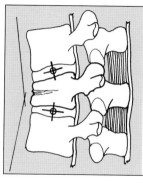

Compression fractures. Simple compression fractures are common, stable injuries involving the anterior column only. Hyperflexion of the spine round an axis passing through the disc space leads to mechanical failure of bone with either anterior (**left**) or lateral wedging. The height of the posterior part of the vertebral body is maintained. Note that *severe* wedging (e.g. more than 15–20°) often indicates damage to the other columns and a burst fracture or fracture–dislocation.

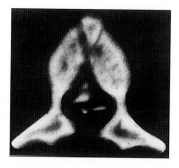

Burst fractures. Axial loading of the spine may cause failure of the anterior and middle columns. One or both vertebral body end plates may be involved, and bone fragments may be extruded into the spinal canal, compromising the neurological structures and causing neurological instability. Radiographs may show the vertebral body fracture, loss of vertebral height and in the AP, laminar fractures and separation of the pedicles. A CAT scan is invaluable in showing bony extrusion (**left**); myelography is also sometimes of help.

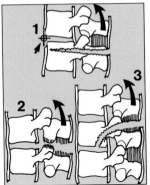

Seat belt type injuries. Rapid deceleration causes the spine to jack-knife round an axis brought forward by a lap type seatbelt, and *tension* forces lead to failure of the posterior and middle columns. The spine is unstable in flexion. Failure may occur entirely through bone (Chance fracture) (**1**), or ligaments (**2**), or a combination (**3**), involving either one (**1 & 2**) or two (**3**) levels of the spine. Injuries of this pattern may be seen in situations outside road traffic accidents, but the essential element is tension failure.

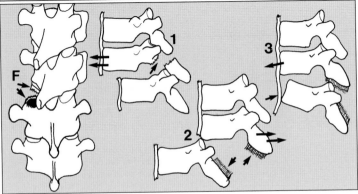

Fracture–dislocations. All three columns fail, and there is loss of the normal constraints, so that dislocation or subluxation may occur. Suspect if: (i) there are multiple rib or transverse process fractures; (ii) there is a slight increase in the height of a disc or a fracture of an articular process. *Types: (a) Flexion–rotation fracture–dislocation.* There is often a fracture of an articular process on one side (**F**), or a slicing fracture through a vertebral body, leading to rotation and subluxation of the spine. *(b) Shear types of fracture–dislocation.* In the posteroanterior type of fracture–dislocation the upper segment is sheared forwards, often with fracture of the posterior arch at one or two levels (**1**). In the anteroposterior type there is complete ligamentous disruption, but often no fracture (**2**). *(c) Flexion–distraction fracture–dislocation.* This is a tension type of injury as in the seatbelt lesion, but there is an anterior annular tear with stripping of the anterior longitudinal ligament, allowing anterior subluxation (**3**).

CERVICAL SPINE INJURIES
Diagnosis
Suspect involvement of the cervical spine where the patient: (a) complains of neck, occipital or shoulder pain after trauma; (b) has a torticollis and complains of restriction of neck movements or supports the head with the hands, or (c) is found unconscious after a head injury, especially in road traffic accidents. In all cases, radiographic investigation is essential.

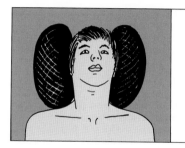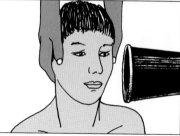

Initial management

If you suspect that the cervical spine has been injured, your first move should be to safeguard the cord by controlling neck movements. The simplest way is to apply a cervical collar, and at the roadside one may be fashioned from rolled newspapers pushed into a nylon stocking and wrapped round the neck. Various substantial splints are carried by the emergency services. If the patient is on a trolley, the head may be supported by sandbags (above left). *Do not allow the head to flex forwards, and do not hyperextend: keep in a neutral position.*

Wherever possible, quickly check that there is active movement in all limbs and that the peripheral sensation is intact.

Especially if there is some evidence of neurological involvement, *do not* check the range of movements in the cervical spine. Accompany the patient to the X-ray department, supporting the head during the positioning of the tube (above right) and making sure that the spine is not forced into flexion. For initial screening an AP, lateral and a through-the-mouth projection of C1 and C2 should be taken.

If these films appear normal, you may proceed in reasonable safety to: (i) further examination of the neck for localising tenderness, restriction of active movements and protective spasm, and (ii) a more thorough neurological examination. If these are normal, apply a cervical collar and arrange a follow-up review in 1 week.

If there is persistent material limitation of movements or neurological disturbance, further investigation is necessary. The following additional films should be taken: (a) two more lateral projections, one in flexion and one in extension; these again should be supervised; (b) right and left oblique projections. The commonest difficulty is the technical one of visualising the lower cervical vertebrae in a stocky patient. The upper border of T1 *must* be seen. *Accept* that detail may be poor. *Do not accept* that the spine cannot be shown in sufficient detail to exclude dislocation of one vertebra over another. If necessary, assist the radiographer by arranging for traction to be applied to the arms—one in adduction and the other in abduction; slight angulation of the tube and an increased exposure may be helpful. A CAT scan may provide valuable additional information. Apart from confirming a fracture (especially of the neural arches and facet joints which may be poorly visualised on normal films), this can give useful additional information on any encroachments on the neural canal, especially in the case of bursting fractures. In some cases screening of the cervical spine movements may be useful.

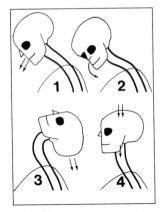

Classification of *cervical spine injuries*

Injuries of the cervical spine may be additionally grouped according to the mechanism of injury: (1) flexion injuries; (2) flexion and rotation injuries; (3) extension injuries; (4) compression injuries.

Causes of flexion and flexion/rotation injuries.
These may result from: (a) falls on the back of the head leading to flexion of the neck—e.g. in motor cycle spills, diving in shallow water, pole vaulting and rugby football; (b) blows on the back of the head from falling objects (e.g. in the building and mining industries); (c) rapid decelerations in head-on car accidents.

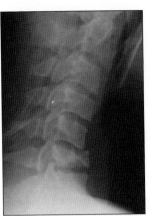

Flexion injuries: stable anterior wedge fracture
The vertebral body is wedged anteriorly, while the posterior part is generally intact. Before being declared stable, there must be: (i) no evidence of injury to the posterior ligament complex; (ii) no damage to the neural arches or facets; and (iii) flexion and extension laterals must show no vertebral instability. If these criteria are satisfied, neurological disturbance is rare and the prognosis excellent. Treat with a cervical collar for 6 weeks. Rarely, when there is lateral wedging there may be troublesome nerve root involvement. *If instability is at all suspected, treat as a cervical dislocation.*

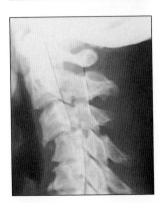

Flexion/rotation injuries: unilateral dislocation with a locked facet joint
One facet joint dislocates, so that in the lateral projection of the cervical spine, one vertebral body is seen to overlap the one below by about a third. The AP view may not be helpful, or it may show malalignment of spinous processes. There is often little difference between the laterals taken in flexion and extension.

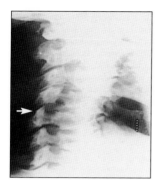

Oblique projections will confirm the diagnosis. The columnar arrangement of bodies, foramina and facet joints will be broken on one side only (**left**). Damage to the posterior ligament complex is variable: *after reduction* the dislocation may be quite stable, but note—if there is an associated fracture involving a facet joint, the injury is *most certainly unstable* and fusion will be required after reduction. On clinical examination of the patient with a unilateral dislocation, the head is slightly rotated and inclined to the side away from the locked facet. There is often great pain with radiation due to nerve root pressure.

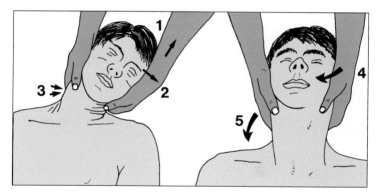

Treatment. This may proceed if there is no neurological defect (otherwise see later). The initial aim in treatment is to reduce the dislocation, and the secret of this is well-controlled traction. While some prefer to do this in the conscious patient so that the neurological status may be constantly observed, general anaesthesia is more common. During induction and intubation (which must be carried out without undue extension of the neck), the head must be well supported. X-ray facilities (preferably an image intensifier) should be available. The surgeon must have freedom to manipulate the head and may do this with the patient fully on the table, or pulled up till the head is supported in the lap of the surgeon seated at the top end of the table.

Place the thumbs under the jaw, clasp the fingers behind the occiput, and apply firm traction (**1**) in *lateral flexion* (**2**) away from the side of the locked facet (**3**), i.e. in the direction the head is usually inclined. Maintaining traction, bring the head into the midline position, correcting the rotation element (**4**) *before* lateral flexion (**5**). Release the traction and support the head (e.g. with foam plastic blocks) while check radiographs are taken. If reduction has not been achieved, repeat the manoeuvre with greater anaesthetic relaxation. Screening may be used. If reduction fails (which is rare), or if preferred, use carefully monitored skull traction.

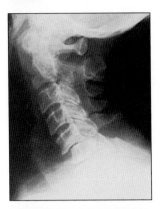

Once reduction has been achieved, a cervical collar should be applied and worn continuously for 6 weeks. Fortnightly radiographs of the neck should be taken, and flexion and extension laterals at the end of the 6 weeks' fixation. *If there is any evidence of late subluxation* (**left**), the patient should be admitted for reduction by continuous traction followed by a local cervical fusion.

Flexion/rotation injuries: unstable injuries

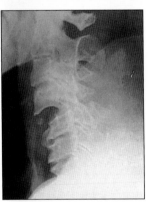

The commonest injury of this type is one where there is a pure cervical dislocation without fracture. Displacement may be severe, and there is frequently locking of both facets (**left**). Damage to the posterior ligament complex is always present, and is generally obvious from the degree of vertebral displacement.

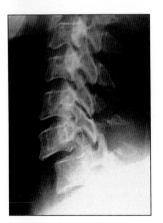

There may be other evidence of instability associated with disruption of the posterior ligament complex. This includes: (1) avulsion pattern spinous process fracture(s) (**left**); (2) widening of the gap between two spinous processes; (3) *evidence of forward slip on the flexion lateral of the spine compared with the extension lateral.* Proceed to treatment if there is no gross neurological defect (otherwise see later).

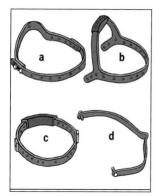

Treatment. Unstable injuries without fracture require fusion, and skull traction will be required to achieve and maintain reduction; this should be applied without delay. It may be carried out using a halo (which at a later stage may be attached to a vest or plaster jacket for continued support). The Bremer range includes (a) adjustable rings; (b) halo-crown devices; (c) small, large and custom built paediatric rings; (d) traction hoops. With the latter, manual or weight traction may be applied to a halo.

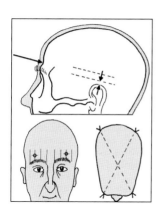

Halo traction pin sites. Palpate the groove between the superciliary ridge and the frontal prominence: the anterior pins should lie on this line, caudal to the maximal circumference of the skull and about 1 cm above the orbital margin. Each should lie in the line of the outer half of the eyebrow (e.g. at the junction of the middle and outer thirds). The posterior pins should be sited diagonally opposite (b), at such a level that the halo band clears the ear by about a half centimetre.

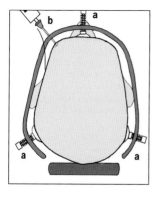

Halo application. Support the head manually throughout the procedure. The head of the supine patient should be just clear of the bed, with a board between the shoulder blades extending up to the occiput. Shave and prep the skin round the areas of the proposed pin sites. Slide the halo into place, and hold it with 3–4 suction cups screwed into the halo (a), positioned away from the skull pin sites. These may then be infiltrated (through the holes in the halo) with local anaesthetic (b).

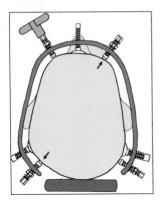

Adjust the suction cups to ensure the halo is centred. Using the fingers at first, screw in opposite pairs of skull pins, before repeating this with the other pair. (At this stage some make small skin incisions to avoid indentation of the skin.) Now tighten them in stages (again in a diametrically opposed sequence) to a maximum torque of 8 inch/pounds (0.90 Newton/metre), using a torque wrench or torque-limiting caps. Then attach a traction hoop. Some prefer to use six pins rather than four, as the loading on each pin is then less and the risks of loosening are reduced. A traction hoop is then attached to the halo.

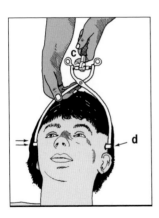

Applying skull tongs. Where use of a halo-vest or halo-pelvic device will not be required, or if suitable halos are not available, skull tongs may be used. Several types are available, including the Cone' pattern illustrated. Shave the skin on each side about 6 cm above the external auditory meatus, infiltrate with local anaesthetic and make a small incision (about 1 cm in length) down to bone (**a**). Bleeding is usually brisk, but generally controllable by firm local pressure applied for a few moments; if not, secure and tie off any remaining bleeding points. Now insinuate one point holder through the temporalis muscle fibres until it is in contact with the skull (**b**).

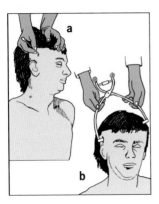

Keep the point holder pressed firmly against the skull; straighten out the calliper and close it with the turnbuckle spanner (**c**). Guide the second point holder through the skin wound; oscillate the calliper slightly to allow its tapered end to part the temporalis fibres on the second side. Close the calliper until both point holders are in firm but not hard contact with the skull.

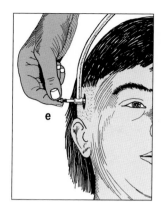

Now screw the points in (**e**). You should check that their protrusion is limited to about 3 mm, to penetrate the outer cortex only; tighten them with a key. If the points fail to enter, either they are blunt or the bone unduly hard. In these circumstances, a small awl may be used as a starter, taking great care to avoid penetration of the inner cortex. Now seal the wound with strips of gauze soaked in Nobecutane™ or a similar preparation.

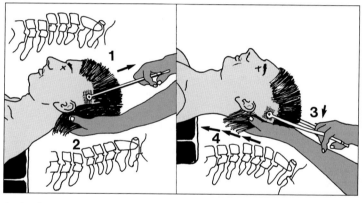

Reduction

By manipulation. If reduction is required, many surgeons prefer to do this manually under general anaesthesia with good relaxation. X-ray facilities are essential, and great care must be taken during induction and throughout the procedure to avoid uncontrolled movements of the head.

(a) When all is ready, the head is supported and the end of the table dropped.
(b) Firm traction is applied in the neutral position or slight flexion (**1**) to unlock the facets (**2**).
(c) Maintaining firm traction the neck is slowly extended (**3**). The hand supporting the occiput may be moved in anticipation down the neck to act as a fulcrum (**4**).
(d) The traction is then slowly reduced and the table end raised.
(e) While maintaining a little controlling traction, the position is checked with radiographs.

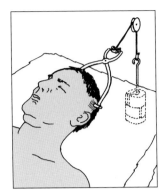 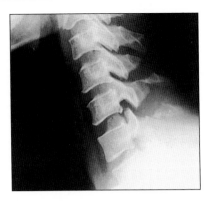

By traction. Continuous (weight) traction may be used to overcome muscle tension and unlock overriding facets. The *amount* of traction can be adjusted by the weights. The *direction* of traction may be controlled by altering the position of the traction pulley, or by the use of pads under the head or shoulders. The *duration* of maximal traction is monitored by radiographs. (With suitable apparatus, traction may also be applied with the patient in a sitting-up position.) The *weight* required will be found to vary from about 7 kg (15 lb) for a light adult woman to 14 kg (30 lb) + for a heavy man. The direction of traction should start in the neutral position or slight flexion. The patient should be sedated, *and in the recently injured patient radiographs to check progress should be taken every 15 minutes.* As soon as the neck has been stretched sufficiently to allow the locked facets just to clear one another **(right above)**, it should be extended to complete the reduction. If the injury is long-standing (say of 1–3 weeks), progress will be much slower, and in extreme cases can extend to days. As soon as check radiographs confirm the reduction, the traction should be reduced to about 2.5 kg (6 lb). *On no account should the neck be allowed to over distract.*

Reduction failure. This is unusual in recent injuries, but assuming that there is not complete paraplegia, open reduction should be attempted by local trimming of those parts of the facets which are blocking reduction (facetectomy). In very long-standing dislocations, spinal stability is more important than accurate reduction, and the spine may be fused in the dislocated position if reduction fails.

Fracture–dislocations with an acute neurological defect. In about 10% of cervical spine dislocations, posterior extrusion of intervertebral disc material can compromise the cord, and there is a risk that the situation can be aggravated if reduction is undertaken without prior decompression. A thorough neurological examination should be carried out on admission, and if there is evidence of neurological involvement (particularly of the cord) then further investigation of the state of the relevant intervertebral disc should be undertaken. This is best done by a carefully supervised MRI scan; failing this, myelography with a postmyelography CAT scan should be carried out. If there is evidence of cord compression, then a decompression by the anterior route *before* reduction is advocated.

Post reduction after care. Where there is dislocation of the cervical spine without fracture, the posterior ligament complex never regains its former strength irrespective of the method of reduction or after care. Spontaneous recurrence is inevitable unless posterior fusion is carried out. The decision about surgery depends on the neurological picture, and may be deferred until this is reasonably clear. In the interval, traction should be maintained. The following situations are common: (a) If there is no neurological disturbance, spinal fusion should be carried out as a carefully planned procedure after a few days. (b) If there is an incomplete paraplegia, there may be a reasonable delay of 1–2 weeks. (c) If paraplegia is complete, there is less indication for fusion. Traction may be discontinued and a collar substituted after 4–6 weeks. (d) Where the injury is accompanied by fracture, and union in this fracture may result in stability (e.g. fracture of the *base* of a spinous process), traction (or support with a halo vest) may be continued until union occurs (say after 8 weeks). Final stability should always be checked by flexion and extension laterals.

Extension injuries
Mechanisms of injury. Extension injuries of the cervical spine are commonly seen in: • forward falls downstairs, when the forehead strikes against the ground • in rear impact car accidents in which the neck extends due to the inertia of the head • in head-on pattern car accidents, where the forehead strikes the car roof, fascia or bonnet (see also 'Soft tissue injuries of the neck—whiplash injuries', p. 386).

Pathology. These injuries are particularly common in the middle aged and elderly who suffer from cervical spondylosis. Osteoarthritic rigidity in the spine may lead to excessive concentration of violence at any area of the spine retaining mobility. A similar predisposition is found in those suffering from ankylosing spondylitis, severe rheumatoid arthritis or congenital deformity of the spine with localised areas of fusion (e.g. Klippel–Feil syndrome).

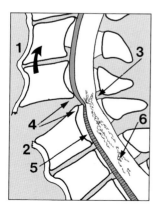

The neck hyperextends (**1**), tearing or avulsing the anterior longitudinal ligament (**2**) and perhaps stretching the cord at the level of the vertebral lesion (**3**). At the same time, or when the vertebrae snap together again, the cord may be nipped by backward-projecting osteophytes where there is spondylosis (**4**). Stretching and kinking of spinal vessels may lead to spreading thrombosis (**5**). The cord damage is often diffuse and may not correspond exactly with the level of injury (**6**). Spreading thrombosis may lead to a deteriorating neurological picture. Sole involvement of the central cord area is rare, but when it occurs the effect is: • motor loss, if present, tends to be greater in the arms than in the legs • temperature and pain conduction are more likely to be affected than proprioception and light touch, which are frequently spared.

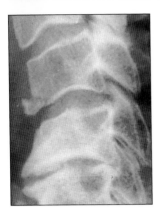

Diagnosis. The history of the injury, pain in the neck and complaint of weakness in the arms are suggestive, especially if seen with bruising or laceration of the forehead.

Radiographs. As spontaneous reduction is the rule, the radiographs *may be quite normal*. Nevertheless, plain films may show: (1) an avulsion fracture of an osteophyte or the edge of a vertebral body **(left)** (by the anterior longitudinal ligament); (2) displacement of the pharyngeal shadow by haemorrhage; (3) fractures of the laminae or spinous processes, or (4) tearing open of a vertebral body. MRI imaging is of great value in showing anterior longitudinal ligament ruptures in doubtful cases.

Treatment. Extension injuries of the spine are stable. *Local treatment* consists of the judicious use of a collar until local pain and cervical muscle spasm settle. *The general treatment* is that of the accompanying neurological problem, which may be minor or profound.

Compression fractures of the cervical spine
Mechanisms of injury. These may be caused by: (a) heavy objects falling on the head, (b) the vertex striking the ground as in falls, diving and other athletic accidents, (c) the head striking the roof in head-on car accidents.

Diagnosis. The history of injury may be suggestive. There may be tell-tale lacerations on the crown of the head. Complaint of pain in the neck is an indication for X-ray investigation.

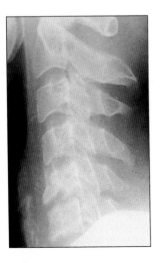

Radiographs. The appearances are dependent on the degree of causal violence. When the forces are moderate, a fissure fracture of the vertebral body may be produced, most obvious in the AP projection. Where the deformity is greater, lateral displacement of the pedicles may be obvious. In more severe injuries the vertebral body may be comminuted and flattened. Fragments of the vertebral body may be extruded in any direction; when this occurs the cord may be endangered. (The radiograph on the **left** shows a compression fracture of C5; note the encroachment on the neural canal by the posterior part of the body.) *CAT scanning is of particular value in clarifying the extent of fractures of this type.*

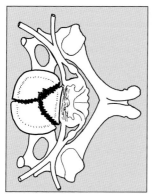

Neurological assessment. The most vulnerable part of the cord lies anteriorly, affecting firstly the motor supply of the upper limbs *before* the motor pathways to the lower limbs: hence paralysis tends to be maximal in the upper limbs. Next to be involved are the spinothalamic tracts carrying pain and temperature, and lastly the posterior columns (proprioception and light touch). On admission, carry out a full neurological examination including: all the main muscle groups in the upper and lower limbs, the skin and tendon reflexes, sensation to pin prick and light touch, and proprioception.

If the paralysis is bilateral, symmetrical and complete, testing should be repeated meticulously at 6 hours, 12 hours and 24 hours post-injury. No recovery after 24 hours in injuries at cervical level almost certainly indicates a hopeless prognosis. *Be careful to note, however, that a profound neurological loss cannot be declared complete unless proprioception and light touch have been carefully assessed.*

Treatment. As the posterior ligament complex is intact, there is no tendency to subsequent displacement once these fractures have healed. They are generally best treated by cervical traction for 6 weeks until cancellous union has occurred. Traction also minimises the chances of backward displacement of bone fragments.

Surgical removal of backward projecting bone fragments which are interfering with cord function may be carried out. This is often recommended in the face of the following criteria: (i) an incomplete cord lesion; (ii) a deteriorating neurological picture; (iii) a local block on myelography; (iv) confirmatory evidence on CAT or MRI scan of spinal encroachment. The indications are less clear when the neurological condition is static or complete. Where on exploration there is evidence of marked spinal instability, internal fixation is advisable.

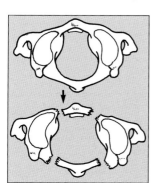

THE UPPER TWO CERVICAL VERTEBRAE
Atlanto-occipital subluxations and dislocations
Traumatic lesions at this level are usually fatal. In those that survive, reduction by traction is indicated.

Fractures of the atlas
The usual pattern of fracture is *quadripartite* (**left**) and is produced as a result of severe downward pressure of the occipital condyles on the atlas. Such force may result from: • a weight falling on the head (e.g. in the construction industry) • the head striking the roof of a car in a road traffic accident • a fall from a height on to the heels.

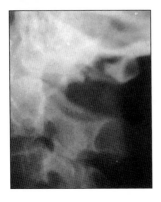

The conscious patient may resent sitting up and supports the head with the hands. There may be complaint of severe occipital pain due to local pressure on the great occipital nerve.

Radiographs. The *lateral* radiograph may show the fracture of the posterior arch **(left)**. The plain AP view is generally unhelpful. A through-the-mouth projection should reveal the displacement of the lateral masses; but if this cannot be taken, a CAT scan is invaluable. Congenital absence of part of the posterior arch may cause confusion, but is of no significance, being a stable condition.

Treatment. These cannot be reduced; with *slight* displacement, a well-fitting collar for 6 weeks with observation in hospital for 2–3 weeks *at least* is desirable. With more severe displacements, 6 weeks' skull traction is advisable.

Transverse ligament lesions

The transverse ligament which retains the odontoid peg may be torn in sudden flexion injuries. (It may become attenuated or rupture in rheumatoid arthritis or in soft-tissue infections of the neck in children.) In either case, the risk to the cord is great, as it becomes pinched between the posterior arch of the atlas and the odontoid peg.

Diagnosis. The condition may be suspected from the history, by pain in the neck *and the head*, and by the presence of marked cervical spasm.

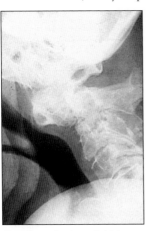

Radiographs. The diagnosis is established by radiographs. Note: (i) the gap between the posterior face of the anterior arch and the odontoid in the lateral. In the adult, the upper limit of normal is 4 mm **(Left, gross shift in an arthritic spine).** (ii) A through-the-mouth view may show an asymmetrical location of the odontoid peg relative to the lateral masses of the atlas. (iii) If there is remaining doubt, flexion and extension laterals should be taken under close supervision. Abnormal excursion of the odontoid peg is diagnostic. CAT scans may be used to clarify the relationship between the odontoid peg and the anterior arch of the atlas.

Treatment. As an initial measure, skull traction of about 3 kg (6–7 lb) in extension should be set up. In children, a period of 6 weeks' traction may suffice to restore stability to the spine, especially where the subluxation has been due to a local infection.

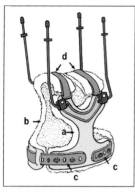

If the dislocation is due to recent trauma, conservative treatment may be carried out for 8 weeks, with the halo attached by vertical bars to an off-the-shelf 'vest'. The Bremer vest has anterior (a) and posterior shells (b) with soft replaceable liners. They are linked inferiorly with thoracic bands (c) secured to locking posts. Shoulder pads are secured in front with webbing straps (d). A pelvic girdle attachment may be fixed to the vest for additional stability. In default, the halo supports may be incorporated in a plaster jacket (lower left). *After-care.* (1) Re-tighten the halo pins after 36 hours. Subsequently a loose pin may be tightened if resistance is met—otherwise insert a new pin, tighten it and remove the old. (2) Clean the areas round the pins daily with soap and water, and remove any crusting with hydrogen peroxide. (3) Treat infected pin tracks with antibiotics and intensified site care. If there is no improvement, introduce a new pin at a fresh site before removing the old, and if necessary carrying out a local debridement. *Other problems* include osteomyelitis of the skull, extradural haematoma and extradural, subdural and cerebral abscess. Symptoms include headache, pyrexia, fits, hemiplegia and coma. Treat the complication, abandon skull traction and use an alternative such as a Minerva plaster. (In a number of patients, a Minerva plaster may be a viable alternative to a halo-pelvic system.)

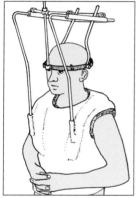

When the device is finally removed, stability must be assessed with flexion and extension laterals; if there is evidence of persisting instability, fusion will be needed. Where the pathology is secondary to rheumatoid arthritis, local cervical fusion is generally advised to prevent subluxation of C1 on C2.

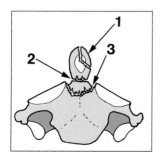

Odontoid fractures
These may be classified as follows:

Type I fractures (1) involve the tip of the peg, are generally stable and have a good prognosis; they require symptomatic treatment only with a collar.

Type II fractures (2) involve the junction of odontoid peg with the body, and are the commonest of these fractures.

Type III fractures (3) fail to unite in about a quarter of cases, so they must be handled as carefully as Type II fractures.

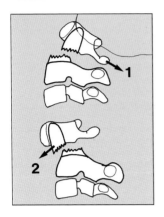

Odontoid fracture mechanisms.
Fracture may result from sudden severe extension (**1**) or flexion (**2**) of the neck (extension and flexion fractures).

Diagnosis. The injury may be suspected from the history, the site of pain and muscle spasm. Occasionally, the injury may be overlooked and discovered only on investigation of an advancing ataxia or other neurological disturbance.

Radiographs. The fracture may show clearly in the through-the-mouth AP projection and/or in the standard lateral view. Carefully supervised flexion and extension laterals or CAT scans should be taken only if there is doubt.

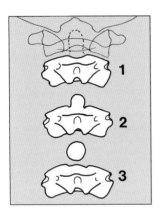

Congenital abnormalities
These can cause confusion and include: (**1**) complete absence of the odontoid process (predisposing to dislocation); (**2**) hypoplasia; (**3**) non-fusion of the odontoid process (persistent os odontoideum). Note that the ossification centre for the apex normally appears at 2 years, with fusion occurring by age 12. Rounded edges and a separate articulation with the atlas may help to distinguish it from a fracture (even though it may behave as such).

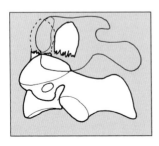

Extension injuries
The atlas and the odontoid fragment displace posteriorly in relation to C2. This pattern of injury is commoner in the elderly and is a relatively stable lesion.

Treatment. If the *shift is slight*, a collar for 8 weeks should suffice. If the *displacement is marked*, apply traction in slight flexion with callipers, *but slacken off the weight as soon as reduction has been achieved to avoid distraction.* After 2–4 weeks, a collar may be substituted.

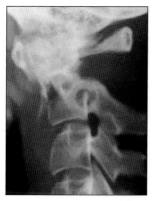

Flexion injuries

C1 and C2 displace anteriorly **(left)**, and this shows well in flexion and extension laterals. The incidence of non-union in junctional fractures is about 60%, with risk of progressive subluxation and neurological involvement.

Treatment. In spite of the risks of complications, these injuries are frequently treated conservatively, especially in children. *Method:* (1) Reduce by applying traction in extension, using skull traction. In the older patient, aim for a good reduction to lessen the risks of non-union. In the younger patient, persistent displacement can in fact re-model.

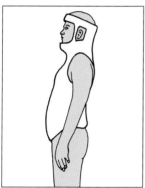

(2) After 1–2 weeks in traction, it may be possible to mobilise the patient. This is especially desirable in the elderly. A stout well-fitting cervical collar may be used. In the young patient, better support will be afforded with a Minerva plaster **(left)** or with a halo-vest device. In all instances, external support should be continued without interruption for 8 weeks.
(3) Stability should then be assessed with flexion and extension laterals.

Fusion of C1 and C2 is indicated: • if conservative treatment fails • if the case presents late • if a good reduction cannot be obtained • where the delays and complications of conservative management are thought to present a greater hazard than the risks of primary surgery.

Treat displacements of the os odontoideum conservatively, unless the forward slip is extensive or there are severe or progressive neurological signs.

Fractures of the odontoid process in adults may be treated by the experienced surgeon with screw fixation and grafting, using an anteromedial approach.

Fractures of the pedicles of C2

These may occur in two distinct ways: (1) by simultaneous *extension and distraction* of the neck, e.g. by hanging or when a cyclist is caught under the chin by a tree branch or a rope. If not immediately fatal, the neurological disturbance is usually profound. (2) Radiologically identical fractures may be produced by forcible *extension and compression*; this may occur in road traffic accidents if the head strikes the vehicle roof and ricochets into extension. Neurological involvement here is rare. These two types of injury may be distinguished by the history, site of bruising (neck or forehead) and the neurological disturbance.

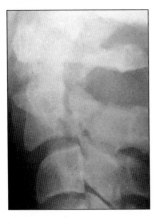

Radiographs. These normally show the fracture clearly (**left**). Occasionally there is a spondylolisthesis of C2 on C3.

Treatment

Extension injuries with distraction. Skull traction for a period of 4–6 weeks is advocated to maintain position only. There is always the risk in this type of injury of further distraction, and it is therefore important to limit traction to a maximum of 2 kg (5 lb). If radiographs suggest distraction, or if neurological signs are advancing, traction must be abandoned. This would be an indication for local fusion.

Extension injuries with compression. If the injury appears stable and there is no neurological disturbance, a well-fitting collar should be worn for 6 weeks. If there is neurological involvement, a 6-week period of cervical (skull) traction should be advised. Thereafter, if there is any evidence of instability, fusion is indicated.

Isolated spinous process fractures

Fracture of the spinous process of C7 or T1 (clay shoveller's fracture) may result from sudden muscular contraction and is an avulsion fracture. This is a stable injury, and symptomatic treatment only is required (e.g. a cervical collar for 2–3 weeks). It must be carefully distinguished from a cervical dislocation with associated fracture. (If in doubt, flexion and extension laterals should be taken.)

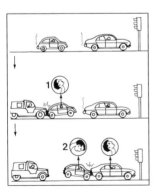

SOFT-TISSUE INJURIES OF THE NECK (WHIPLASH INJURIES)

Whiplash injuries of the neck occur most frequently in road traffic accidents. In the classical incident, the spine is hyperextended following a rear impact collision (**1**) and then rapidly flexed as the vehicle in which the patient is travelling hits an object in front—usually another car (**2**). 'Whiplash injury' is a somewhat emotive term and has been considerably abused, being at times chosen with regrettable imprecision to describe virtually any neck injury unaccompanied by fracture.

It is usually agreed that the extension element is the more important in producing disability: amongst the reasons for this include the observation that flexion is generally limited by the chin contacting the chest, while there is no equivalent restriction placed on extension.

The variety of associated clinical findings, the Whiplash-Associated Disorders, have been classified thus:

Grade I. Complaint of neck pain, stiffness or tenderness only, with no abnormal physical signs.
Grade II. Neck complaint, with musculoskeletal signs (e.g. decreased range of movements or point tenderness).
Grade III. Neck complaint, with positive neurological signs (e.g. reflex disturbance, muscle weakness or sensory defects).

Other symptoms which may be found in all grades include deafness, dizziness, tinnitus, headache, temporary memory loss, dysphagia and temporomandibular pain. (A fourth grade where there is an associated fracture or dislocation has been described but would seem unreasonable to include.) While it has been long recognised that there is little clarity regarding the exact nature of the physical basis for the complaints associated with these disorders, it is now apparent that in very many there is a non-organic element. (For example, it is twice as common in women than men; it is increasing in frequency in spite of the introduction of head restraints and other protective measures; and in certain countries where there is not a climate of litigation, it is virtually unknown.) While there seems little doubt that malingering does occasionally occur, this is considered to be rare. It is thought that in many cases, a significant component of late disability is psychological, even if this is not at conscious level, and that psychological elements and sometimes illness related behaviour are often established within three months of injury.

The prognosis for recovery is adversely affected by the severity of the collision, the age of the patient (the prognosis is poorer in the old) and the position of the passenger in the vehicle (the prognosis being worse for front seat passengers than those in the rear). A high proportion of patients make a full recovery, but in about 10% of cases disability may continue for years or become permanent, sometimes interfering with or preventing return to previous employment. There is uncertainty as to whether a whiplash injury may precipitate arthritic changes in the neck.

Diagnosis. The main symptoms are of pain and stiffness in the neck. In addition there may be radiation of pain and numbness into the shoulder, arm and hand, or to the interscapular region or occiput. In an appreciable number of cases there may be an additional complaint of low back pain, the mechanism of which is uncertain. Clinically, neck movements are generally restricted, and asymmetrical restriction is considered by some to be of particular significance. Widespread cervical tenderness is usual, often with involvement of the anterior cervical muscles, but localisation should be looked for. Objective neurological signs are rare, but again these should always be sought.

Need for further investigation. X-ray examination is indicated if any of the following are present (Hoffman criteria): • posterior mid-line tenderness • intoxication (which may mask the complaints and findings) • lowered alertness • focal neurological signs • other painful, distracting injuries.

This is reliable but not infallible, and if in doubt, further investigation should be pursued.

Radiographs. These may show the following: • loss of the usual cervical curvature or localised kinking • occasionally evidence of hyperextension (anterior osteophytic avulsion) or hyperflexion (flake fracture of a spinous process) • pre-existing osteoarthritic changes in the cervical spine which predispose to injury (by concentrating local stresses).

MRI scans. These may show evidence of disc prolapse or nerve root compression, but the results, however, can be unreliable as abnormalities have been reported in symptomless patients, and vice versa.

Treatment. Treatment is primarily conservative, and to minimise the risks of the superimposition of a non-organic element, a positive approach in the handling of these cases with emphasis of the likelihood of a complete recovery, is strongly advised. Note that some regard the prolonged use of cervical collars as being associated with poorer outcomes, and the following regimes have been suggested:

Grade I. Immediate return to normal activities, with no work restrictions and no medication.

Grade II. To return to normal activities as soon as possible, and preferably within a week. Temporary alteration of work patterns may be required, but the need for these should be reassessed after two weeks unless the clinical circumstances or the working environment are unusual. Non-narcotic analgesics and/or NSAIDs may be prescribed for up to one week only.

Grade III. As in Grade II, but narcotic analgesics may be required for short periods initially. Manipulation may be of transient benefit, but not more than two sessions are recommended. Treatment started by a physiotherapist and continued at home by the patient himself is generally very helpful, with emphasis again being placed on the likelihood of a good recovery.

Cases persisting over three months. Carefully reassess, and if necessary consider the prescription of minor tranquillisers or antidepressants. Grade III patients with progressive neurological deterioration and a proven disc prolapse may be considered for surgery (e.g. an anterior cervical fusion).

The Barré–Lieou syndrome
After a whiplash incident there may be complaint of headache, vertigo, tinnitus, ocular problems and facial pain. It is thought that these may be due to a sympathetic nerve disturbance at the C3–4 level, and in 75% of the cases there is impairment of sensation in the C4 dermatome, with weakness of shoulder and scapular movements. Myelography may show nerve root sleeve disturbances. Good results have been claimed for anterior discectomy combined with a local cervical fusion.

FRACTURES OF THE THORACIC AND LUMBAR SPINE
Mechanisms of injury. These fractures occur most frequently as a result of forces which tend to produce flexion of the spine. A rotational element is often present. They may result from: (a) falls from a height on to the heels, where the normal curvature of the spine results in further flexion; (b) blows across the back and shoulder which cause the spine to jack-knife at the thoracolumbar junction—e.g. injuries in the mining and construction industries; (c) flexion and rotational forces transmitted to the spine in car and motor cycle accidents; (d) heavy lifting, especially in the middle-aged and elderly, where there is often a degree of osteoporosis or osteomalacia, and less commonly malignancy (especially metastatic deposits). The causal force then may be minimal.

Diagnosis. Suspect a history of back pain after trauma, especially if there is local spinal tenderness, pain on spinal percussion, and particularly if there is an angular kyphosis. Thoracic or abdominal radicular pain may wrongly divert attention to the chest or abdomen, and in the elderly there may be no convincing history of injury; any suspicion merits X-ray examination.

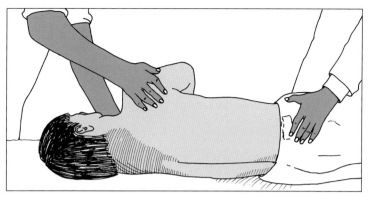

Radiographs. AP and lateral radiographs only should be taken in the first instance. In the obviously seriously injured patient there may be difficulty in obtaining a lateral because of severe pain, or through fear of causing cord damage. In these circumstances, a shoot-through lateral may be taken, using a fixed grid or chest bucky. If these measures are unsatisfactory, you should *personally* supervise the turning of the patient on his side in order to obtain a lateral projection; in essence you should see that the patient is turned gently and smoothly in such a way that the upper part of the spine with the shoulders is rotated in step with the pelvis, and that the patient remains well supported (e.g. by pillows) when he is on his side.

Note: As previously stated, the most important decision to make in any spinal injury is whether it is stable, as this profoundly influences treatment. The commonest spinal injury *by far* is the wedge compression fracture, and consequently in practice the most frequent problem is to decide whether such a fracture is stable or not. (Other patterns of injury are most often unstable.)

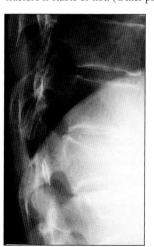

Stable wedge fractures

Wedge fractures are most commonly observed in the lateral radiographs (anterior wedge fractures) and are caused by pure flexion forces. (On the **left** is a wedge fracture of D11; note the difference in height between the anterior and posterior margins of the vertebral body.) Less commonly, when there is an added rotational element, vertebral wedging may be apparent in the AP projection (lateral wedging). This form of wedging is often associated with root compression on the narrowed side, and these injuries have a poorer prognosis regarding ultimate functional recovery and freedom from pain.

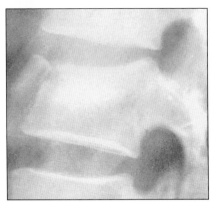 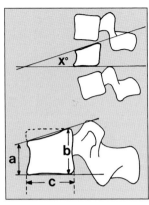

Interpreting the radiographs. Note the following points:

- In anterior wedge fractures, the anterior border of the vertebra will measure less than the posterior border. The anterior border may be quite regular, or show marginal shearing **(left)**. Decrease in height of the *posterior* margin is evidence of greater violence, and a possible burst fracture, with the risk of bony fragments encroaching the vertebral canal. If this is suspected, a CAT scan is recommended.
- The amount of wedging should be assessed **(right)**. The fracture is likely to be stable if the height of the anterior margin **(a)** still amounts to two-thirds or more of the posterior margin **(b)** or if the degree of wedging **(x)** is 15° or less, or if the depth of the body **(c)** divided by the difference in the heights is greater than 3.75.
- Each of the upper thoracic vertebrae is linked by ribs to the sternum, and *appreciable* wedging cannot take place without involvement of these structures.
- In the thoracic spine, fracture of a single vertebra will often lead to localised angulation of the spine (gibbus). Multiple fractures will lead to a regular kyphosis. In either of these circumstances, the increased thoracic curvature will tend to produce an increased lumbar lordosis and/or hyperextension in the hip joints.

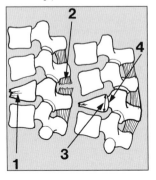

Unstable fractures

Marked wedging (20° or more, or collapse of the anterior margin to less than half the posterior) **(1)** is likely to denote instability (as it is probably associated with posterior ligament complex rupture **(2)**). If the posterior margin is reduced in height **(3)**, a greater degree of wedging is possible without rupture of the posterior ligament complex, but indicates an element of bursting. Posterior *lumbar* bulging **(4)** is less serious than in the dorsal spine where the canal is narrow.

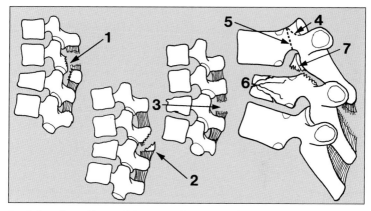

Look for other evidence of damage to the posterior ligament complex and associated structures fundamental to spinal stability. Note an avulsion fracture of a spinous process (1), or of its tip (2), or wide separation of the vertebral spines due to tearing of the interspinous ligament (3). Look for evidence of fractures at the level of the facet joints (4) or pedicles (5). A comminuted fracture of a vertebral body (6) with involvement of these structures (e.g. facet joint fracture, 7) is generally unstable; bilateral pedicle fractures are *invariably* unstable. If there is any doubt regarding the integrity of the articular processes, CAT scans may give valuable additional information.

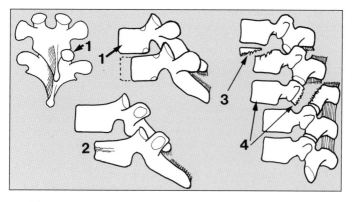

Look for *vertebral shift*, an invariable sign of instability. The patterns include the following: (1) unilateral facet joint displacement, giving in the lateral a forward shift of about a third or less; (2) bilateral dislocated facet joints, often with fracture and more displacement; (3) shearing fracture of a vertebral body; (4) bilateral neural arch fractures and traumatic spondylolisthesis. *Note in all these injuries there is damage to the posterior complex.* If still in doubt take oblique projections, a further lateral (*supervised*) in slight flexion, and a CAT scan.

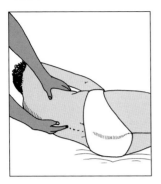

The spinal radiographs may give unequivocal evidence of instability. In other cases where there is the *slightest* suspicion of the posterior ligament complex being involved, that structure must be carefully examined clinically. Press firmly between successive spines, preferably in slight flexion. If the interspinous ligaments are torn, the examining finger will encounter a boggy softness instead of the normal resistance to pressure.

Treatment

Stable fractures. (1) Admit for complete bed rest in recumbency with one pillow. (2) Give analgesics as required. (3) When the acute symptoms have settled (say after 1 week), extension exercises should be commenced and vigorously practised. (4) The patient can be allowed up and home at 6 weeks, the time it takes a fracture of cancellous bone to unite. This programme may be compressed if wedging is minimal.

Unstable fractures, with either no neurological lesion or an incomplete neurological lesion. The aims are to reduce any displacement that is present and to prevent any recurrence of displacement (with the risk of a neurological disaster) until stability is regained. *Stability* may be achieved by:
• spontaneous anterior fusion • healing of the torn posterior ligament complex (an unreliable event especially in cases uncomplicated by fracture) • internal fixation and fusion.

Where a fracture is present, as a rule stability returns as the fracture unites and the injury may be treated conservatively throughout. Initially, in many other cases, conservative treatment may also be undertaken to give the patient time to recover from the immediate effects of the acute trauma, and to allow a thorough assessment; surgical treatment may then be undertaken as an elective procedure.

Reduction can generally be achieved by gently extending the spine with a pillow or a sandbag at the level of injury. (If this is unsuccessful, or if there are locked facets, open reduction will be required.) After reduction, further care is dependent on the nature of the injury and the availability of equipment.

- The patient may be nursed in a Stryker frame. This allows rotation from the supine to the prone position with minimal nursing effort.
- Alternatively, where instability is minimal *or* as a follow up to a period in a Stryker frame (e.g. after 6 weeks), a POP jacket may be applied with the spine in extension.
- If the fracture cannot be reduced by simple measures (e.g. if there are locked facets), open reduction will be required and the opportunity may then be taken to internally splint the spine. A number of devices are available, but in most cases a local spinal fusion will also be required (immediate or delayed).

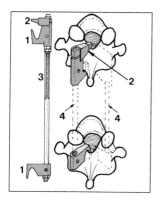

Most forms of internal fixation for spinal fractures fall into three categories: (i) hook and rod systems; (ii) plates and screws; (iii) internal fixators with pedicle or vertebral body screws. Typical examples include:

The *AO locking hook rod system* (left) which may be used between T3 and T10. The hooks (1) snug against the laminae, and can be locked to them as required (2). They in turn are locked to paired partially threaded rods (3, 4), which may be bent to fit the contours of the spine.

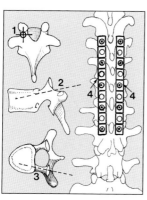

In the case of *plates and screws*, sound anchorage may be obtained for the screws if they are passed through the pedicles into the vertebral bodies. The entry point (1) is below the facet close to the upper margin of the transverse process, with the track through the pedicle inclined downwards (2) and medially (3) at an angle which varies with the vertebral level. Great care must be taken (by probing and image intensifier control) to see that the spinal canal is not entered. *AO notched plates* (4), which can be bent in all three planes to fit, and 4.5 mm screws may be used between T6 and S1.

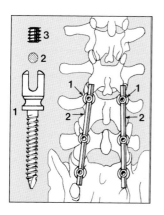

The *Oswestry pedicle screw system* can be used from T10 to S1, and employs rigid self-tapping pedicle screws (1). These are inserted after the accuracy of their proposed paths has been confirmed with probing and the use of plain and twisted wire pedicle markers (for side discrimination), using an image intensifier. The pedicle screws are linked with connecting bars (2) which can be bent to suit the local contours, before being locked with grub screws (3) in the threaded ends of the pedicle screws.

Generally bone grafting is used in conjunction with the above systems.

Unstable fractures with a complete, irrecoverable cord lesion.
If the spine is grossly unstable, internal fixation may be indicated on the following grounds:

- to facilitate nursing
- to prevent or minimise spinal deformity which if marked may compromise respiratory function and the ability to sit up, to use a wheelchair, and complete a satisfactory programme of rehabilitation
- to permit earlier mobilisation
- to reduce the risks of chronic back pain from nerve root involvement.

If the spine is not wildly unstable, and first-class nursing is available, there is less need for internal fixation, and the treatment is then of the paraplegia.

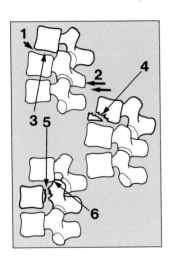
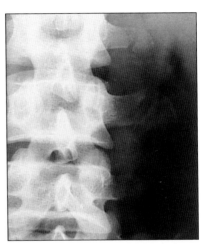

OTHER INJURIES OF THE SPINE
Retrospondylolisthesis
Retrospondylolisthesis (1) occurs especially at T12–L1 and may follow a distally sited blow (2). There may be shearing through the disc (3), the vertebral body (4) or the pedicles (5) so that the body of the vertebra above impinges on the articular processes of the one below (6). Any neurological involvement is seldom complete, but as the posterior ligament complex is damaged, instability may be present; these injuries should be treated with respect.

Fractured transverse processes
In the lumbar region these may result from direct trauma or avulsion (from sudden contraction of quadratus lumborum). (Note transverse process fractures above right.) They may be associated like multiple rib fractures with fracture–dislocation of the spine. Even without spinal instability, multiple fractures may be complicated by retroperitoneal haemorrhage, shock, paralytic ileus or renal damage, all of which will require appropriate treatment. No treatment apart from rest is needed for uncomplicated fractures.

NEUROLOGICAL ASSESSMENT OF SPINAL INJURIES

Where there is *evidence of a deficit*, a thorough neurological examination is required on admission. This must include as a minimum:

- Testing for evidence of muscle activity and its power in all muscle groups below the level of injury.
- Testing sensation of pin prick and light touch over the entire area affected.
- Testing proprioception.
- Testing the reflexes—the tendon reflexes, the plantar responses; the anal reflex (stimulation of the perineum leading to contraction of the external anal sphincter) and the glansbulbar reflex (compression of the glans leading to perineal muscle contraction).

If the findings indicate a complete spinal lesion, the examination should be repeated after 6 hours, 12 hours and 24 hours.

The common lesions

- Spinal concussion causes a temporary arrest of conduction within the cord; its effects are patchy and recovery is rapid. If, for example, there is a *complete* spinal lesion on first examination, spinal concussion is an unlikely but possible cause. If after 12 hours the lesion remains complete, spinal concussion is *not* the cause.
- If there is *any* evidence of voluntary motor activity, skin sensation or proprioception below the level of the lesion, the cord has *not* been transected (and further recovery is possible).
- After an injury to the cord, the reflexes generally disappear for at least some hours, and sometimes for as long as 2 weeks. Return of reflex activity with continued absence of all sensation and voluntary muscle contraction confirms a *transection of the cord*.
- Where the injury is at a level where there is potential damage to lumbar nerve roots or the cauda equina (e.g. injuries at the thoracolumbar junction), persistent absence of reflexes would confirm such damage.
- Note that cord transection is irrecoverable, but there is potential recovery where there is involvement of nerve roots and the cauda equina.

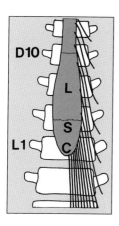

Neurological lesion in spinal injuries

Note the following:

- The spinal cord ends at **L1**; any injury distal to this can involve the cauda but not the cord.
- All the lumbar, sacral and coccygeal segments of the cord lie between **D10** and **L1** only.
- Injuries at the thoracolumbar junction produce a great variety of neurological disturbances as: (a) the cord may or may not be transected, (b) the nerve roots may be undamaged, partly divided or completely divided. Cord or root damage is reflected in disturbance of myotomes or dermatomes.

Cervical cord: special features

The phrenic nerve arises from C4, with minor contributions from C3 and C5. Cord section proximal to the phrenic nerve will lead to rapid death from respiratory paralysis. Lesions at C4–5, and more distal, may permit respiration without external support. C2 and C3 supply the vertex and occiput (accounting for pain here in upper cervical lesions).

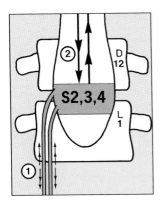

Neurological control of the bladder

Autonomic fibres controlling the detrusor muscle of the bladder and the internal sphincter travel from cord segments S2, 3 and 4 to the bladder via the cauda equina (**1**). Normally bladder sensation and voluntary emptying are mediated through pathways stretching between the brain and the sacral centres (**2**).

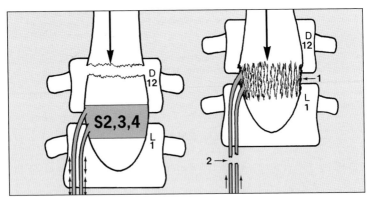

If the cord is transected above the S2, 3, 4 segments (**left**) voluntary control is lost, but the potential for coordinated contraction of the bladder wall, relaxation of the sphincter and complete emptying remains. (Normally 200–400 ml of urine is passed every 2–4 hours, the reflex activity being triggered by rising bladder pressure or skin stimulation — the automatic bladder or cord bladder.) Injuries which damage the sacral centres or the cauda (**right**) prevent coordinated reflex control. Bladder emptying is always incomplete and irregular, and occurs only as a result of distension. Its efficiency varies with the patient's state of health, urinary infection and muscle spasms. (Autonomous or isolated atonic bladder.)

TREATMENT OF SPINAL PARALYSIS

The aim of treatment is maximal physical recovery and mental readjustment with, ideally, complete physical independence and return to full-time employment.

These ideals can be most fully realised through the special resources and environment of a paraplegic unit, and no effort should be spared in having the patient transferred to such a unit at the earliest convenience. Pending transfer, and assuming the injury has been dealt with in an appropriate fashion, it is vital that attention is paid to the problems of the skin and bladder.

The skin

If pressure is applied to the skin it becomes ischaemic; if pressure is maintained, necrosis from tissue anoxia results. The skin of the elderly is thin, and least able to tolerate pressure. Poorly nourished or abraded skin, and anaemia are also adverse factors. The most important points, both of which are amenable to treatment, are the duration of ischaemia and the amount of pressure applied to the skin.

The *duration of pressure* applied to any one area is in practice regulated by regular turning of the patient. During the initial weeks of treatment it is essential that the patient does not lie for longer than 2 hours in one position. It is important to note that regular turning of the patient should start from the time of injury; irreversible damage may be done on the day of admission when other problems may allow this vital aspect of treatment to be overlooked for perhaps some hours.

The *amount of pressure* is important because if it is locally concentrated, then ischaemia will be complete; in consequence pressure sores tend to commence over bony prominences—the sacrum, the trochanters, the heels, the elbows and the malleoli. Particular attention should be paid to these areas, and local padding over the ankles and elbows may help. To distribute the body weight more evenly, the patient may be nursed on pillows, or on water or sand beds.

The *condition of the skin* should be maintained. If moist, it becomes susceptible to bacterial invasion; if subjected to friction through contact with rough, unyielding surfaces, local abrasions may occur. Local injuries of this nature increase oxygen demands and may initiate the production of pressure sores. To prevent this: (i) Unstarched, soft bed linen should be used and non-porous surfaces avoided. Nursing the patient on sheepskin is sometimes advocated. (ii) The skin should be protected from incontinence. (iii) Skin hygiene should be maintained by frequent, thorough cleansing with soap and water. After washing, the skin must be thoroughly dried; rubbing with alcohol may help this, and at the same time lead to temporary, local vasodilatation. Talcum powder is also used to help drying and reduce friction between the skin and the bed linen.

If pressure sores occur, preventative measures should be tightened up, and any underlying anaemia corrected. Any local sloughs or sequestra should be removed. If the area involved is small, local dressings may achieve healing which will go through the stages of granulation and contraction. If a large area is involved, rotational flaps usually afford the best means of closure. If sores persist, they are frequently followed by progressive anaemia, deterioration in general health and well being, and often amyloid disease.

The bladder

The effects of spinal paralysis on the bladder are dependent on the level of injury. The immediate problem is prevention of over distension while minimising the risks of infection. The methods available include:

- *Intermittent suprapubic cystostomy using plastic tubing.* This method is demanding on staff and facilities, and carries the risk of pelvic infection.
- *Intermittent catheterisation.* If properly performed with a full aseptic ritual, the risks of infection are probably lowest with this method, but it is also very demanding on staff.
- *Indwelling catheterisation.* This is probably the commonest method employed, but is almost invariably accompanied by some degree of urinary infection.

Mechanical emptying of the bladder by one of these methods is usually required for 3–4 weeks, after which, in the appropriate lesions, automatic function will be starting to take over. This should be assessed by trial removal of the catheter; giving copious fluids; and when filling of the bladder is apparent, trying to achieve emptying by stroking the skin in the inner groin area or by applying manual pressure over the bladder.

If these measures fail, recatheterisation will be necessary, and the procedure repeated after a week. Thereafter, the efficiency of emptying should be assessed by measuring the residual urine every 3–6 months. Renal function should be reviewed by a yearly intravenous pyelogram, urine culture and estimation of the serum urea. Failure to establish a satisfactory emptying pattern will require skilled urological investigation and management.

Physiotherapy and occupational therapy

These should be commenced without delay, attention being paid to the following aspects of management:

Chest. The risks and effects of respiratory infection should be minimised by deep-breathing exercises, the development of the accessory muscles of respiration, assisted coughing, percussion and postural drainage.

The joints. Mobility should be preserved in the paralysed joints by passive movements. This must be done with caution; if there is any spasticity; overstretching must be avoided to minimise the risks of myositis ossificans.

The unparalysed muscles. These should be developed for compensatory use— e.g. shoulder girdle exercises to make unaided bed–wheelchair transfers possible. Troublesome muscle spasms may be controlled with diazepam.

Depending on the level of the lesion the patient may require assistance in some or all of the following areas:

- Regaining balance for sitting or standing.
- Tuition in calliper walking (or gait improvement in partial lesions).
- Overcoming problems with dressing.
- Help with alterations and adjustments within the home to permit wheelchair use.
- Industrial retraining or other measures to help return to employment.

Regional injuries: fractures of the pelvis, hip and femoral neck

Fractures of the pelvis 400
Complications of pelvic
fractures 412
Traumatic dislocation of the
hip 415
Fractures of the femoral neck
423

FRACTURES OF THE PELVIS
General principles
The two wings of the pelvis are joined to the sacrum by the sacroiliac ligaments, and in front they are united by the symphysis pubis. This arrangement forms a cylinder of bone, the pelvic ring which *protects the pelvic organs* and *transfers the body weight* from the spine to the limbs.

If the ring is broken at two levels, the pelvis may be free to open out, or for (generally) one half to displace proximally, carrying the limb with it: these are the so-called *unstable fractures*. Isolated injuries of the ring do not have this tendency and are described as *stable fractures*.

The pelvis is richly supplied with blood vessels which are frequently damaged by fractures. *Internal haemorrhage is often severe, leading to shock which can be rapidly fatal.* Control of blood loss is often the first and main consideration in dealing with pelvic fractures.

The urogenital diaphragm is attached to the pubic rami, and fractures of the pelvis may damage the membranous urethra which pierces it, or the bladder which lies behind it. Less commonly there may be damage to the rectum. (See later for other features of pelvic fractures and complications.)

Tile classification of pelvic fractures
Three clear categories are defined:

- Type A fractures are *stable* and are subdivided into two groups:
  A1: fractures of the pelvis not involving the pelvic ring
  A2: stable, minimally displaced fractures of the pelvic ring.
- Type B fractures are *rotationally unstable but vertically stable*:
  B1: anteroposterior compression fractures (open book fractures)
  B2: lateral compression fractures, ipsilateral
  B3: lateral compression fractures, contralateral.
- Type C fractures are *both rotationally and vertically unstable*:
  C1: unilateral
  C2: bilateral
  C3: associated with acetabular fracture.

Diagnosis
Fractures of the pelvis commonly occur in falls from a height and from crushing injuries.

Screening films of the pelvis should be taken:
- in every case of multiple trauma (especially in the unconscious patient)
- where there is unexplained shock following a traumatic incident, or a blunt abdominal injury
- where there is a femoral shaft fracture.

Instability is best assessed by pelvic inlet and outlet films, and by CAT scans. If the software for 3-D imaging is available, this greatly facilitates interpretation of the exact relationships of the bony elements involved.

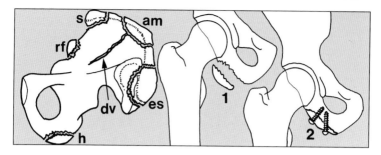

A1: Stable fractures not involving the ring

Sudden muscle contraction, especially in athletes, may avulse the anterior superior spine (sartorius, **s**), the anterior inferior spine (rectus femoris, **rf**), the ischial tuberosity (hamstrings, **h**), the posterior spine (erector spinae, **es**) and the iliac crest (abdominal muscles, **am**). The crest and blade may also be fractured by direct violence (**dv**). In all cases there is localised tenderness, and symptomatic treatment is all that is usually required. In the case of the ischial tuberosity, however, non-union is an appreciable risk, leading to chronic pain and disability. If there is much separation (**1**) of the fragments (2 cm or more), open reduction and internal fixation (**2**) may be advocated.

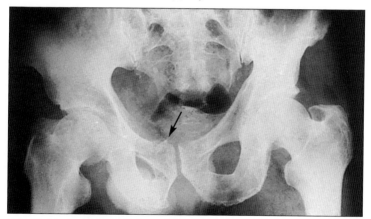

A2: Stable fractures of the pelvic ring

By far the *commonest fracture* is one involving the superior pubic ramus. This is seen frequently in the elderly patient following a fall on the side, and osteoporosis may be a contributory factor. *This injury is often missed* and should always be suspected if there is difficulty in walking after a fall, and a femoral neck fracture has been excluded. Radiographs of the hip may fail to visualise the area and full pelvic films are required. Clinically, there will be tenderness over the superior ramus and pain on side-to-side compression of the pelvis; movements of the hips may be relatively pain-free. Treatment is by bed rest for 2–3 weeks until the pain settles.

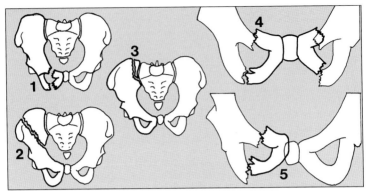

Other stable fractures of the pelvic ring include: fractures of two rami on one side (**1**); fracture of the ilium running into the sciatic notch (**2**); fracture of the ilium or sacrum involving the sacroiliac joint (**3**). Many quadripartite (butterfly) fractures (**4**) of the pelvis and double fractures of the rami with involvement of the symphysis (**5**) are also stable injuries. They usually result from AP compression of the pelvis which is insufficient to disrupt the anterior sacroiliac ligaments: the posterior part of the pelvic ring remains intact and rigid, while the loose anterior fragment is only slightly displaced. *Anticipate shock and damage to the urethra*, but otherwise treat with 6 weeks' recumbency.

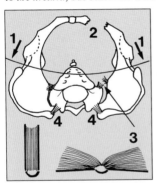
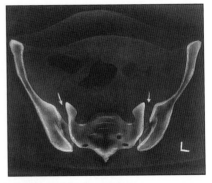

B1: Rotationally unstable, vertically stable fractures— anteroposterior compression fractures

These frequently result from run-over incidents where the wheel of a motor vehicle forces the anterior superior iliac spines backwards and outwards (**1**); they may also occur when the pelvis is compressed by falling rock or masonry which pins the patient to the ground. The ring fails *anteriorly* (e.g. at the symphysis or through two rami) (**2**), *and posteriorly,* with tearing of the sacrospinous and sacrotuberous ligaments (**3**). The pelvis opens out (hence the term *open-book fractures*) and CAT scans may show the resulting anterior widening of the sacroiliac joints. The posterior sacroiliac ligaments (**4**) remain intact, so that there is no vertical instability.

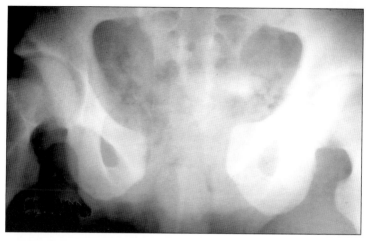

Treatment

Where the posterior damage is minimal and the anterior gap does not exceed 2.5 cm, treat by bed rest until the pain settles; monitor the symphyseal separation by repeated radiographs.

Where the separation exceeds 2.5 cm (**above**), more active treatment is required. The symphyseal gap may be narrowed by manipulation and held with an external fixator. These devices differ in their rigidity and the placement of the fixing pins required.

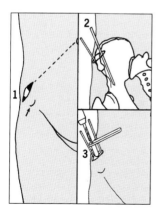

When performed formally, the procedure is usually carried out under general anaesthesia using an image intensifier, but the method described below can be carried out in the emergency room without one. Two or three pins are inserted. To do this, a 1.5 cm incision, directed towards the umbilicus, is made over the iliac crest 2.5 cm posterior to the anterior iliac spine (**1**). With blunt forceps-dissection the inner and outer tables are identified. K-wires are worked down on either side in contact with bone so that the plane of the pelvic wall can be correctly determined (**2**). The crest is then drilled between them, using a guide to protect the soft tissues (**3**).

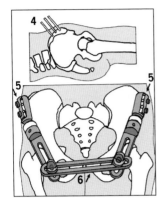

The pins may be self-drilling, threaded Schanz pins of 5–6 mm in diameter, and are inclined at an angle of 45° to the body axis (4). The wounds are closed, the pin tracks sealed and the two sets of pins joined with a rigid connector. With the Orthofix® (illustrated), the ends of the fixation pins are firmly held with clamps (5) and joined with a connecting bar (6) which stands well clear of the abdomen. Before the connector screws are tightened, the fracture should be reduced (the book closed), e.g. by side-to-side manual compression by turning the patient on his side if his condition will permit or by pulling on the crossed ends of a rolled-up towel passed under and round the pelvis.

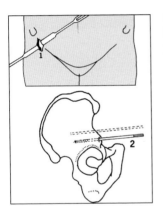

Stronger and more secure fixation, allowing greater purchase, may be obtained using long, heavy duty 6 mm screws. To insert these, a 2 cm incision, 3 cm distal and slightly medial to the anterior superior spine (1), is made, dissecting bluntly down to bone while taking care to avoid damaging the lateral femoral cutaneous nerve. A K-wire inserted close to bone may be used as a guide (2). The screw should lie above the acetabulum and its position checked with an intensifier. Second screws, parallel to the first, may also be used for additional grip. (Holding these with distancing forceps may allow manipulation under intensifier control.)

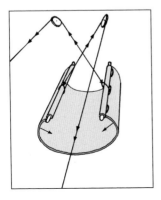

These injuries may also be treated conservatively using a canvas pelvic sling, with weights to apply side-to-side compression. This treatment should be continued for 6 weeks, taking the usual precautions over skin care. Weight bearing can generally be allowed after 8 weeks.
   Where there is symphyseal disruption, and an abdominal exploration is required, the opportunity may be taken to consider internal fixation. In some cases this procedure can be followed by a disabling osteitis of the symphysis and is contraindicated if there is faecal or urinary contamination.

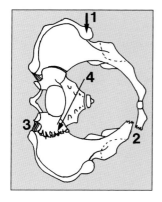

B2: Ipsilateral lateral compression injuries

Violence to the side of the pelvis (1) may cause fracture of the rami (2) or overlapping of the pubic bones; the posterior sacroiliac ligaments remain intact (3), and the hemipelvis hinges round them, often with crushing of the anterior margin of the sacroiliac joint (4). If tissue elasticity leads to spontaneous reduction, no fixation is needed; otherwise an external fixator may be used to control any instability. (Open reduction is required in the rare tilt fracture, where bone protrudes in the perineum.)

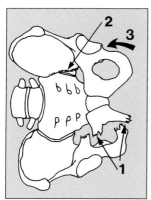

B3: Contralateral compression injuries (bucket handle fractures)

Two rami fracture (1) on the opposite side from the posterior injury (2). In some cases the anterior fracture is of butterfly pattern. The hemipelvis rotates (3), causing leg shortening without vertical migration of the hemipelvis. The majority are stable injuries and best accepted; only if the deformity is gross, the leg shortening in excess of 1.5 cm and the risks of intervention discussed, should more active treatment be considered. Reduction of the rotational deformity may be attempted using a pelvic fixator.

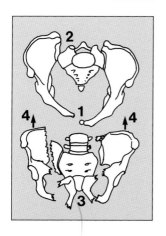

C1 & C2: Rotationally and vertically unstable injuries

The pelvic ring is completely disrupted at two or more levels. *Anteriorly*, in the unilateral (C1) injury the symphysis is disrupted (1) or the rami fractured. *Posteriorly*, there is total loss of continuity between the sacrum and ilium. This may result from complete ligamentous rupture and dislocation of the sacroiliac joint (2); or it may involve fractures of the posterior iliac spines, the ilium at other levels or the sacrum. In bilateral (C2) injuries, there is extensive disruption (often with an anterior butterfly fracture (3)) involving both sides of the pelvis, so that both are free to migrate proximally (4, 4).

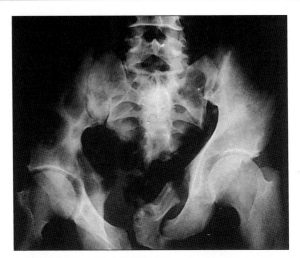

Radiographs of C1 & C2 injuries. The most obvious sign of vertical instability is the proximal migration of a hemipelvis. In addition, there may be avulsion of the transverse process of L5, and avulsion of the tip of the ischial spine. In the CAT scan, posterior displacement of a hemipelvis by more than 1 cm is diagnostic. Note in the **above** radiograph (of a C2 injury) there is gross vertical instability on the left (right side of the radiograph), with fracture of both rami and dislocation of the sacroiliac joint. There is in addition disruption of the symphysis pubis and a fracture through the sacrum on the right (most noticeable at the inferior margin of the sacroiliac joint). Although not clearly shown, both transverse processes of L5 are fractured.

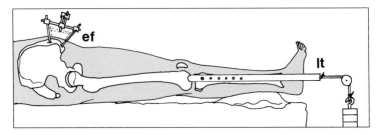

Treatment. These serious injuries are the ones most frequently associated with life-threatening internal haemorrhage, many other complications and permanent disability. Prompt application of an external fixator (**ef**), avoiding a formal procedure may give satisfactory control of blood loss. Proximal migration of a hemipelvis may be counteracted by leg traction (**lt**).

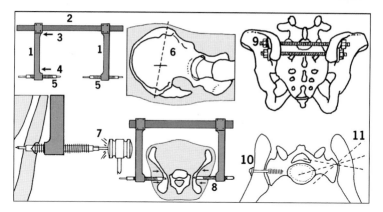

In others, sacroiliac disruption and its associated haemorrhage may be controlled by use of an anti-shock pelvic C-clamp. This has side arms (**1**) which can slide along a cross bar (**2**) when force is applied proximally (**3**), but lock when the force is distal (**4**). Hollow bolts (**5**) are screwed into the cross arms. These are inserted through small incisions made 6 cm from the posterior superior iliac spine (on a line connecting this with the anterior spine) (**6**). The bolts are anchored on each side by hammering a Steinman pin for a depth of 1 cm into bone (**7**). The bolts are then tightened with a spanner to close the disrupted sacroiliac joints (**8**).

Definitive surgical treatment

In the case of definitive as opposed to emergency treatment of the disrupted sacroiliac joint, there are a number of procedures available. The posterior parts of the pelvis may be linked by sacral bars (**9**) inserted through small posterior incisions. The sacroiliac joint may also be stabilised using screws running into the lateral masses (ala) of the sacrum (**10**). Their position must be determined with great accuracy, and the use of an image intensifier is mandatory. Guide wires and cannulated screws are particularly useful. Where the sacrum is fractured, the fixing screws must engage the body of the sacrum (central dotted line, **11**), and broaching the sacral canal or pelvis must be scrupulously avoided.

As regards other pelvic fractures, as a general rule open surgery (especially in acute injuries) should wherever possible be avoided. Most of these procedures carry a high morbidity due to problems which include uncontrollable haemorrhage, wound breakdown (especially in the case of posterior wounds), neurological damage and infection. The technical difficulties are often great, and pelvic reconstructive surgery should only be undertaken by the highly experienced. Nevertheless, open reduction and internal fixation may be considered if advantage can be taken of existing wounds in the affected area (so long as they are not in the perineum). Surgery should also be carefully considered if there is an irreducible dislocation of a sacroiliac joint, for this injury carries the highest risk of causing permanent disability.

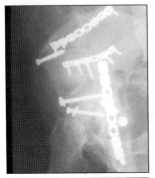

Note that in *Type C3 injuries*, the acetabular injury takes priority in management and should generally be reconstructed if it is thought that a reasonable functional restoration is possible; even if it is not possible to fully repair the articular surfaces it may render a later hip replacement procedure feasible. In the example on the **left**, the acetabulum has been rebuilt using a combination of implants including reconstruction plates, well-contoured plates and lag screws.

Fracture of the sacrum

These may be transverse (**A**) or involve the ala (**B**). Most sacral fractures result from falls from a height on to hard surfaces. There may be some lateral or anterior displacement. In some there may be involvement of sacral nerve roots, leading to sensory disturbance, weakness in the leg(s) or saddle anaesthesia and incontinence.

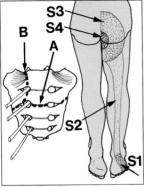

Treatment. The fracture may be treated with 2–3 weeks' bed rest. In the majority of cases the neurological disturbance is transitory, but if there is failure to improve (usually in gross displacements only) laminectomy may be advised.

Coccygeal injuries

These usually result from a fall in a seated position, and there is local pain (often on defecation) and tenderness. The main patterns of injury are: (1) fracture of the coccyx, with a varying degree of anteversion, (2) anterior subluxation of the coccyx, (3) anterior displacement of the coccyx secondary to fracture of the end piece of the sacrum, (4) rarely, posterior subluxation of the coccyx.

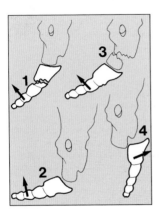

Treatment. Primarily, use of an inflatable rubber ring for sitting on and avoidance of constipation. If symptoms become chronic, local SWD or ultrasound may be tried, or the painful area injected with Bupivaine hydrochloride. If all conservative measures fail, consider excision of the coccyx.

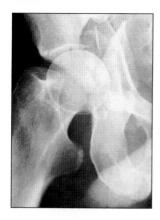

Central dislocation of the hip/fracture of the acetabulum

Here force transmitted through the femoral head fractures the pelvis. This may be from violence which is direct, such as a fall on the side, or indirect, as in a fall on the feet or from the impact of the knee on a car dashboard.

Diagnosis. Routine radiographs usually show characteristic disturbance of the acetabulum (**left**). There are, however, many patterns of injury due to variations in the amount and direction of the causal force. Pending full assessment, the patient should be treated for any accompanying shock, and skin traction (*c.* 4 kg) applied to the limb.

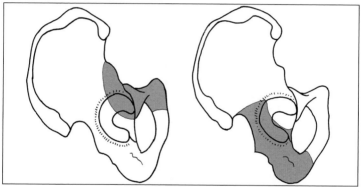

Assessment. When the hip joint is seriously disorganised, open reduction and internal fixation of the fragments can give good results. A very careful analysis is necessary to select the few cases suitable for this type of treatment. The first screening procedures should be a standard AP projection of the *pelvis* showing both hips on the one film, along with a lateral. If there is any significant displacement of the fragments or of the femoral head, oblique projections or preferably a CAT scan will be required.

First assess the integrity of the anterior and posterior columns. (The anterior column (**left**) is the mass of bone which stretches downwards from the anterior inferior iliac spine and includes the pubis and the anterior part of the acetabular floor. The posterior column (**right**) stretches upwards from the ischial tuberosity to the sciatic notch and includes the posterior part of the acetabular floor.) The particular column involved dictates the nature of any surgical approach. Secondly, you should assess the state of the floor of the acetabulum. (If this is highly fragmented, the chances of restoring it surgically are poor, so that in this particular group of fractures, conservative treatment is normally advised so long as the disruption does not exclude a subsequent hip replacement.)

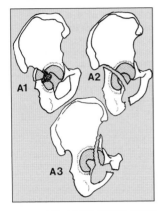

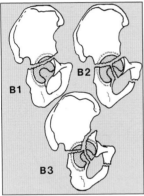

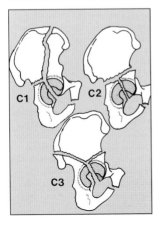

AO Classification of acetabular fractures.

Having assessed the state of the columns and the acetabular floor, you may find it helpful to relate your findings to the AO Classification of acetabular fractures.

In *Type A* fractures, one column only is involved, the other remaining intact.

A1: fractures of the posterior wall and variations; these injuries may be associated with posterior dislocation of the hip.

A2: fractures of the posterior column and variations.

A3: fractures of the anterior column and variations.

In *Type B* fractures, the main fracture line lies transversely. Part of the acetabular roof always remains in continuity with the ilium.

B1: transverse fracture, with or without involvement of the posterior acetabular wall.

B2: a vertical fracture added to the transverse fracture forms a T-fracture, of which there are several variations.

B3: a vertical fracture added to the transverse fracture involves the anterior column.

In *Type C* fractures, both columns are involved and no part of the acetabulum remains in continuity with the ilium.

C1: the portion of the fracture involving the anterior column extends to the iliac crest.

C2: the portion of the fracture involving the anterior column extends to the anterior border of the ilium.

C3: the fracture involves the sacroiliac joint.

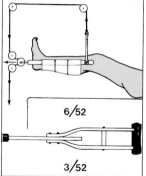

6/52

3/52

Treatment. If the displacement of the fracture is minimal or if the acetabular floor is highly fragmented, the injury may be treated conservatively with traction (e.g. Hamilton–Russell of 3 kg) for 6 weeks. Active hip movements should be pursued energetically during this period. Weight-bearing may be permitted after a further 3 weeks. Some loss of hip movements is inevitable, but overall function is often very good. Further treatment will only be required if secondary osteoarthritis supervenes.

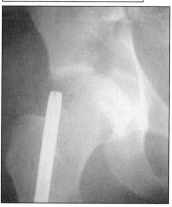

If the main weight-carrying part of the acetabulum is intact but the femoral head displaced, and if the disruption of the acetabulum is such that reduction and fixation of the main fragments is likely to be technically feasible, then surgical reconstruction and internal fixation are indicated. (The radiograph on the **left** shows a fracture of both columns, with an associated fracture of the femoral shaft which has been treated by intramedullary nailing.)

Open reduction of acetabular fractures is seldom easy. An extensive exposure is always required, and attendant haemorrhage is a common problem. There is often great difficulty in obtaining a substantial improvement in the position of the bone fragments and in holding them, so that operating time can be very long, increasing the risks of infection and other complications. Such surgery is contraindicated in the elderly or the unfit.

As these fractures involve highly vascular cancellous bone, the vigorous processes of repair may render reduction impossible if surgery is delayed for much longer than a week or so.

Assuming the patient is considered fit and suitable for surgery, that substantial blood replacement facilities are available and that the surgeon has the necessary skills and familiarity with the region, the choice of surgical exposure depends on which columns and which parts of the acetabulum have been involved. Surgical approaches include the Moore or Kocher for the posterior column, a Smith–Petersen or iliofemoral approach for the anterior column, and a Carnesale or Reinert for both. Once the fracture has been exposed, reduction may be facilitated by traction applied in the line of the femoral neck. Once this is achieved, the fragments may be held by the most appropriate methods which include cancellous screws and reconstruction plates.

COMPLICATIONS OF PELVIC FRACTURES

Haemorrhage

Substantial internal haemorrhage is common, particularly where there is disruption of the pelvic ring and proximal migration of the hemipelvis. Shock must be anticipated in all but the most minor of fractures by: • routine blood grouping and cross-matching • setting up a good intravenous line • monitoring the pulse rate, blood pressure and, where applicable, the urinary output. Replacement requirements are frequently substantial (transfusion in excess of 5 litres of whole blood is not uncommon) and additional measures for monitoring response (such as measuring central venous pressure) may be required. The effects of massive transfusion must be kept in mind and appropriate precautions taken (e.g. blood warming, addition of calcium, etc.).

In many cases, internal haemorrhage may be greatly reduced by the prompt stabilisation of the pelvic fracture by application of an external fixator as an emergency procedure. Where there is unstable disruption of the sacroiliac joint, an anti-shock C-clamp may also be helpful. The use of an anti-shock pneumatic garment has also been advocated.

Bruising appearing in the scrotum or buttock, or spreading diffusely along the line of the inguinal ligament are indications of major internal haemorrhage. In the abdomen, a large retroperitoneal haemorrhage may be felt as a discrete mass on palpation. If the peritoneum on the posterior abdominal wall has been broached, blood may escape into the abdominal cavity. Intraperitoneal haemorrhage may also result (rarely) from the tearing of mesenteric vessels. This is a serious complication and may be suspected by loss of bowel sounds, abdominal guarding, a progressive increase in abdominal girth, a blood-stained peritoneal tap and by ultrasound examination; it is an indication for abdominal exploration. Where haemorrhage is extraperitoneal, exploration is generally unprofitable and likely to aggravate blood loss; treatment in the first instance should be by fluid replacement.

Ischaemia in one leg is a grave sign and may be due to rupture or intimal damage to an iliac artery. If the patient's condition will permit, exploration of the vessel involved is indicated.

In the uncommon situation where the pelvic fracture has been stabilised and a massive transfusion programme has been carried out, yet the blood loss continues to gain over replacement, small-bore arterial bleeding may sometimes be brought under control by selective embolisation, using image intensifier angiography. Exploration may also be reconsidered. It is seldom that a single bleeding source can be found, the haemorrhage generally arising from massive disruption of the pelvic venous plexus, but occasionally successful results have been claimed from ligation of one or both internal iliac arteries.

Damage to the urethra and bladder

Out of every hundred fractures of the pelvis, roughly five are likely to have a urinary tract complication; more than two-thirds involve the urethra. Butterfly fractures are the main cause of urethral damage, while displaced fractures of the hemipelvis are generally responsible for the sharp edge of a superior public ramus rupturing the bladder.

Types of injury

Rupture of the membranous urethra. In the majority of cases the rupture is partial, with an intact portion of the urethral wall connected to the bladder. Less commonly there is complete rupture.

Extraperitoneal rupture of the bladder. This is usually caused by a sharp spike of bone penetrating the anterior wall.

Intraperitoneal rupture of the bladder. This may result from the same mechanism, but only occurs if the bladder is full at the time of injury.

Rupture of the penile urethra. Injuries of this type generally follow a fall astride a bar or similar object.

Diagnosis

- Suspicion should be aroused if the radiographs show either of the fracture patterns described.
- The presence of perineal bruising is highly suggestive.
- The presence of blood at the tip of the penis is diagnostic.
- If there is no penile blood, and damage to the bladder or urethra thought possible but not probable, the patient should be asked to attempt to pass urine. If the urine is clear, no further investigation or treatment is required. If after several tries he fails, try to palpate the bladder and consider catheterisation.
- Catheterisation carries the risk of converting a partial urethral tear into a complete one, and of introducing infection. A diagnostic catheterisation with a fine catheter should be abandoned if the catheter cannot be introduced with ease. If the tap is dry, this suggests intraperitoneal rupture of the bladder; blood-stained urine suggests an extraperitoneal tear of the bladder or a partial tear of the urethra; blood only suggests a major tear of the posterior urethra.
- If significant damage to the bladder or urethra is likely (e.g. penile blood), a urethrogram should be performed in preference to catheterisation.

Treatment

Intraperitoneal rupture of the bladder. The bladder is explored and the tear located and sutured. The bladder is then drained with a Foley catheter.

Extraperitoneal rupture of the bladder. The bladder is explored and the rupture repaired and drained by suprapubic catheterisation.

Incomplete tear of the urethra. If there is evidence of tearing of the membranous urethra, but the bladder is undisplaced, it is likely that some urethral tissue remains in continuity; a suprapubic drain is inserted and the urethrogram repeated after 10 days. If the circumstances are favourable, a Foley catheter may be introduced at this stage and the suprapubic catheter withdrawn. Later serial bouginage may be required.

Complete rupture of the urethra. If the bladder is floating free it must be drawn back down into position. This may be achieved by opening the bladder and rail-roading a Foley catheter downwards. After the balloon has been inflated, the catheter may be used for applying gentle traction. The bladder is drained by a suprapubic catheter which is kept in position for several days. The retropubic space may require separate drainage.

Rupture of the penile urethra. An incision is made over the tip of a catheter passed to the level of the obstruction. The catheter is then passed into the bladder through the other end of the urethra. If this cannot be located, the bladder will require opening. The urethra is then repaired, using the catheter as a stent.

Other complications

Injury to the bowel. The rectum may be torn in open fractures with perineal involvement, and rarely in closed injuries. Small bowel mesenteric or shearing tears (leading to infarction or perforation) may result from crushing injuries of the pelvis. Suspect this complication if there is abdominal rigidity, loss of bowel sounds, loss of liver dullness and distension. Exploration and a defunctioning colostomy are essential.

Rupture of the diaphragm. Routine chest radiographs should be taken in all major fractures of the pelvis as this complication is often overlooked. If a rupture is confirmed, a thoraco-abdominal repair through the bed of the eighth rib should be undertaken.

Paralytic ileus. This may result from disturbance of the autonomic outflow to the bowel due to the accumulation of a retroperitoneal haematoma. Treatment by nasogastric suction and intravenous fluids usually brings rapid resolution within 2–3 days.

Limb shortening. Shortening of one leg may result from persistent proximal displacement or rotation of the hemipelvis. Clinical measurement of the amount of shortening in these cases is often difficult, but examination of the radiographs may show the discrepancy in the level of the iliac crests. A correction (raise) should be made to the footwear if there is shortening of over 1.25 cm (1/2″).

Neurological damage. Neurological damage may involve: • the lumbosacral trunk at the triangle of Marcille in fractures involving displacement of the hemipelvis • isolated sacral nerves where the sacrum is fractured • the sciatic nerve as it passes behind the hip. Lesions in continuity predominate, and exploration is seldom indicated although some persistent disability is the rule. Impotence occurs in about a sixth of major pelvic fractures, and in about half of those cases in which there is rupture of the urethra. It is frequently permanent.

Obstetrical difficulties. Even in the case of quite marked post-fracture pelvic distortion, natural childbirth is rarely affected to the extent that caesarian section will be required. Where there has been a symphyseal disruption, this may recur, persist and warrant surgery.

Persistent sacroiliac joint pain. Sacroiliac pain is a common complication of pelvic fractures (especially where there has been clear involvement of a sacroiliac joint) and may be permanent. Where there has been a frank sacroiliac joint dislocation, the risks of severe, disabling pain are particularly high and are related to the degree of displacement. In some cases local fusion may be merited.

Persistent symphyseal instability. This is a rare complication and an indication for internal fixation; screening may be of help in confirming the diagnosis.

Osteoarthritis of the hip. This may follow central dislocation of the hip. It is dealt with along routine lines. Many cases may come to and are suitable for total hip replacement, and prior reduction of a major displacement will render this easier.

Myositis ossificans. This is seen most frequently after operative intervention or where there is an accompanying head injury. The treatment is along the lines previously indicated.

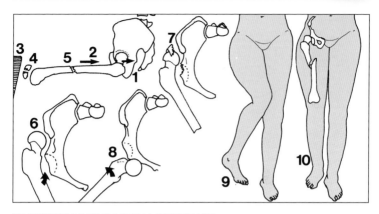

TRAUMATIC DISLOCATION OF THE HIP

The hip may dislocate (1) as a result of forces transmitted up the femoral shaft (2); this often occurs from dashboard impact (3) in road traffic accidents. *Note that this mechanism may be responsible for simultaneous fracture of the patella (4) or of the femoral shaft (5).* The hip may also dislocate from falls from a height, or a blow on the back of someone kneeling. If the leg is flexed at the hip and *adducted* at the time of impact, the femur dislocates posteriorly, and internally rotates (6). In some cases, the posterior lip of the acetabulum is fractured (7). If the hip is *abducted*, the hip may dislocate anteriorly and externally rotate (8).

Diagnosis. In a typical posterior dislocation, the hip is held slightly flexed, adducted and internally rotated (9). The leg appears short. Few other injuries are associated with the agony accompanying posterior dislocation, and this is almost as diagnostic as the deformity. Pain is less severe if the acetabulum is fractured, and the deformity may be concealed if there is an associated femoral fracture (10). Look for evidence of sciatic nerve involvement.

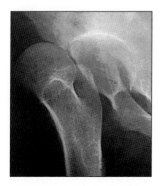

Radiographs. The deformity is usually obvious on the AP projection, but *dislocation cannot be excluded with one view.* A lateral projection is also helpful in confirming the distinction between an anterior and a posterior dislocation, and is *essential* if no abnormality is obvious on the AP film. The radiograph on the **left** shows an obvious posterior dislocation. An acetabular rim fracture should also be looked for. If a large or comminuted acetabular fracture is found, there is an increased risk of sciatic nerve palsy, instability after reduction and secondary osteoarthritis.

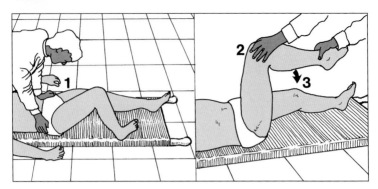

Reduction. Reduction should be carried out as soon as possible as the complication rate is lowest in those treated within 6 hours of the injury. The key to success is *complete* muscle relaxation; the anaesthetist should be reminded of this and of the need to lower the patient to the floor. An assistant should kneel at the side and steady the pelvis (1). When the patient is fully relaxed (and the administration of a muscle relaxant just prior to manipulation is invaluable) the knee and hip (2) are flexed gently to a right angle, at the same time gently correcting the adduction and internal rotation deformities (3). (*Note:* in the illustration the assistant's hands have been omitted for clarity.)

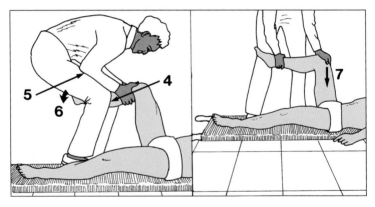

The head of the femur should now be lying directly behind the acetabulum and just requires to be lifted forwards. The force required is variable, but great leverage can be obtained by gripping the leg between the knees (4), resting your forearms on your thighs (5) and flexing your knees (6). The assistant keeps the pelvis from lifting by downward pressure. Reduction usually occurs with an obvious 'clunk'. It is often less striking when there is a rim fracture, and if one is present (as the radiographs will have shown), the stability of the reduction should always be checked by downward pressure on the femur (7). Gross instability is an indication for open reduction and internal fixation of the rim fracture.

Check radiographs. These should be taken in two planes, and some advocate post-manipulation CAT scans. The following possibilities arise: (a) The dislocation has been fully reduced. (b) The dislocation and a rim fracture have both been reduced, and the hip is stable clinically. *In both (a) and (b), further treatment is conservative.* (c) Although the femoral head is concentric with the acetabulum, the joint space is increased. This should be investigated, preferably by a CAT scan. Persistent displacement may be due to a trapped bone fragment or infolding of the labrum. The former should be removed by surgery, as if left it will lead to rapid onset osteoarthritis. A trapped labrum may also be excised, but there is some justification for a 'wait-and-see' approach. (d) There is persistent displacement of a fracture of the rim and the hip is unstable. (e) There is a displaced fracture of the rim with a persisting sciatic palsy. Operative reduction and internal (screw) fixation of the fragment are indicated in (d) and (e).

After-care. With a view to reducing complications, the hip may be rested in a Thomas splint for 4 weeks, with bed mobilisation for a further 2 weeks before weight-bearing. Many advocate much shorter periods of recumbency. If there is a rim fracture, weight-bearing should be deferred until about 8 weeks post-injury.

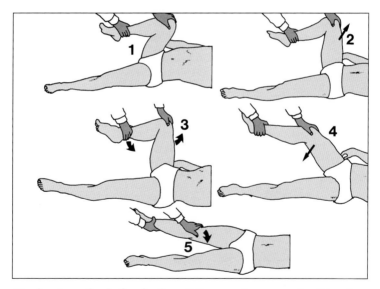

Bigelow's method of reduction. Failure to reduce a posterior dislocation of the hip by the method described is uncommon, and is generally due to insufficient muscle relaxation. If failure occurs, Bigelow's method may be tried. In essence, the hip is reduced by a continuous movement of circumduction which may be broken down into five stages: the hip is fully flexed (1) and then abducted (2); the joint is smoothly externally rotated (3) and then gradually extended (4). As extension of the hip progresses, the externally rotated limb is turned into the neutral position (5).

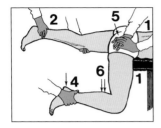

Stimson's method. This is occasionally attempted when a general anaesthetic must be withheld or where there is an associated femoral fracture. The patient is turned into the prone position (**1**) over the end of the table which supports the pelvis. The good leg is held by an assistant (**2**). The affected leg is flexed at the knee and held at the ankle in the neutral position (**4**). The hip may be reduced by direct pressure over the head of the femur (**5**) or, if the femur is intact, by downward pressure on the upper calf (**6**). This may be done manually or by the stockinged foot; the latter procedure allows simultaneous application of pressure over the head of the femur as at (**5**).

Anterior dislocation of the hip
The leg is usually held in abduction and external rotation, and there may be swelling and later bruising in the groin. Anterior dislocation may be complicated by femoral vein compression (with the risks of thrombosis and embolism), by femoral nerve paralysis or by femoral artery compression.

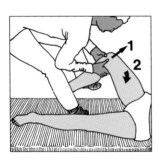

Reduction: standard method (upper illustration). An assistant steadies the pelvis of the well-anaesthetised patient. Flexing the hip (**1**) and correcting the abduction and external rotation (**2**) convert an anterior dislocation into a posterior dislocation. At the end of this procedure the head of the femur is lifted up as before into the acetabulum. (*Note*: Persistent absence of the peripheral pulses after reduction is an indication for exploration.)

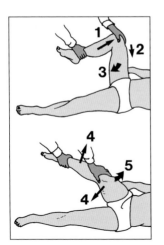

Reduction: Bigelow's method (lower two illustrations). This method is less reliable for routine use, but may be tried in the difficult case. Circumduction of the hip is again carried out in the following order of movements:

(1) fully flex the hip
(2) adduct the hip
(3) internally rotate
(4) extend the knee and hip
(5) bring the hip into the neutral position.

Complications of dislocation of the hip

Irreducible dislocation. This may result from in-turning of the labrum or by bony fragments trapped in the acetabulum. Open reduction is necessary, *but be certain* that the patient has been completely relaxed during the attempts at closed reduction.

Fracture of the femoral head. An osteochondral fracture of the femoral head may remain displaced after reduction of the hip. Small fragments should be excised, but large fragments should be replaced and fixed.

Intracapsular fracture of the femoral neck. The risks of avascular necrosis are extremely high, and the following treatment should be considered: • in the elderly, excision of the femoral head, and replacement with a Thomson or similar prosthesis • in the middle-aged, total hip replacement • in the young, open reduction and internal fixation through a posterolateral approach.

Slipped upper femoral epiphysis complicating hip dislocation. Treat by open reduction and internal fixation through a posterolateral approach.

Extracapsular fracture of the femoral neck. The fracture should be dealt with first by open reduction and the insertion of a pin and plate or similar device. The dislocation may then be reduced by manipulation.

Fracture of the femoral shaft. It is sometimes possible to treat both injuries conservatively, reducing the hip dislocation by Stimson's method and treating the femoral fracture in a Thomas splint. If Stimson's method fails, it may be possible to apply sufficient traction to the upper fragment by a substantial threaded screw inserted percutaneously into the greater trochanter: but it is more satisfactory to expose the femoral shaft and reduce the dislocation by means of a heavy duty bone clamp applied directly to the upper fragment. Thereafter the femoral shaft may be internally fixed.

Fracture of the patella and other knee injuries. The dislocation should be reduced by any of the methods described and the knee injury treated as if it were an isolated one.

Sciatic nerve palsy. This complicates about 10% of dislocations of the hip. Fortunately, three out of four are incomplete, and about half recover completely. If no improvement follows reduction of the hip, exploration is indicated within the first 24 hours of injury *only* if there is a large or comminuted rim fracture which may possibly be causing persistent local pressure on the nerve. Otherwise this complication should be managed conservatively. When the patient is mobilised, a drop foot splint may be required, with precautions to avoid trophic ulceration.

Avascular necrosis. The inevitable tearing of the hip joint capsule accompanying dislocation of the hip may disturb the blood supply to the femoral head; in about 10% of cases this may lead to avascular necrosis. X-ray changes are usually, but not always, seen within 12 months of injury. Clinically, persistent discomfort in the groin and restriction and pain on internal rotation are suggestive of the presence of this complication.

Secondary osteoarthritis of the hip. This is the inevitable sequel to avascular necrosis, but may also occur when dislocation of the hip is accompanied by a fracture involving the articular surfaces. It is also seen as late as 5–10 years after injury; the cause then is less clear, but it may possibly arise from articular cartilage damage concurrent with the initial injury. (An MRI scan at an early stage may sometimes confirm potentially harmful articular cartilage damage.) In the young patient, hip fusion may be considered, but generally total hip replacement is the treatment of choice.

Recurrent dislocation. This complication is rare; operative fixation of a large acetabular rim fragment in a hip which is demonstrated to be unstable clinically may largely avoid it. Otherwise, a bone–block type of repair may have to be considered.

Myositis ossificans. This is seen most frequently following exploration of the hip or when the dislocation is accompanied by a head injury. It may lead to virtual fusion of the hip. The risk of this complication may be minimised in the following ways: • avoid surgery if possible • splint the hip following reduction • avoid passive movements of the hip in the head injury case with limb spasticity. Late excision (say after 1 year) of a discrete bone mass may restore function, but the recurrence rate in other circumstances is high.

Late diagnosed dislocation. This is a euphemism for a dislocation that has been missed. Always suspect that a dislocation of the hip may be accompanying a fracture of the patella or femur. If discovered within a week of injury, manipulation may be attempted. *After a week and up to several months,* good results have been claimed by heavy (up to 18 kg) skeletal traction under sedation for up to 3 weeks: when the radiographs show the femoral head level with the acetabulum, the leg is placed in abduction and the traction decreased. If this fails, open reduction may be attempted; in either case a good result is achieved in many cases. *After a year* open reduction is unlikely to be possible, and an upper femoral (Schanz) osteotomy may have to be considered.

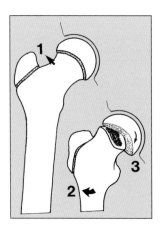

Slipped upper femoral epiphysis

The term is misleading, as in fact it is the femoral shaft which moves proximally (1) and externally rotates (2) on the epiphysis. Only occasionally is there movement of the epiphysis relative to the acetabulum (3). There is never any juxtaepiphyseal fracture (i.e. it is a Salter–Harris type I lesion). It occurs in adolescence, and hormonal factors may play a part in the aetiology. It is commoner in males, occurs at adolescence and those affected are often adipose and sexually immature, or are very tall and thin. It is often bilateral, and there is a history of injury in less than 30%.

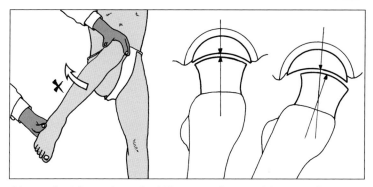

Diagnosis. The condition should be *suspected* in any adolescent with a history of limp and occasional groin or knee pain, especially if belonging to one of the body types described. On clinical examination the leg is usually held externally rotated at the hip, and movements of internal rotation are restricted (**left above**).

Radiographs. A *lateral projection* is essential as the earliest signs are more obvious than in the AP. A line drawn up the centre of the neck and shaft should normally bisect the epiphyseal base of the head. In a grade 1 shift, the resulting angle is less than 30°; grade 2 is between 30° and 60°; and grade 3 over 60°.

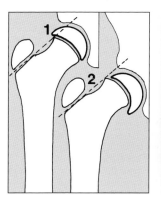

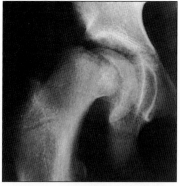

In the AP view, slip is less obvious but nevertheless may be detected with experience. In the normal hip (**1**) a tangent to the neck should cut through a portion of the epiphysis. When slip is present (**2**) this is no longer the case. In the radiographs, also look for evidence of new bone formation (buttressing) at the inferior and posterior aspects of the neck, signifying chronicity. In an *acute slip*, the history is short (less than 3 weeks) and the radiographs show slipping without buttressing (**above right**). Where an *acute slip is superimposed on a degree of chronic slip*, there is often a history of intermittent limp and discomfort for several weeks, with recent sudden deterioration; any buttressing is slight. With a *chronic slip*, the history is of many weeks' duration, and buttressing is a feature.

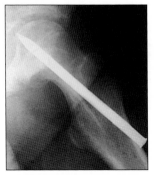

Treatment. Avascular necrosis, chondrolyis and coxa vara are the main complications of this condition, and every step must be taken to avoid them. Avascular necrosis may follow forcible manipulation but other causal factors have not yet been fully elucidated. To avoid any inherent risk in manipulation, all grade 1 and grade 2 slips should be internally fixed in situ (usually with a single screw). This should be done whether the slips are acute or chronic, or stable or unstable. (Unstable slips may be diagnosed by the patient's inability to weight bear.) Grade 3 slips are technically difficult to fix in situ, as little of the epiphysis is available to take the screw. As the risks of manipulation seem minimal if performed within the first 24 hours of an acute slip, this should be considered. (The procedure is carried out on an orthopaedic table with *light* traction, turning the leg into 20° of internal rotation and moving it into 20–30° of abduction. If fresh films confirm that the position has thereby been improved, the slip should then be fixed in situ; if not, a corrective wedge osteotomy should be performed.) If a grade 3 case is first seen 24 hours or more after an acute slip, admit and apply light traction for 3 weeks—after which a decision should be made regards pinning in situ or a wedge osteotomy.

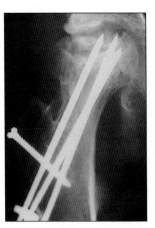

Avascular necrosis **(left)** is the most serious complication in the adolescent, and every attempt must be made to avoid it by: • prompt diagnosis • rejection of any attempt to reduce the deformity by forcible manipulation • avoidance of unsuitable internal fixation device • meticulous handling of the epiphysis and its vascular supply during any (now rarely performed) operative intervention. *Treatment:* in the established case, a choice may have to be made between: (i) the uncertain results of osteotomy; (ii) the difficulty of hip arthrodesis and the risks of late secondary osteoarthritis in the knee, other hip and spine; (iii) the risks and long-term uncertainties of total hip replacement.

Involvement of other hip
In keeping with the aetiology, the other hip may be affected at any time. This is particularly liable to be overlooked if the patient is being rested in bed during treatment of the primary complaint. Routine repeated X-rays of both hips is advised, particularly in the recumbent patient. If the second hip is involved, treatment is pursued along the lines already described.

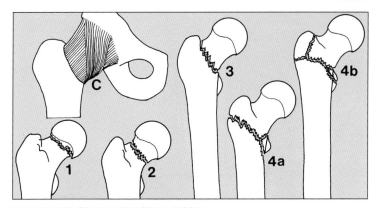

FRACTURES OF THE FEMORAL NECK

Level of fracture. Four sites are well recognised, the most important being
(1) subcapital and (2) transcervical. The distinction between these two is rather
blurred, as rotation in the plane of the X-rays may be misleading. Both,
however, lie clearly within the joint capsule (C) and are well described as
intracapsular fractures. The other common sites are *extracapsular.* In the
intertrochanteric or basal fracture (3), the fracture line runs along the base of the
femoral neck, between the trochanters. In pertrochanteric fractures (4), the
fracture line involves the trochanters, one (a) or both (b) of which may be
fractured or separated, so that in effect this is often a comminuted fracture.

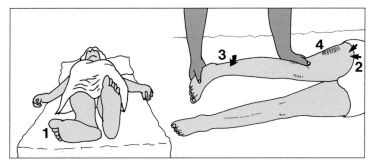

Aetiology. The incidence increases with age, and in later life is much
commoner in women, where osteoporosis is an important factor. Below the age
of 60, femoral neck fractures (usually extracapsular) are commoner in men.

Diagnosis. Inability to bear weight in an elderly patient after a fall is most
likely to be due to this common fracture, which must always be excluded.
External rotation of the limb is a valuable (but not invariable) sign (1). *Tenderness*
will be found over the femoral neck anteriorly (2) or laterally in extracapsular
fractures. *Pain* is produced by rotation of the hip (3). *Bruising* (4) is a *late* sign in
extracapsular fractures, and is absent in acute injuries and in intracapsular
fractures. Rarely, with an undisplaced fracture, weight-bearing may be possible.

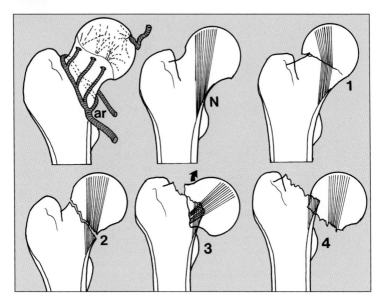

Intracapsular fractures

Features. There are two main problems associated with intracapsular fractures of the femoral neck. Firstly, the blood supply to the femoral head (which is derived principally from an arterial ring **(ar)** at the base of the neck) may be seriously disturbed, leading to *avascular necrosis*. Secondly, the head fragment is often a shell containing fragile cancellous bone which affords poor anchorage for any fixation device. Difficulty in obtaining good fixation and persisting mobility at the fracture site may lead to *non-union*. It follows that complications are most frequent in *proximally situated and displaced fractures*.

Garden classification. Any displacement should be assessed along the lines laid down by Garden which amongst other things take into account the disturbance of the weight-carrying trabeculae radiating from the calcar femorale. (**N** = normal.)

Type 1 fractures. The inferior cortex is not completely broken, but the trabeculae are angulated (abduction fracture).

Type 2 fractures. The fracture line is complete and the inferior cortex is clearly broken. The trabecular lines are interrupted but are not angulated. In both type 1 and type 2 fractures there is no obvious displacement of the major fragments relative to one another.

Type 3 fractures. Here the fracture line is obviously complete. There is rotation of the femoral head in the acetabulum, the proximal fragment being abducted and internally rotated. This may be apparent from the disturbance in the trabecular pattern. The fracture is *slightly displaced*.

Type 4 fracture. In this, the severest grade, the fracture is fully displaced, and the femoral head tends to lie in the neutral position in the acetabulum. Garden type 3 and 4 fractures of the femoral neck carry the worst prognosis.

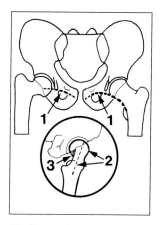
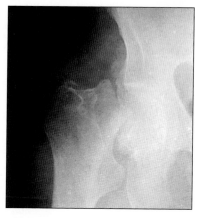

Radiographs. An AP radiograph of the pelvis with a lateral of the affected hip are best for screening of this area. Generally, the fracture line is obvious, but if not look for asymmetry in Shenton's lines **(1)** and in the lateral, angulation of the head with respect to the neck **(2)** or fragmentation **(3)**. If there is any remaining doubt, a localised AP view should be taken; if this appears negative, re-examine by bone scan after 48 hours, or repeat the plain films after 1–2 weeks. The radiograph on the **right** shows a typical subcapital Garden type 4 fracture. The femoral head is lying in the neutral position relative to the acetabulum.

Treatment of intracapsular fracture
General principles. Intracapsular fractures may be treated by:

- reduction and internal fixation
- by primary replacement of the femoral head (hemiarthroplasty or bi-polar arthroplasty)
- total hip replacement
- conservative measures.

Methods
Young and middle-aged adults. Most centres advocate closed reduction and internal fixation of all grades of intracapsular fracture.

Elderly patients. Those with Type 2 fractures are also usually treated by closed reduction and internal fixation. Type 1 fractures are generally treated in the same way in order to avoid the risks of disimpaction, but in a very few centres are managed conservatively. In the elderly fit patient, internal fixation is usually extended to include fractures of types 3 and often type 4, the view being that if the complications of avascular necrosis or non-union supervene, the patient will be able to tolerate a later, secondary procedure (usually a total hip replacement).

Where the risks of either of these complications are considered in the otherwise fit elderly patient to be particularly high (e.g. a badly displaced, proximally situated type 4 fracture), then a primary total hip replacement procedure may be considered. Where the patient is less fit, with a life expectancy of perhaps a few but not many years and the risks of complication are also thought to be high, a hemiarthroplasty may be considered.

Investigations. A few days' delay prior to fixation of the fracture seems to have only a marginal effect on the prognosis, and this interval may be employed with profit to bring the patient into the optimal medical state. The following investigations may prove invaluable in assessment and are performed routinely in many centres:

- chest radiograph and, if there is a productive cough, a sputum film and culture
- electrocardiograph
- full blood count, with at some stage grouping and cross-matching of blood for surgery
- estimation of the serum urea and electrolytes
- routine charting of fluid input and output.

General treatment

- *Preliminary skin traction* (3–4 kg) may help to relieve initial pain and minimise further displacement of the fracture.
- *Analgesics, tranquillisers and hypnotics* appropriate to the patient's pain, age and mental state should be prescribed.
- *Intravenous fluids* are given routinely in many units (with caution where there are concurrent respiratory and cardiovascular problems) to combat dehydration and minimise the risks of anaemia. (A raised serum urea is clearly associated with a poor prognosis in femoral neck fractures.) Whole blood or packed cells may be required if the patient is markedly anaemic. The type and quantity of replacement are determined by the urinary output, the urea, electrolyte and haemoglobin levels, and the respiratory and cardiac state. Oral fluids are encouraged.
- *The physiotherapist* may give valuable assistance in the management of the moist chest.
- *Nursing* of the highest standard is required if, in particular, pressure sores are to be avoided, especially in the heavy patient who is afraid to move because of pain.
- *Antibiotics* may be prescribed where there is a heavy purulent spit or frank urinary tract infection; although treatment may be started immediately, bacteriological confirmation must be sought.

Fixation. A large number of systems have been developed for the internal fixation of intracapsular fracture. None meet all criteria that are desirable in this exacting situation. Most of the design problems relate to the softness of the bone and restricted size of the proximal fragment; it is often difficult to grip it in a manner that will not further imperil its dubious blood supply, while at the same time holding the fragments in close, reliable and continuing proximity, without penetration of the femoral head or extrusion of the device.

The AO dynamic hip screw (DHS) addresses most of the difficulties, and it and its variations are in widespread use for the treatment of most femoral neck fractures. It is inserted in a *blind procedure;* the fracture site is not exposed, but its reduction and the placement of the device are visualised with an image intensifier.

After-care. One of the aims of internal fixation is rapid mobilisation, and in most cases on the day following surgery the patient can be allowed out of bed to sit. Early (i.e. within the first week) weight-bearing does not seem to affect the union of intracapsular fractures in a material way and should therefore be encouraged as soon as the patient's general condition will permit. After the wound has healed, the patient may often be allowed home, depending on her mobility and social circumstances. A domiciliary domestic assessment by an occupational therapist is often invaluable in making a decision in this respect.

Out-patient attendances, with check radiographs every 4–6 weeks, should be arranged until the patient is independent; thereafter, she should be seen at intervals of 6 months to 1 year for a total of 3 years to allow detection of avascular necrosis which may be late in declaring itself.

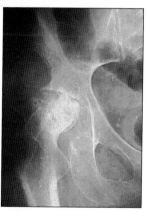

Complications

(1) Avascular necrosis. The cause is disruption of the blood supply by the fracture at the time of injury. There is complaint of increasing pain, a limp and deteriorating function. In some cases there may be a good period of several months before the condition declares itself.

Radiological changes: these are usually present within the first year, but may not show for as long as 3 years. The whole femoral head may be involved, with increased density, loss of sphericity, joint space narrowing and secondary OA lipping **(left)**. In less severe cases, changes may show only in the weight-bearing portion of the head ('superior segmental necrosis').

Treatment: mild symptoms may be controlled with analgesics. In severe cases in the young patient, a MacMurray osteotomy should be considered; in the older patient, a total hip replacement is usually advised.

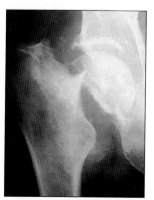

(2) Non-union. This is most often seen in grade 3 and 4 fractures. In the young patient, bone grafting may be considered. In the older patient, especially where an untreated fracture has come seriously adrift **(left)** or where there is rounding of the bone ends, sclerosis or marked cystic changes in the neck, prosthetic replacement of the femoral head (hemiarthroplasty) or total hip replacement are the treatments of choice. A Pauwel's osteotomy is a useful procedure both in the young and in the old (up to the age of 70) for whom a total hip replacement is a fall-back procedure.

Alternative treatments of intracapsular fractures

Non-operative management. All impacted fractures (Garden 1 and some Garden 2) may be treated conservatively, and this is an important consideration, especially where in an ageing population these fractures are on the increase, and where surgical time is in heavy demand. Overall a lower mortality rate has been claimed in those treated conservatively as opposed to surgically. *Method:* (1) The leg is rested in a gutter splint until pain settles (usually after about a week). (2) Partial weight-bearing with crutches is then commenced and continued for 8 weeks, after which full unsupported weight-bearing may be allowed. (3) Check radiographs are taken 2 days after the start of mobilisation, and thereafter every 2 weeks until the eighth week. (4) If the fracture disimpacts and becomes unstable (a 14% incidence only is claimed) then active treatment becomes necessary, when a hemi- or total arthroplasty may be performed. Disimpaction is seen most often in those over age 70, especially those in poor general health, or in the younger patient with a low life expectancy. The problems of prolonged recumbency in the elderly may nevertheless follow this line of treatment.

Hemiarthroplasty. A Thompson prosthesis or similar device may be used with or without cement, especially in the elderly patient with a fracture which has a high risk of non-union or avascular necrosis. There is a tendency to late, slow erosion of the acetabulum, so that it is best reserved for the patient who is not likely to have a long or very active life. The use of a bi-polar prosthesis is sometimes preferred for the slightly fitter elderly patient.

Total hip replacement. If successful, this affords the patient the greatest chance of returning to her pre-fracture state. This more major procedure is fully justified if the patient is in good health, physically and mentally active, and the unit's mortality and morbidity figures are low.

Other fixation methods. These include: • Three or more Moore or Knowles pins. These are of particular value in children, as they have the least effect on the blood supply of the head; they may be inserted percutaneously. • Three or four self-tapping cannulated screws (e.g. MAGNA-Fx™, AO).

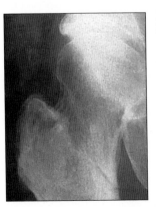

Intertrochanteric basal neck fractures

Fractures of this type (**left**) are extracapsular and in the adult are not associated with avascular necrosis. Good internal fixation can usually be achieved with a dynamic hip screw (DHS) and plate (see following page).

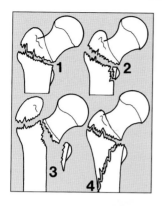

Pertrochanteric fractures

These lie distal to the intertrochanteric line and several patterns are common. The fracture line may pass through the mass of the greater trochanter and run to the lesser trochanter without (1) or with (2) its separation. They are often highly fragmented, with separation of the greater and usually the lesser trochanter (3). The fracture may be continuous with a spiral fracture of the proximal femoral shaft (4).

Treatment. Where there is little or no fragmentation, stability is not a problem, and a dynamic hip screw with a long plate will give adequate fixation.

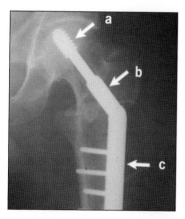

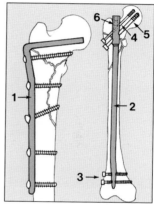

In the unstable fracture, it is difficult to obtain strong reliable fixation although an AO dynamic hip screw (**above, a**), tensioned in a sleeve (**b**) and attached to the shaft with a long plate (**c**), is often employed. Alternative devices include the AO dynamic condylar screw (1), a rigid all-in-one device screwed to the femoral shaft. With further involvement of the shaft, a Russell–Taylor reconstruction (locking) nail (2) offers considerable versatility. This has slots distally (3) for locking screws. There are proximal slots for cancellous screws (4, 5) which can be locked with a separate screw (6). A Gamma nail and external fixators may also be used. Non-weight-bearing on crutches can usually be started after 48 hours, and union on average takes 16 weeks.

Intertrochanteric and pertrochanteric fractures may also be treated by bed rest and skeletal traction, with a Thomas splint for additional support. Indications include unfitness for anaesthesia and problems with other injuries; but the period of immobilisation will always be long.

After-care. In stable fractures with high quality internal fixation, the patient may be mobilised early, with weight-bearing at any stage. In less stable injuries, the decision when to permit weight-bearing is dependent on the rigidity of the form of fixation employed. In the very unstable fracture, premature weight-bearing may lead to mechanical failure of the internal fixation device, and it is often wise to advocate non-weight-bearing with crutches until callus appears and is seen to be offering appreciable local reinforcing support.

Complications. The commonest complication is failure of fixation with drift into coxa vara (usually secondary to cutting out of the fixation device). If this occurs before much callous has appeared, it can usually be corrected by returning the patient to bed and applying skeletal traction of 5–7 kg. This is maintained till union is established. If coxa vara is discovered late, the position has usually to be accepted.

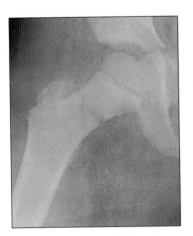 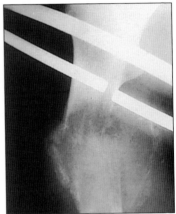

Fractures of the femoral neck in children
These rare injuries result from severe violence, the undisplaced transcervical fracture (**left**) being commonest.

Treatment. *All undisplaced fractures* should be treated with a hip spica till united. Complications are low in this group. In *displaced fractures* under age 10 years, reduce by manipulation and fix with Knowles pins. If reduction fails or if the child is over 10, primary subtrochanteric osteotomy with plaster fixation is advised to reduce the incidence of non-union and coxa vara. Open reduction is undertaken in *subcapital fracture–dislocations* where the capital epiphysis has been extruded from the joint, but avascular necrosis is virtually inevitable.

Subtrochanteric fractures. These are often due to metastases. If the patient's general condition is very poor, pain relief may be obtained by traction in a Thomas splint (right). In all other cases, internal fixation is advocated, using for example, a Russell–Taylor Reconstruction nail, with acrylic cement packed into any large osteolytic defect. Immediate mobilisation may then be possible.

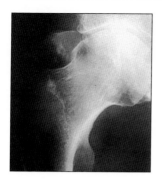

Trochanteric fractures. Isolated fractures of the greater **(left)** or lesser trochanters may result from sudden muscle contraction (i.e. avulsion of the insertions of gluteus medius or iliopsoas). Fractures of the greater trochanter may also be caused by direct violence. Only symptomatic treatment is required, and the patient may be mobilised after a few days' bed rest. Some, however, advocate internal fixation of a severely displaced trochanter to reduce the risks of a Trendelenberg limp.

General principles: femoral
    fractures 434
Conservative treatment 434
Non-conservative treatment
    of femoral fractures 444
Complications of fractures of
    the femur 450
General treatment
    guidelines: femoral
    fractures 451
Injuries of the patella and
    extensor mechanism of
    the knee 452
Medial, lateral and cruciate
    ligament injuries 457
Meniscus injuries 459
Fractures of the tibial tables
    461

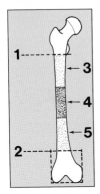

GENERAL PRINCIPLES: FEMORAL FRACTURES
Classification of femoral shaft fractures.
In the AO system the femoral shaft is defined as, in effect, stretching between the inferior margin of the lesser trochanter (1) and the upper border (2) of a square containing the distal end of the femur. For descriptive purposes, the shaft (or diaphyseal segment) may in turn be divided into proximal (3), middle (4) and distal thirds (5). The proximal third is sometimes referred to as the subtrochanteric zone.

Causes of fracture. Considerable violence is usually required, and the common causes include road traffic accidents, falls from a height and crushing injuries. Osteoporosis, metastatic deposits and bone erosions at the stems of hip replacements may cause pathological fractures.

Fluid loss. In a *simple* (closed) fracture, blood loss of 0.5–1.0 litre into the tissues is common. Open fractures are accompanied by greater blood loss, and this is generally greatest in those *open from without in*. Blood replacement is often required in closed fractures and is normally essential in open ones; grouping, cross-matching and setting up of an intravenous line should be done routinely (except in children). In the transport of patients to hospital, temporary splintage will help reduce local bleeding and shock.

Diagnosis. Weight-bearing is impossible and there is abnormal mobility at the level of the fracture. The leg is often externally rotated, abducted and shortened. Radiographs confirm the diagnosis. *It is most important to exclude concurrent fracture of the patella, and anterior, posterior and central dislocations of the hip.*

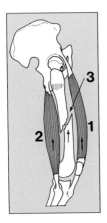

CONSERVATIVE TREATMENT
The first principle to appreciate is that the large muscle masses of the quadriceps (1) and hamstrings (2) tend to produce displacement and shortening (3). Traction can overcome this, and is the basis of most conservative methods of treatment.

Traction methods
Skin traction with adhesive strapping. This is used in children and young adults. There are occasional problems with skin sensitivity and pustular infections under the strapping.

Skeletal traction. A Steinman pin through the tibial tuberosity is usually employed. This is preferred in the older patient with inelastic skin and where heavy traction is required. There are occasional problems with pin-track infections.

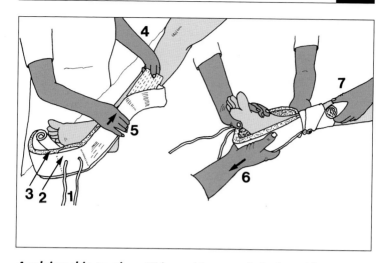

Applying skin traction. With care this can usually be done without an anaesthetic. Begin by shaving the skin. It is then traditional to swab or spray the skin with a mildly antiseptic solution of balsam of Peru in alcohol. This may facilitate the adhesion of the strapping.

Commercial traction sets use adhesive tapes which can stretch from side to side but not longitudinally. They come supplied with traction cords (1) and a spreader bar (2) with foam protection for the malleoli (3). Begin by applying the tape to the medial side of leg—do this by peeling off the protective backing with one hand (4) while pressing the tape down and advancing the other (5). The leg is then internally rotated and the tape applied to the outside of the leg, preferably being sited a little more posteriorly than on the medial side. *The tapes should extend up the leg as far as possible, irrespective of the site of the fracture.* Now apply traction to the leg (6) and finally secure the tapes throughout their length with encircling crepe bandages (7).

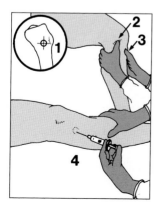

Applying skeletal traction. The preferred site is the upper tibia, a little under 2 cm (1″) posterior to the prominence of the tibial tuberosity (1). It is important to avoid the knee joint and, in children, the growth plate: so begin by carefully identifying the knee joint itself by flexing the knee (2) and noting its relationship to the tuberosity (3). If a general anaesthetic is not being employed, infiltrate the skin and tissue down to periosteum with local anaesthetic (e.g. 2–3 ml of 1% lignocaine) (4).

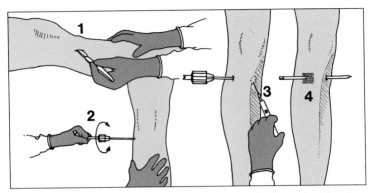

Now make a small incision in the skin (1), enough to take the traction pin only; insert it until the point strikes bone. Drive the pin through the lateral tibial cortex by applying firm pressure and twisting the chuck handle (2); insert the pin at right angles to the leg. You should feel it penetrate the bone and pass quickly with little resistance till it meets the medial cortex. Stop at this stage. Infiltrate down to periosteum on the medial side, using the lie of the pin to guide you to the expected exit area (3). Drive the pin through the medial cortex; make a small incision over the tenting skin to allow it to come through. Protect the openings with gauze strips soaked in Nobecutane or a similar sealant (4).

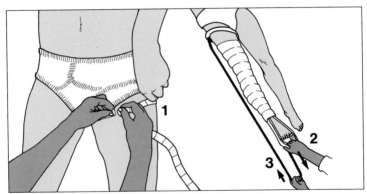

Traction systems: skin traction in a Thomas splint

The most important decision in selecting a Thomas splint is the *ring* size. To save time (e.g. before anaesthesia), the uninjured leg may be measured (1) and an allowance made for swelling, present and anticipated. It is nevertheless wise to have readily available a size above and below the estimate. Then, applying traction with one hand on the spreader bar (2), the selected splint is pushed up the leg (3). It should reach the ischial tuberosity (or more likely the perineum), and it should be possible to pass one finger beneath the ring round its complete circumference. If the ring is too large or too small, maintain traction while the next size is tried.

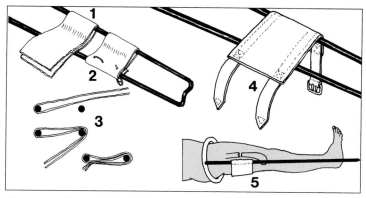

Thomas splint soft furnishings. There is much choice. Slings to bridge the side irons may be formed from strips of 15 cm (6″) wide calico bandage (1). It is traditional to secure these with large safety pins inserted from below, close to the outer iron (2). Sometimes spring clips are used. Alternatively, a double bandage thickness ensures greater rigidity (3). The sling placed directly beneath the fracture should preferably be unyielding, and one of canvas with web and buckle fastenings is often favoured (4). It is customary to apply the splint with the master sling (5) in position; the other slings are then attached and adjusted to the contours of the limb. Less satisfactorily, the splint is applied with all the slings already in position.

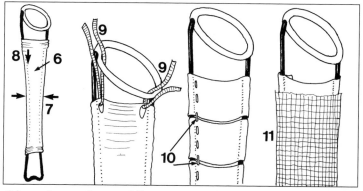

Calico and canvas slings can drift, separate or ruck, and many prefer the smoothness of an unbroken double thickness circular bandage (e.g. 'Tubigrip' (6)). This may 'waist' the splint (7), be less than firm under the fracture and may drift distally (8). The last may be prevented by anchoring it to the ring with ribbon gauze or bandage (9). If separate slings are used, their tendency to separate may be minimised by pinning each to its neighbour (10). Nevertheless, a layer of wool should be placed between them and the limb to smooth out any unevenness (11) (not necessary with circular woven bandage). In all cases, a large pad (e.g. of gamgee) should be placed directly beneath the fracture to act as a fulcrum.

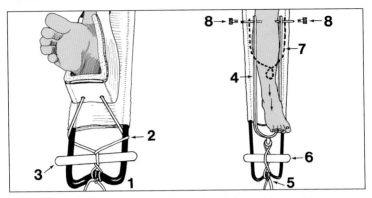

Traction details. In long oblique fractures and those with apposition, no manipulation will be needed and the traction system may be completed by tying the cords to the end of the splint (**1**). The convention of passing the medial cord under the corresponding iron helps to control the tendency to lateral rotation (**2**). A Chinese windlass, using a spatula or a metal rod may be used to take up slack (**3**). With skeletal traction, a Tulloch–Brown loop (**4**) permits a direct pull in the line of the limb. The loop may be tied to the end of the Thomas splint (**5**) and also tensioned with a windlass (**6**). A stirrup may be employed to prevent springing of the loop (**7**). Protect the sharp ends of the pin with caps (**8**) or corks.

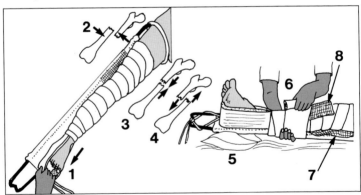

Manipulation. With the exception of the young child, manipulation is advisable if there is loss of bony apposition. With the splint in position, an assistant applies strong traction (**1**) while pressure is applied in the directions deduced from the radiographs (**2**). When the traction is eased off, the limb remains the same length if a hitch has been obtained (**3**), but telescopes if not (**4**). After the traction cords have been attached, raise the end of the splint on a pillow (**5**) while the limb is bandaged to the splint, using for example 15 cm (6″) crepe bandages (**6**). Note gamgee or wool padding behind the fracture to act as a fulcrum and behind the knee to keep it in slight flexion (**7**); and along the shin to avoid sores (**8**).

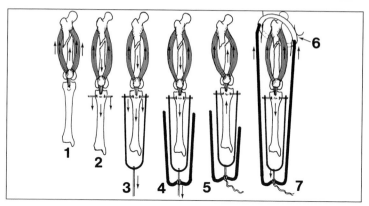

Fixed traction. The system described is referred to as fixed traction in a Thomas splint. It is important to understand the simple basic principles. Muscle tension (mainly quads and hams) tends to produce shortening (1); this can be overcome by traction, for example through a Steinman pin (2) aided by a loop and traction cord (3). If the traction cord is tied to a (theoretical) ringless Thomas splint, the reduction is maintained so long as a pull is kept on the cord (4); redisplacement occurs if the cord is released (5). This proximal migration is normally prevented by the ring (6) so that the reduction is maintained even when the traction cord is released (7). Note that muscle tone = tension in the traction cord = ring pressure.

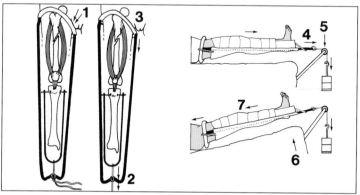

This pressure of the ring of the Thomas splint tends to produce sores (1) (especially in the perineal, groin and ischial tuberosity regions) and must be relieved (3). This is done by applying traction (*c.* 3 kg/8 lb) to the anchored cords (2). If ring pressure is unrelieved, *increase the traction weights.* The traction weights have a tendency to pull the patient down towards the foot of the bed (4). This may continue till the splint comes to rest on the traction pulley (5). This may be countered if it becomes a problem by raising the foot of the bed (6), when the traction weight is balanced by the upward component of the patient's body weight (7).

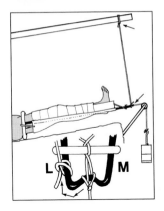

Supporting the limb and the splint
Fixed support. To allow the patient to move about the bed and prevent pressure on the heel, it is desirable to support the splint; this may be done most simply by tying a cord from the end of the splint to an overhead bar of the Balkan beam bed. The position of the suspension cord may be adjusted from near the midline to either side. (The illustration shows a lateral (**L**) attachment of the cord to help control the tendency to external rotation.) (**M** = medial.)

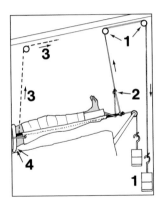

Lively supports. Some prefer a lively system which can be achieved in various ways, e.g. by weights and a system of pulleys (**1**). The suspension cord may be arranged in Y-fashion to straddle both irons of the Thomas splint (**2**). Support for the proximal end of the splint (**3**) is less clearly an advantage, although often pursued—it may cause extra pressure beneath the ring (**4**).

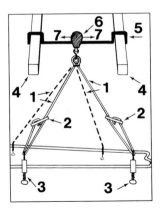

An alternative form of lively splint support ('the octopus') consists of elastic Bunjee cord (**1**), which can be adjusted with tensioners (**2**). The cords are attached to the splint with G-clamps (**3**) and to cross members of the Balkan beam (**4**) by means of a bar (**5**) along which a pulley (**6**) is free to move, allowing easy movement up and down the bed (**7**).

Check radiographs. These should be taken after the application of a Thomas splint, after any major adjustment, and thereafter at fortnightly intervals till union.

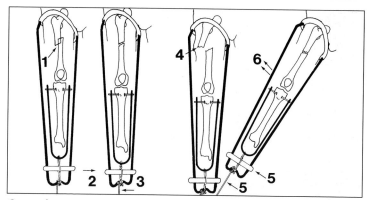

Corrections

Shortening. If there is persistent shortening (**1**), tighten the windlass in a fixed traction system (**2**). This will inevitably increase ring pressure and must be compensated by increasing the traction weight (**3**). (Soft tissue between the bone ends may nevertheless thwart reduction.)

Abduction. Where the proximal fragment is abducted (**4**), the situation may be improved by increasing the traction (**5**) and abducting the leg (**6**). The position of the ring traction pulley and the splint supports will require appropriate adjustment.

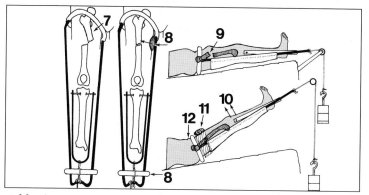

Adduction. If the proximal fragment is adducted (**7**), it may be helpful to apply a side thrust with a pad placed between the leg and the medial side iron, and increasing traction (**8**).

Flexion. This may be coupled with abduction and result from unresisted psoas and gluteal action (**9**); it is often a very painful complication. In the young patient, raising the splint (**10**) and/or abducting the leg and bandaging a local pad in position (**11**) may bring the fragments into alignment, but beware of pressure in the region of the anterior superior iliac spine (**12**). In the older patient, internal fixation is often preferred for femoral fractures of this type.

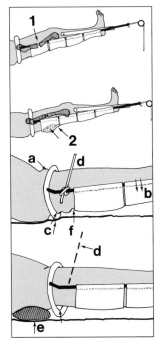

Posterior angulation. Backward sag at the fracture site (**1**) is perhaps the commonest residual deformity which is readily amenable to correction. If a continuous posterior support is used, the padding behind the fracture should be increased in thickness. If separate slings are used, the sling behind the fracture should be tightened and/or the padding behind the fracture increased (**2**).

After-care
The following items should be checked daily:

- *The ring area.* Tightness of the ring from swelling is especially common during the first 72 hours. (Normally it should be easy to put a finger under the ring at any point.) To avoid having to change the splint, split the ring with a hacksaw. Look also for impending pressure sores: if in the perineum, increase the ring traction weight; if at the anterior spine (**a**), lower the splint (**b**); if there is pressure behind the ring (**c**) decrease or remove any support weight (**d**) and place a pillow *above* the ring (**e**); pad the edge of the upper sling if needed (**f**).

- Look also for impending pressure sores and take appropriate action: *in the Achilles tendon region* if the slings stop at this level; *under the heel*, if the heel is included; and *over the malleoli.*
- Check for weakness of ankle dorsiflexion, indicative of common peroneal nerve palsy and necessitating careful inspection of the neck of the fibula where the cause is generally felting of the wool padding, transmitting pressure from the side iron. Repad, and fit a Sinclair foot support if the palsy is complete: expect recovery in 6 weeks.
- In those cases where skeletal traction is employed, look for: *loosening of the Steinman pin*—apart from recentring, other treatment is seldom required, so that traction may be continued; *pin-track infection*—a wound swab should be sent for bacteriological examination and the appropriate antibiotic administered. If infection is marked, the traction site may have to be abandoned; shifting and digging-in of the loop—adjust with padding.

The patient while in bed should practise quadriceps and general maintenance exercises. Splintage in children should be continued till union (6–12 weeks). In adults, where there is abundant callus and the fracture cannot be sprung, splintage may be discarded and the knee mobilised till there is sufficient mature callus to allow weight-bearing. Mobilisation of the knee joint and/or the patient may also be possible before union is complete. Methods include the use of a Pearson knee flexion piece, or where appropriate the application of a cast brace.

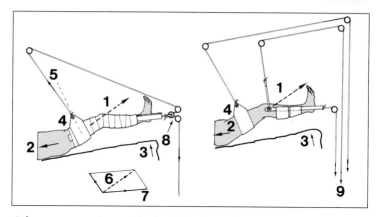

Other conservative methods of treatment

Hamilton–Russell traction. This is a form of balanced traction where the pull on the limb (1) is countered by the body weight (2) through the bed being raised (3). The fracture is supported by a padded canvas sling (4), angled slightly towards the head (5) to counter a tendency to distal drift. The theory behind the classical arrangement is that the line of pull on the femur is the resultant (6) of a parallelogram of forces, where the horizontal component (7) is doubled because of the pulley arrangement (8). Friction losses spoil the theory, and many prefer direct control of all forces (9). Balanced traction can be carried out using a Thomas splint bandaged to the limb, but unattached to any of the traction cords.

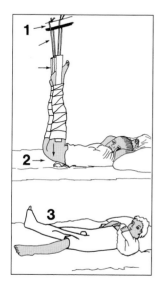

Gallows traction. Children up to the age of 3 years (or 4 if light) are ideally treated by this method, which may sometimes be used at home if the circumstances are suitable. Traction tapes are applied to both legs and fixed to an overhead beam (1) so that the child's buttocks are just clear of the bed (2), making nursing easy. The body weight is responsible for the traction. Gallows traction should not be used in the older child as there is the risk of vascular spasm and peripheral gangrene.

Hip spica. Stable femoral shaft fractures may be supported by a plaster hip spica; this must include the injured leg to the toes, the other leg to above the knee and extend to above the nipple line (3). A hip spica may be used for the fretful child where good nursing care is available at home (with fortnightly out-patient reviews) or for the badly infected open fracture in the adult.

NON-CONSERVATIVE TREATMENT OF FEMORAL FRACTURES
Intramedullary nailing
In many centres, internal fixation by intramedullary nailing is considered the preferred treatment for femoral shaft fractures in the adult. The prime advantage is that it generally permits early mobilisation of the patient, lessening the risks of pulmonary, circulatory, renal, joint stiffness and other complications, while promoting muscle activity and functional recovery. It may also alleviate problems of bed occupancy (which is the historic reason for its introduction).

Intramedullary nailing is of particular value in cases of multiple injuries, where its use is advocated if the patient's general condition will allow. The main patterns of nail include the following:

- Plain intramedullary nails (Küntscher, clover-leaf and other patterns) which are inserted without preliminary reaming, or with reaming limited to removal of any medullary tight spots which might interfere with their passage.

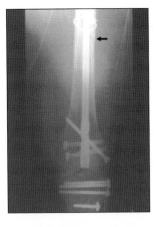

- AO (or other intramedullary nails of similar tubular pattern) which are inserted after a thorough reaming, which is carried out to ensure that the nail has a tight fit throughout the length of the medullary canal.
- Interlocking nails (e.g. Russell–Taylor, AO and others) where rotation of the upper, lower, or both bone fragments is prevented by horizontal screws which are passed through slots in the intramedullary nail to engage cortical bone on both sides. The use of interlocking nails is advocated in all unstable or potentially unstable fractures.

Nailing is usually carried out by a blind (closed) technique from above, with the fracture not being exposed unless reduction cannot otherwise be obtained. In the illustration, the nail has been inserted from *below* (the retrograde technique), the fracture requiring exposure and holding with a cerclage wire. Proximal tibial fractures are held with cross screws.

In the older child where remodelling is less certain, paired flexible (Nancy) intramedullary nails may be used. These are flattened at one end (1) to engage in cancellous bone and control rotation, and rounded at the other (2) to avoid catching the soft tissues. They may be inserted from below through 2 cm incisions for mid-shaft fractures, and from above for fractures in the distal third. The patient can usually be mobilised with crutches after 10 days.

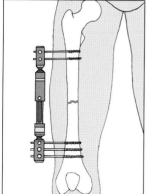

External fixators may be used, but due to the magnitude of the stresses to which the pins are subjected, the support offered is less rigid than would be the case in similarly treated tibial shaft fractures. Nevertheless, the technique is of particular value in the treatment of heavily contaminated open fractures, and under suitable circumstances may be replaced at up to 10 days post-trauma with an intramedullary nail. Instead of using rigid pins, some cases may be treated by multiple thin wires held under tension in encircling ring-shaped frames which are linked together (Ilizarov method).

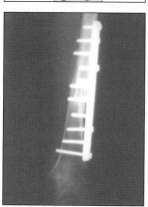

Plating may be used for rapid, rigid fixation of a femoral shaft fracture, particularly where this is required as a preliminary to a vascular repair. It is often commonly used along with bone grafting in cases of non-union. There are many patterns of plate but the most satisfactory are of a heavy duty pattern. A minimum engagement of 8 cortices above the fracture and 8 below is recommended, preferably with an interfragmentary screw and attention to bone compression at the fracture site to increase rigidity and encourage healing.

After-care. After-care is dependent on the quality of fixation. If a tight-fitting, large-diameter nail is used, and if torsion is well controlled by interdigitating fragments or cross-screws, no additional splintage is necessary. The knee may be mobilised and the patient allowed up on crutches. To avoid the risks of the nail bending or of fatigue fractures, many prefer to defer weight-bearing until some callus appears. If fixation is less sound, a period of a few weeks with the leg cradled in a Thomas splint may be thought desirable.

After union of the fracture, removal of an intramedullary nail is usually advised in all but the very old and frail to reduce the risk of a comparatively minor injury causing a fracture of the femoral neck (from local stress concentrations). Where the bone has been plated this is usually retained unless the patient is under the age of 40 or it is the source of symptoms.

Special situations

Ipsilateral fracture of the femur and tibia. The complication rate for these combined injuries is high, irrespective of treatment. To allow early mobilisation, internal fixation (e.g. by intramedullary nailing) of both fractures is often preferred. Where conservative treatment is indicated (e.g. in children), a Steinman pin is inserted in the proximal tibia, the tibial fracture manipulated and a below-knee cast applied, incorporating the pin. Traction on the pin in a Thomas splint is used to control the femoral fracture.

Fracture in the confused patient. Where there is a head injury or a senile confusional state, a patient being treated conservatively may try to remove his own splint; it is possible to prevent this by encircling it with plaster bandages laid on top of the normal crepe bandages (Tobruk splint). This procedure may also be used to give extra security when a patient is being transported.

Metastatic fracture. If death is not imminent, intramedullary nailing is advised to relieve pain. Acrylic cement packed round any defect may give sufficient support to allow the patient to bear weight.

Femoral shaft fracture with (acute) ischaemia of the foot. Nearly all will respond to reduction of the fracture. If the femoral artery is in fact divided, internal fixation will be required prior to vessel repair.

Femoral shaft fracture with nerve palsy. The majority are lesions in continuity, the common peroneal element being most often affected. If there is reason to believe that there may be nerve *division*, exploration and internal fixation may have to be undertaken.

Fracture of the femoral neck and shaft. If the shaft fracture is proximal, both fractures may be treated by a dynamic hip screw and long plate.

Femoral shaft fracture with dislocation of the hip. See under complications of dislocation of the hip (pp. 419–422).

Fractures of the femoral shaft and patella. Note the following:

- early mobilisation of the knee is essential for retention of function
- avoid patellar excision when mobilisation of the knee is going to be delayed
- avoid if possible exposure of the femoral fracture and the creation of tethering adhesions between the femur and quadriceps.

The ideal treatment of the femoral fracture is closed nailing (see later for details of fixation of patellar fractures). If the femoral fracture must be treated conservatively, it is best to leave even badly displaced or comminuted patellar fractures to unite by fibrous union; mobilise the knee as early as possible. Excision of the patella can then be carried out as a late secondary procedure when no further flexion can be gained.

Open fractures. If internal fixation is indicated (especially with multiple injuries), the infection rate in grade I and grade II injuries is said to be no greater after a meticulous debridement and blind nailing than in closed fractures. Grade IIIA fractures with good skin cover and no medullary contamination can be nailed in reasonable safety, although some regard that reaming should be avoided. Grade III B & C open fractures are perhaps best treated conservatively or with an external fixator.

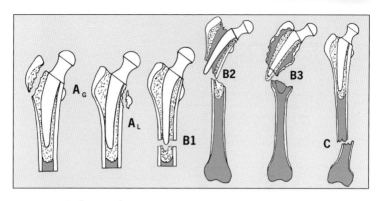

Fractures in hip replacements

A number of fracture types are described, and as a rule operative treatment is advised except in the case of undisplaced trochanteric fractures or if the patient's condition is poor.

Types A_G and A_L include all displaced fractures of the trochanters and may be fixed with cerclage wires, supplemented if need be with screws or plates.

Type B1 fractures occur at the tip of well-held stems. If spiral, they may be held with cerclage wires alone, but transverse fractures require to be splinted with one or two onlay grafts or plates held in position with screws and cerclage wires. **In Type B2**, the prosthesis is loose but the proximal bone stock is good; a revision prosthesis with a long stem which by-passes the fracture is needed, with as required additional plates and/or bone grafts held with screws and/or cerclage wires.

In Type B3, the bone stock is poor and treatment particularly difficult. A custom-made prosthesis or methods similar to those used in B2 fractures may be required.

Type C fractures lie entirely distal to the stem of the prosthesis and may be managed using standard methods without having to consider the prosthesis above.

Pending such procedures light traction may be applied and the leg cradled in a Thomas splint.

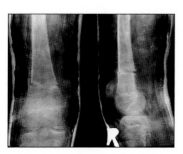

Supracondylar fractures

Children. Fractures in the distal third of the femur are frequently only minimally displaced in children and may be successfully treated by the application of a cylinder (pipe-stem) plaster. Weight-bearing should not be permitted till evidence of early union appears on the radiographs, but during this period the patient may be mobilised with crutches.

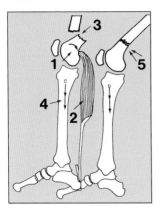
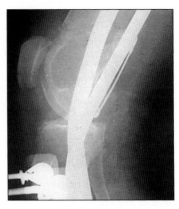

Adults. In the adult especially, supracondylar fractures have a strong tendency for the distal fragment to rotate **(1)** under the continuous pull of the gastrocnemius **(2)** into a position of posterior angulation **(3)**. This cannot be controlled by traction in the line of the limb **(4)**: it is necessary to flex the knee and maintain the traction over a fulcrum **(5)**. The necessary degree of knee flexion may be obtained using a Pearson knee flexion piece, or better still by bending the Thomas splint at the level of the fracture **(right)**. Mobilisation of the knee should be started as early as possible, as the risks of knee stiffness from the development of tethering adhesions (between the quadriceps muscle and the fracture) is high. *To allow early mobilisation of the knee and lessen the risks of stiffness, many prefer internal fixation of these potentially difficult fractures.* If the fracture is proximally situated, an interlocking intramedullary nail may be used. Otherwise, good fixation may be achieved with a condylar blade-plate or a dynamic condylar screw.

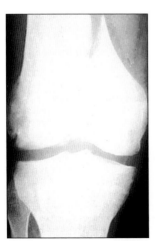

Unicondylar fractures

If the displacement is slight **(left)**, these injuries may be treated conservatively. A straight Thomas splint may be used for the first 1–2 weeks, but thereafter mobilisation should be started, either with a Pearson knee flexion piece or with Hamilton–Russell traction.

Many, however, prefer to treat all fractures of this pattern (especially shearing fractures which are entirely intra-articular) by internal fixation, especially if displacement has disturbed the contours of the articular surfaces. Methods include the use of cancellous screws and buttress plates.

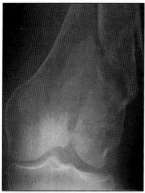

T- and Y-condylar fractures

Undisplaced fractures may be treated conservatively or surgically. *Displaced fractures without gross fragmentation* are generally best treated by open reduction and internal fixation of the fragments (e.g. with a dynamic condylar screw). *In displaced fractures with gross comminution*, open reduction is likely to be unrewarding and the aim should be to restore the alignment of the knee and mobilise it as early as possible—e.g. by using Hamilton–Russell traction. Alternatively, in the elderly, primary joint replacement may be considered.

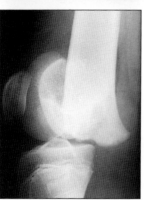

Displaced femoral epiphysis

This injury usually results from hyperextension of the knee, and there is risk of vascular complications; reduction should be carried out expeditiously by applying traction, flexing the knee to a right angle and pressing the epiphysis backwards into position. The knee should be kept in flexion for 3 weeks in a plaster slab, and for a further 3–5 weeks in a plaster cylinder in a more neutral position.

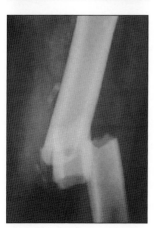

Segmental (double) fractures

These are uncommon in the femur, but are associated with a high incidence of non-union at one level. Fracture exposure may lose the tenuous blood supply to the intermediate segment. Although they may be treated conservatively (dealing with each complication as it arises), closed nailing (if reduction can be accomplished) is a more attractive alternative. A nail, locked at both ends, should be used. Static nailing may be converted at a later stage to dynamic nailing if union is delayed.

COMPLICATIONS OF FRACTURES OF THE FEMUR

Among the many complications which may accompany fractures of the femur, the following should be noted:

Oligaemic shock
Fat embolism
Slow or delayed union. These are common, and in conservatively treated fractures may result in permanent restriction of knee movements. Where the fracture is being treated by an intramedullary locked nail, conversion from static to dynamic locking may encourage union.

Non-union. In fractures being treated conservatively, this is generally dealt with as soon as it is confidently diagnosed, by intramedullary nailing and bone grafting. If non-union occurs in a fracture which has been treated by intramedullary nailing, bone grafting will usually be required. The quality of the fixation must also be reviewed and if necessary improved.

Malunion. Persistent lateral angulation is the commonest deformity in shaft fractures, and if it is 25° or more then correction by osteotomy and intramedullary nailing should be considered. Angulation near the knee may give rise to instability, difficulty in walking and secondary osteoarthritis in the joint.

Limb shortening. Shortening in the adult should be corrected by shoe alteration to within 1–2 cm (1/2″) of the limb discrepancy. In children, any difference in leg length usually corrects (or indeed overcorrects) spontaneously within 6–18 months of the injury.

Knee stiffness. This is a common complication of femoral and tibial fractures, and of injuries to the extensor mechanism of the knee. The causal factors include:

- *Quadriceps tethering.* If the quadriceps becomes adherent to a femoral shaft fracture, it becomes unable to glide over the smooth distal shaft in the normal fashion, thereby fixing the patella and restricting knee movements. The closer the fracture is to the knee, the more important this effect.
- *Fractures involving the knee joint.* Fractures which involve the articular surfaces may give rise to intra-articular and periarticular adhesions, or may form a mechanical block to movement. Early mobilisation is especially desirable where a fracture involves the joint.
- *Prolonged immobilisation.* Fixation of the knee for an undesirably long period may lead to stiffness and this effect is particularly marked in the elderly.

Infection. Infection may sometimes supervene in femoral shaft fractures treated by intramedullary nailing, especially in open injuries. The course of treatment must be individually determined, but the following guidelines usually apply:

1. The causal organism should be isolated and the appropriate antibiotic administered in effective doses for an adequate length of time.
2. If the infection has become established, it is unlikely to respond unless the fracture is firmly supported, and a most thorough debridement carried out under antibiotic cover.
3. If the fixation afforded by the nail remains good, the nail should be retained.
4. If the nail fixation is not good, and provided the debridement does not entail extensive bone removal, then consider using a larger diameter nail with locking screws.
5. If the fixation offered by the nail is poor, and much bone stock has to be removed, remove the nail and use an external fixator.

GENERAL TREATMENT GUIDELINES: FEMORAL FRACTURES

Quadriceps exercises. Stability in the knee and extension power are dependent on a good quadriceps. It is important that the muscle is not allowed to waste, and quadriceps exercises should be started as soon after injury as possible.

Flexion exercises. Commence these as soon as the fracture is adequately supported. Flexion should not be permitted unless stress on the fracture can be reduced to a safe level or where healing can be more or less guaranteed.

Discarding walking aids. Walking without the support of sticks or crutches is frequently followed by an improvement in flexion, and such supports should be discontinued as soon as the state of union and the patient's balance will allow.

Physiotherapy. Ideally quadriceps and flexion exercises should be supervised by a physiotherapist with access to aids and facilities such as weights, slings, local heat and hydrotherapy, but basically the patient should be instructed in quadriceps and flexion exercises. The importance of performing these frequently should be stressed. Passive mobilisation of the patella in appropriate cases may also be helpful. Physiotherapy should be continued until an acceptable functional range has been achieved, or until a static position has been reached: and it is therefore necessary to record the range of movements in the knee— initially at weekly and then at monthly intervals. A measurable gain in the range, no matter how small, encourages the patient to further effort; and on the other hand, the absence of any improvement should make it clear that to continue treatment is unjustifiable.

Additional notes

Acceptable functional range. What is acceptable obviously varies considerably from case to case, being dependent on the gravity of the injury, the age of the patient, his occupation, athletic or outdoor pursuits, hobbies, etc., but the basic aim is a stable knee which places little restraint on normal everyday activities.

Lack of extension. Loss of extension, both active and passive, may be found— e.g. in an angulated supracondylar fracture of the femur, or where there has been previous osteoarthritis in the knee. Such losses are seldom severe enough to cause appreciable disability, usually being compensated at hip and ankle. If the knee can be passively but not actively extended, this is known as an *extension lag*. Extension lag frequently gives rise to 'giving way' of the knee. It is common after patellectomy, but usually recovers if quadriceps exercises are intensified. Where extension lag is due to quadriceps tethering, quadriceps exercises should also be encouraged. In most cases of persistent lag, the patient compensates for the disability by using the hip extensors to keep the knee straight while standing.

Lack of flexion. Appreciable disability follows if flexion to 100° cannot be obtained. Flexion to 80–90° will permit sitting in inside seats (i.e. non-aisle seats) in public transport, cinemas, etc., but will not allow the patient to kneel. Less than 100° will cause difficulty with steps, deep tread and narrow stairs, and if both knees are affected, rising from armless chairs. Where flexion has just become static at less than 100°, manipulation of the knee under general anaesthesia should be considered. However, this is best avoided after patellectomy (and quadriceps tendon and patellar ligament repairs) because of the risks of secondary rupture. Gains in flexion by manipulation are seldom high, and late manipulations are usually unrewarding. Where 80° or less flexion is possible and the position is static, the patient's disability and functional requirements should be carefully assessed. If there is a marked deficit, quadricepsplasty should be considered. This often gives a useful gain (often in the region of 40°), although sometimes this is at the expense of an extension lag, and always with some loss of power.

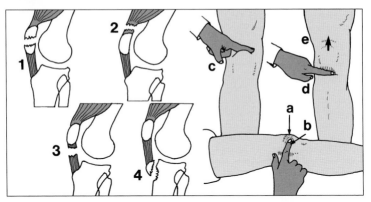

INJURIES OF THE PATELLA AND EXTENSOR MECHANISM OF THE KNEE

Mechanisms. The patella may be fractured by *direct violence*, e.g. if the knee contacts a hard surface (such as the edge of a step or a car fascia), or if the knee is struck by a heavy object (such as a falling rock). The patella may also be fractured by *indirect violence*, i.e. as a result of a sudden muscular contraction (1). This same mechanism may also cause rupture of the quadriceps tendon (2), rupture of the patellar ligament (3) or avulsion of the tibial tubercle (4).

Diagnosis. Fracture of the patella should be suspected when there is a history of direct violence to the knee; fracture of the patella and other injuries to the extensor mechanism should be suspected when there is difficulty in standing after a sudden muscular effort (especially when there is a snapping sensation within the knee). In most cases, *there is inability to extend the knee.* Note clinically any of the following: **(a)** bruising and abrasions; **(b)** the presence and site of tenderness; any palpable gap **(c)** above or **(d)** below the patella; **(e)** any obvious proximal displacement of the patella.

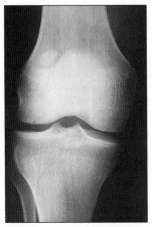

Radiographs. In all cases, radiographs are essential for clarification. An AP projection and a lateral (preferably in extension) will generally suffice. In the acute case, tangential projections cannot usually be obtained because of pain, but these views are often of value in those which present late. In doubtful cases, oblique projections may be helpful. Do not mistake a congenital bipartite patella **(left)** for a fracture. This anomaly generally affects the *upper* and *outer* quadrant; it may be obvious in one view only. The edges are usually rounded, and this may help to differentiate it from a fracture. Other anomalies, such as tripartite patella, may also be distinguished by similar rounding and absence of local tenderness.

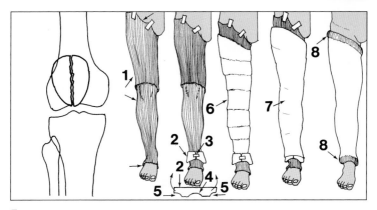

Treatment

Vertical fractures. Fractures of this type (**above, left**) are usually undisplaced and stable. They do not show in the lateral radiographs. In the AP view, the overlapping femoral shadow may make them difficult to detect, and they are frequently missed. Treat conservatively with a 6-week period in a cylinder plaster. *Method:* apply a layer of stockingette (two pieces) from the hind foot to the groin (**1**). Protect the malleoli with a piece of felt (**2**), butt-joining the ends with adhesive tape (**3**); note the concavities for the Achilles tendon (**4**) and the dorsum of the foot (**5**). Pad the leg with wool (**6**). The knee is normally kept in full extension (but not in recurvatum or hyperextension) while 20 cm (8″) plaster bandages are applied (**7**). A slab is not necessary. The edges of the stockingette are turned back before completion (**8**). Crutches are usually advised for the first 2 weeks, with a total of 6 weeks in plaster.

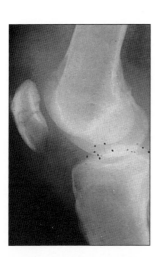

Undisplaced horizontal fractures.
Undisplaced horizontal fractures (even with some comminution, **left**) may also be treated conservatively in a cylinder plaster. However, radiographs should be taken at weekly intervals for the first 2–3 weeks to exclude late separation of the fragments. After removal of the plaster at 6 weeks, physiotherapy will be required and crutches may be needed again for the first few weeks till confidence is regained.

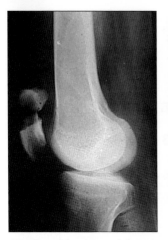 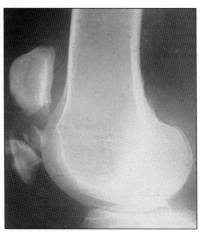

Displaced horizontal fractures. Fractures of this type should be explored so that the exact nature of the pathology may be determined and the appropriate treatment carried out:

- If the degree of comminution is slight **(above left)** so that the fracture can be reduced and the articular surface restored, then internal fixation should be performed (e.g. by tension band or Pyrford wiring).
- If the joint surfaces cannot be restored, but the damage is confined to one pole of the patella **(above right)** then good results can be obtained by partial patellectomy.
- If there is major fragmentation and an accurate reduction is not feasible, patellectomy should be carried out, with repair of the quadriceps insertion and lateral expansions.

Knee function after patellectomy is often excellent, but may fall a little short of perfect; although a full range of movements may be regained, there is often a feeling of instability while descending steep slopes, and there may be some weakness in rising from the squatting position.

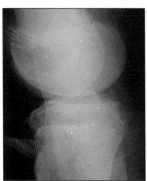

Avulsion fractures of the tibial tubercle. In the *adult* or *adolescent* near skeletal maturity **(left)**, the displacement if marked should be reduced and the tubercle fixed with a screw. If displacement is slight, a 6-week period in a plaster cylinder should suffice.

In *children*, surgery should be avoided if at all possible because of the risks of premature epiphyseal fusion. If, however, manipulative reduction fails, open reduction and fixing with a suture may become necessary.

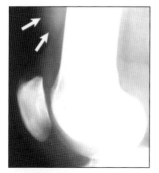

Rupture of the quadriceps tendon.

The diagnosis is essentially a clinical one, but examination of the soft-tissue shadows in the lateral radiograph (**left**) may sometimes confirm this. An MRI scan may also be helpful.

Treatment: the tendon must be re-attached surgically, and it is often necessary to drill the patella to provide anchorage for the sutures. Thereafter, a plaster cylinder is applied. Quadriceps exercises are commenced at 2 weeks, weight-bearing at 4 weeks and knee flexion at 6 weeks.

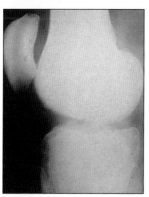

Rupture of the patellar ligament.

This is also essentially a clinical diagnosis, although proximal displacement of the patella in the plain films (e.g. left) may be suggestive. Again, an MRI scan may give confirmation.

Treatment: these injuries may be treated surgically as in the case of quadriceps tendon ruptures. When there is avulsion of the distal tip of the patella, the bony fragment should be removed. The patellar ligament may be re-attached using holes drilled through the patella for anchorage.

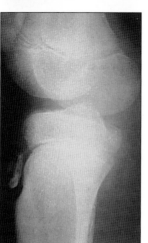

Osgood–Schlatter's disease.

In children, sudden or repeated quadriceps contraction may be responsible for this condition, which is characterised by recurrent pain, tenderness and swelling over the tibial tubercle. In some cases the onset may be acute and be associated with a fracture of the tongue-like downward projecting proximal tibial epiphysis. In these circumstances a 2-week period in a cylinder plaster may be helpful. While slow spontaneous resolution is the rule, severe persistent symptoms occasionally merit excision of the detached fragment.

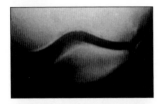

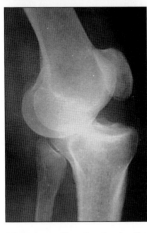

Acute lateral dislocation of the patella. This may occur as a result of a sudden muscular contraction or a blow on the side of the knee. It may be reduced with firm lateral pressure (anaesthesia is seldom required). If a first incident, a 6-week period of plaster fixation is advised; if not, apply a pressure bandage for 1–2 weeks. Lateral dislocation commonly occurs as a first or subsequent incident in the course of recurrent dislocation of the patella (see Ch. 11). A marginal osteochondral fracture in the tangential projection (**left above**) is usually diagnostic of an incident of lateral dislocation, but this may not be obvious for some weeks.

Dislocation of the knee. This injury may follow comparatively minor trauma. Most commonly the tibia is displaced anteriorly (**left, below**), but medial, lateral, posterior and rotational displacements are also found. There is inevitably major damage to the ligaments of the knee; all or most may be torn, along with the joint capsule. Sometimes there is displacement of the menisci, fractures of the tibial spines, common peroneal nerve palsy and, most seriously, popliteal artery damage.

Treatment. Closed reduction by traction and the application of pressure over the displaced tibia is generally easy and often gives good results. Thereafter, the leg may be supported by light traction (2–3 kg/6 lb) in a Thomas splint for 3–4 weeks, followed by a further 4 weeks in a plaster cylinder before mobilisation is commenced. Alternatively, primary surgical repair of all the damaged structures is favoured by many, and exploration is certainly indicated if closed reduction fails or if there is circulatory impairment from suspected popliteal artery damage which persists after reduction.

Soft-tissue injuries of the knee. When the radiographs are normal, a significant soft-tissue injury should be suspected, especially if there is a haemarthrosis. There is a common clinical picture of pain in the knee, swelling and difficulty in weight-bearing. In every case you should exclude damage to the extensor apparatus, lateral dislocation of the patella with spontaneous reduction and tears of the ligaments or menisci. In some centres, further investigation is pursued in an aggressive fashion: any haemarthrosis is aspirated and the soft-tissue elements examined directly by arthroscopy or indirectly by MRI scan. If there is little to implicate any of the major structures (and this is so in the majority of cases), a provisional diagnosis of 'knee sprain' or 'sprained ligaments with traumatic effusion' may be made, and the case treated appropriately (e.g. with a crepe, Tubigrip or Jones pressure bandage) and re-assessed at weekly intervals thereafter until either the symptoms have settled completely, or a more accurate diagnosis can be established.

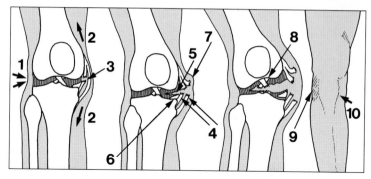

MEDIAL, LATERAL AND CRUCIATE LIGAMENT INJURIES
Medial ligament injuries

The commonest cause is a blow on the lateral side of the knee (1) which forces the joint into valgus (2). With slight force, there is partial tearing of the medial ligament (knee sprain) and the knee remains stable on clinical testing. With greater violence, the deep portion of the ligament ruptures (partial tear) (3), and stressing the knee in 30° flexion with the foot internally rotated causes more opening up of the joint than normal. There may be clinical evidence of rotatory instability. With still greater violence, superficial *and* deep parts of the ligament rupture (4) and the tear rapidly spreads across the posterior ligament (5), so that stressing the joint in extension causes moderate opening out on the medial side. The medial meniscus (6) may also tear. If the edge of the ligament rolls over, it may be felt subcutaneously (7). With severe violence, one or both cruciates rupture (8) and the joint opens widely on stressing. Bruising on the lateral side (9) and medial tenderness (10) are suggestive of medial ligament damage. If there is remaining doubt, repeat the clinical tests after aspiration, or take stress radiographs, comparing one side with the other.

Treatment

Sprain. Crepe bandages or a Jones pressure bandage should be applied and the patient given crutches to use until the acute symptoms have settled.

Isolated tear. Assuming there is no evidence of 'rolling over' of the medial ligament, POP fixation *with the knee at 45° flexion* for 8 weeks, or the use of a limited motion knee brace is advised.

Major tear. If isolated and uncomplicated, conservative management may also be pursued and a good result expected. If there is evidence of involvement of other structures, operative repair should be carried out of both the medial ligament and the secondary structures, preserving the menisci if at all possible.

Complications

Late valgus instability. If this occurs, consider a secondary reconstruction.

Persistent rotatory instability. Improvement may follow a medial capsular repair and pes anserinus transposition, although the late results are often disappointing.

Pelligrini–Stieda disease. A valgus strain of the knee may produce partial avulsion of the medial ligament, with subsequent calcification in the subperiosteal haematoma. There is prolonged pain, local tenderness and limitation of flexion, but no instability. Treat acute cases with immobilisation in a cast for 2–3 weeks, and chronic cases with local hydrocortisone infiltrations.

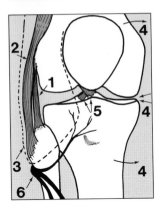

Injuries to the lateral ligament

The lateral ligament (1) is part of a complex which includes the biceps femoris tendon (2) and the fascia lata (3) attached to tibia, fibula and patella. All these structures may be damaged if the knee is subjected to a varus stress (4), and with severe violence, the cruciates (5) will also be torn. The common peroneal nerve (6) may be stretched or torn.

Diagnosis. Test the stability of the knee by applying a varus stress with the knee in extension. Look for evidence of common peroneal involvement. Examine radiographs of the knee for avulsion fracture of the head of the fibula.

Treatment. If the knee is clinically stable (i.e. if the diagnosis is one of a sprain), symptomatic treatment only is required (e.g. a crepe bandage and crutches). If there is instability, operative repair is indicated, unless there is a definite, undisplaced fracture which seems likely to go on to union. In such circumstances, a plaster cylinder should be applied and retained for 6–8 weeks before mobilisation. If there is a common peroneal nerve palsy, this is likely to be due either to a lesion in continuity or a complete disruption of the nerve over an extensive area. In neither case is exploration indicated for the neurological injury alone, although if the ligament is being repaired, the opportunity should be taken to inspect the nerve. In both cases, treatment for drop foot should be started. With a lesion in continuity, recovery usually starts within 6 weeks, but a disruptive lesion carries a poor prognosis.

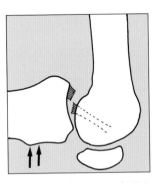

Posterior cruciate ligament injuries

The mechanism whereby the posterior cruciate ligament is damaged is usually either a fall on some object, or dashboard impact in a road traffic accident which results in the tibia being forced backwards. There is often associated damage to the medial or lateral ligaments.

Diagnosis. In most cases there is a striking alteration in the profile of the knee when placed in flexion, often associated with a false anterior drawer test. The posterior drawer sign may be positive. Radiographs may show avulsion fractures of the posterior cruciate ligament attachments, and MRI scans may help.

Treatment. If untreated, instability often persists, leading to considerable disability and secondary osteoarthritis which progresses rapidly. If there is an undisplaced fracture of the posterior tibial spine representing an avulsion of the posterior attachment of the ligament, the leg should be kept in a plaster cylinder for 6–8 weeks before mobilisation. A displaced tibial spine fracture should be reduced and held with a screw. A detached ligament should be re-attached.

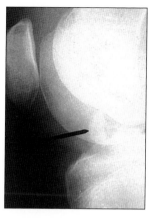

Anterior cruciate ligament tears

Isolated tears are uncommon and usually result from forced flexion or hyperextension of the knee. More frequently there are associated tears of the medial ligament and the medial meniscus (O'Donoghue's triad).

Diagnosis. Excess anterior excursion of the tibia relative to the femur may be confirmed by the drawer and Lachman tests, and the ligament may be visualised by arthroscopy or MRI scan. Plain X-rays may show avulsion of the anterior bony attachment of the ligament (**left**). Check the integrity of the other structures, especially the medial ligament and the medial meniscus.

Treatment. If the anterior tibial spine is fractured but undisplaced, treat with a 6–8 week period of fixation in a plaster cylinder. If displaced, it should be carefully repositioned and internally fixed. If the anterior attachment of the ligament is avulsed, it should be re-attached.

The treatment of isolated tears of the central portion of the ligament is controversial. Good results can follow conservative management, and some advocate this in all cases; minor degrees of residual instability may be dealt with by intensive quadriceps building and the use of a knee brace, with late reconstruction procedures being reserved for more severe cases. Others prefer immediate repair, which usually involves some form of ligament augmentation. In all cases, associated meniscal and medial ligament injuries take precedence in treatment.

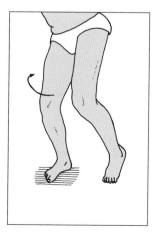

MENISCUS INJURIES

In *infants* and *children* the menisci, instead of being C-shaped, are plate-like structures which completely separate the articular surfaces of the femur and tibia (congenital discoid menisci). If they become detached at the periphery, they may cause permanent loss of full extension.

In the *young adult*, the menisci are generally injured as a result of a rotational stress applied to the flexed, weight bearing knee (**left**). Injury can also result from rapid knee extension (tears of the anterior horn) and by direct violence (cysts).

In the *middle-aged*, horizontal tears may occur within the substance of the meniscus, sometimes without any history of trauma. Tears of this pattern may extend towards the articular surfaces and displace.

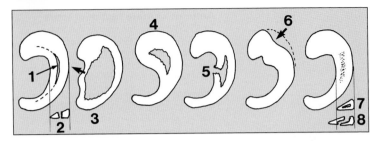

Patterns of meniscal injuries in the adult. The majority of tears commence as vertical splits in the substance of the meniscus ('longitudinal tear') (**1, 2**). The free edge may displace centrally, forming a bucket handle tear (**3**) or a racquet tear of the posterior (**4**) or anterior horns. The central edge may rupture forming a parrot-beak tear (**5**). In peripheral detachments, part (**6**) or all of the meniscus may displace centrally. Horizontal cleavage tears may be confined to the centre of the meniscus (**7**) or extend either superiorly or inferiorly, with displacement (**8**), with potential for mechanical effects.

Diagnosis of meniscus injuries
Note the following points:

- Acute tears in the young adult generally result from a clear-cut incident of weight-bearing stress, often while engaging in an athletic pursuit such as football. There is immediate pain in the knee and difficulty in weight-bearing. Initial disability is usually marked, and if the patient has been playing football, he will be unable to continue. This important aspect of the history should be clarified.
- Meniscus tears are very uncommon in women. Dislocation of the patella or chondromalacia patellae should always be eliminated before the diagnosis of a torn meniscus is contemplated in a female.
- Absence of knee swelling may be deceptive. After peripheral tears there is certainly in most cases a rapidly forming haemarthrosis but there may be no immediate swelling after longitudinal tears (the menisci are avascular). Any reactionary synovitis may appear quite late (e.g. several days) after the initial incident.
- There is almost invariably joint-line tenderness, but as many minor lesions give this finding this is of little diagnostic value apart form localisation to either side of the joint.
- A springy block to full extension is, however, almost diagnostic of a displaced, bucket-handle tear.
- Some days after the first incident, other signs may appear, such as quadriceps wasting and slight oedema in the joint line. When pain subsides, other confirmatory tests such as MacMurray's manoeuvre may give positive results.
- Radiographs should always be taken to exclude other pathology.
- In chronic lesions, positive physical signs are often lacking and further investigation may be required (e.g. by arthroscopy, MRI scan or arthrography).

Treatment of meniscal injuries

Locked knee. If the diagnosis is unequivocal and due to a meniscus tear, admit at an early date for surgical treatment. Pending admission, a pressure bandage support, crutches and analgesics may be prescribed. Attempts to unlock the knee are of questionable value.

Cases where the history and findings suggest a fresh meniscus tear. Treat conservatively. Remember that peripheral detachments can unite, and that many joint injuries may mimic a torn meniscus, yet recover completely. A pressure bandage should be applied, the patient given crutches and advised to practise quadriceps exercises. If the knee fails to settle within 2 weeks, the usual practice is to perform a diagnostic arthroscopy followed by the appropriate procedure (e.g. repair or excision). In general terms, the aim should be to preserve any part of the meniscus that can make a contribution to the proper functioning of the knee.

Meniscus cysts. The cyst should be excised, along with any meniscal extension.

Horizontal cleavage tears. Symptoms may resolve with physiotherapy alone, and meniscectomy may frequently be avoided.

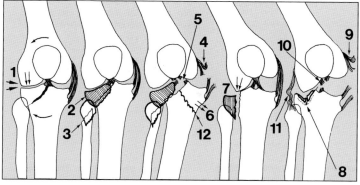

FRACTURES OF THE TIBIAL TABLES

The lateral tibial table. These generally result from a severe valgus stress, and several patterns of injury are found. Impact of the mass of the lateral femoral condyle may be responsible for the 'sliding fracture' which passes downwards and laterally from the tibial spine region, the main articular surface remaining intact (1). With increasing violence, the tibial fragment is depressed (2), and there may be an associated fracture of the fibular neck (3). In severe cases there may be rupture of the medial ligament (4), rupture of the cruciates (5) and medial subluxation of the tibia (6). The 'corner' of the lateral femoral condyle may cause a split fracture (7), or a crush fracture of the tibial table (8). In either of these cases, there may be tearing of the medial ligament (9), or the cruciates (10), relative lengthening of the lateral ligament (11) or crushing of the lateral meniscus. A second fracture line (12) may convert any of these injuries into a bicondylar fracture.

The medial tibial table. Fractures of the medial tibial table are uncommon, but do occur. They may be associated with lateral ligament ruptures and common peroneal nerve palsy. (Their treatment is along similar lines to lateral tibial table injuries).

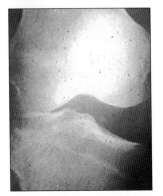

Diagnosis of fractures of the lateral tibial table

The clinical findings include haemarthrosis, lateral bruising and abrasions, and valgus deformity of the knee. Confirmation is by X-ray. In assessing these, note the maximal depression of any fragment relative to neighbouring intact bone. If the medial ligament is suspect (e.g. local tenderness, etc.), stress films (preferably after aspiration and under GA) may be helpful. (**Left:** small split fracture with stress films showing medial ligament tear.) The tibial table may also be assessed by CAT scans.

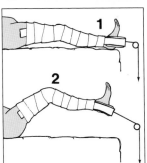

Treatment of fractures of the lateral tibial table
No ligament damage, no tibial subluxation and a depression of less than 10 mm. Apply skin traction of 3 kg (**1**). Commence quadriceps exercises immediately, and flexion exercises as soon as pain will permit (**2**). Traction may often be discontinued after 4 weeks, and weight-bearing begun after 8 weeks. The late results are generally excellent.

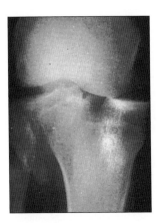

Displaced unicondylar fractures. If the displacement is more than 10 mm, there will be persistent valgus deformity and often some residual instability. Note (**left**) the large lateral fragment and the medial subluxation of the tibia suggesting medial ligament damage. These injuries should be treated by open reduction and internal fixation. When the fracture has been fixed, the medial ligament should be re-tested, and if found to be ruptured it should be repaired. It may also be possible to re-attach any displaced meniscus.

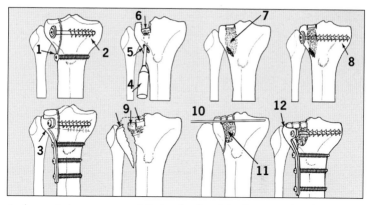

In the surgical management of displaced unicondylar fractures, after the fragment has been elevated, its position can be maintained with a cross screw (**1**), and a cancellous lag screw (**2**) used to close any gap and compress the elements. In some situations, a buttress T-plate (**3**) screwed to the shaft may be preferable. Where part of the articular surface has been depressed (e.g. by the 'corner' of a condyle) a punch (**4**) passed through a hole (**5**) made in the lateral cortex may be used to elevate the fragment (**6**). The resulting bony defect may then be packed with bone chips (**7**) stabilised with a cross screw (**8**). Where the tibial margin and the articular surface have been fractured (**9**), it is sometimes possible to reconstruct the tibial table over a Steinman pin (**10**), pack up the surface with bone grafts (**11**) and hold the reduction with a T-plate and screws (**12**). CAT scans of the fracture area prior to surgical treatment of these fractures can provide valuable information regarding the extent of the problem.

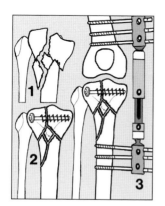

Bicondylar fractures

If undisplaced, injuries of this pattern may be treated conservatively by 6–8 weeks' traction (initially in a Thomas splint), mobilising as soon as the pain settles. If badly displaced (**1**), they may be treated surgically using cancellous screws (**2**). An additional buttress plate (on one side only to reduce the risks of rendering the fragments avascular) may be required. An external fixator (**3**) may be needed to maintain length and reduce deforming pressure on the reconstruction. Later, a hinged link between the pin holders can be introduced to allow early knee movement.

Alternatively, especially if there are more than two main tibial fragments, fixation may be achieved using fine wire methods or a hybrid system of wires and pins.

CHAPTER

26

Regional injuries: fractures of the tibia

Mechanisms of injury 466
Tibial fractures in children 467
Tibial fractures in the adult 470

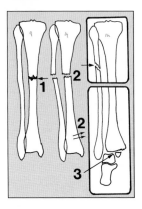

MECHANISMS OF INJURY

The tibia is vulnerable to torsional stresses (e.g. in sporting injuries), to violence transmitted through the feet (e.g. in falls from a height) and from direct blows (e.g. from falling rocks or masonry). Isolated fractures of either the tibia or fibula may occur from direct violence (1), although this is comparatively uncommon. As in the case of the forearm bones, indirect violence leads to fracture of both the tibia and fibula (2). Always obtain radiographs of the whole length of the limb to exclude a distal injury accompanying a proximal fracture (3).

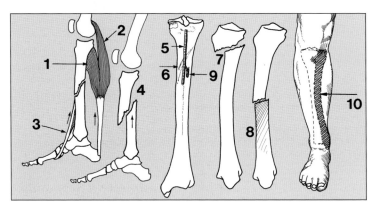

Because of the triangular shape of the tibia in cross-section, and the frequency of injuries caused by torsional forces, oblique and spiral fractures are common. Muscle tone in the soleus (1), gastrocnemius (2) and tibialis anterior (3) tends to produce shortening and displacement (4) in fractures of this type.

The popliteal artery (5) is anchored as it passes under the origin of the soleus at the soleal line (6). It is susceptible to damage in upper tibial fractures (7) and may cause Volkmann's ischaemia of the calf with permanent flexion contracture of the ankle. Fractures of the tibia may be followed by ischaemia of the distal fragment (8) through damage to the nutrient artery (9).

Note also that a third of the tibia is subcutaneous (10), a fact which accounts for the frequency of open fractures in this region.

It is particularly important to correct angulation in fractures of this weight-bearing bone. Unlike angulation in femoral shaft fractures which can be compensated to some extent at the hip, residual angulation in tibial fractures will inevitably throw additional stresses on the ankle and knee.

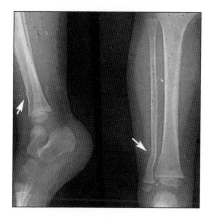 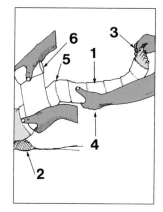

TIBIAL FRACTURES IN CHILDREN
Undisplaced fractures

Owing to the thickness of the subcutaneous fat and periosteum, and the elasticity of the bones, fractures are often of greenstick pattern and closed. In many cases, too, the fractures are minimally displaced. (**Above, left**: greenstick fracture of the distal tibia and fibula, betrayed by fibular kinking and tibial cortical buckling.)

Treatment. When deformity is minimal, apply a long leg plaster immediately over a generous layer of wool (**1**); only mild sedation may be required. A sandbag under the buttocks (**2**) may be helpful, while an assistant holds the toes (**3**) and supports the calf (**4**). The knee is slightly flexed (**5**) and the plaster may be applied in one stage with or without a slab (**6**).

Thereafter, elevation of the leg and a regular, careful check of the circulation is essential, and admission for this is desirable. Non-weight-bearing with crutches can usually be allowed as soon as there is no circulatory risk (say 2–3 days post-injury). The child should then be seen at a fracture clinic every 2–3 weeks (the casualty rate in children's plasters is high). A walking heel can certainly be applied when there is evidence of early callus on the radiographs (e.g. after 3–4 weeks in a child of 9 years). Before that, a heel may be applied if in your assessment there is no risk of displacement or problems from swelling. Any hesitation may sometimes be dispelled by the appearance of the sole of the plaster which often indicates premature successful weight-bearing!

The fracture may be assessed for union after say 4–5 weeks in a child of 4 years, 8 weeks in a child of 8, and 8–12 weeks in a child of 12. On removal of the plaster, no support for the limb is usually required, but confidence may be raised by a crepe bandage. Crutches for the first few days are advocated as the child often shows timidity in commencing weight-bearing: and the parents may require reassurance.

The child should be reviewed 2 weeks after removal of the plaster. In most cases he will be walking unsupported, movements in the knee and ankle will have returned, and the limb lengths will be equal; he may then be discharged. The parents should be reassured that any residual limp will resolve, and advised that athletic activities may be safely resumed say in a further 2 months.

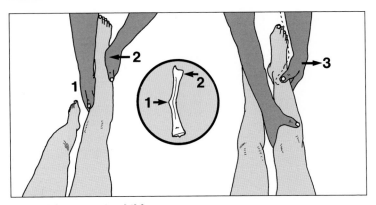

Angled fractures in children

Treatment. These are reduced under general anaesthesia. One hand is placed over the fracture site (**1**) while the other, at the ankle (**2**), is used to correct the angulation. Although the AP plane only is illustrated, naturally any deformity in the lateral plane should be similarly corrected. The pressure of the hand at the ankle should be released (**3**), and any tendency for the deformity to recur noted (indicating springy, intact periosteum). If this is found, particular care must be taken during the application of the plaster to maintain full correction; alternatively, complete tearing of the periosteum may be obtained by over correction of the deformity.

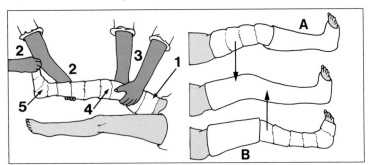

If there is no tendency to recurrence of angulation, the plaster may be applied as follows. Wool roll is wound round the limb from toes to groin (**1**); one assistant supports the fracture and the toes (**2**) while the second takes the weight of the thigh (**3**). The knee is flexed to 15° (**4**) and the ankle maintained at right angles (**5**). The supporting hands are moved during the application of the plaster. Use a sandbag under the buttocks. *If there is a tendency to re-angulation,* the plaster must be moulded while it sets. Except in the smallest of children it is difficult to apply a full length plaster and mould the fracture within the setting time. A two-stage technique may be used: *either* apply a below knee plaster (**A**), mould, and then complete the thigh, *or* (**B**) apply the thigh cuff first, complete the plaster and then mould.

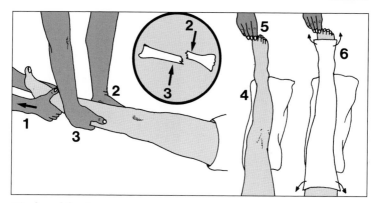

Displaced fractures

An assistant applies strong traction in the line of the limb (**1**), while strong pressure is applied with the heels of the hands above (**2**) and below (**3**) the fracture to correct the displacement. The traction is then slackened off to allow the bone ends to engage.

Checking the reduction clinically can be difficult: try to gauge the position of the main tibial fragments by palpating the subcutaneous border, or in the case of a transverse fracture, confirm there is a hitch by absence of telescoping.

If the reduction is somewhat precarious and slipping is feared during the application of the plaster, place the limb on a firm plaster pillow (**4**), steady the leg by holding the toes (**5**) and apply a thick, *anterior* plaster slab (**6**), tucking the edges well round the limb. When it has set, the leg can then be carefully bandaged into the slab. Ultimately, if necessitated by circumstance, displacement and even off-ending may be accepted in children, but angulation should be corrected.

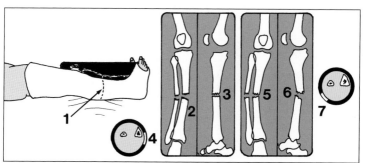

Correction of angulation by wedging of the cast. Begin by marking the plaster circumferentially at the level of the fracture (**1**) using the radiographs as a guide. Now carefully work out where the plaster must hinge to correct the deformity. For example, where there is medial angulation (**2**) and the lateral projection is normal (**3**), the hinge should lie medially (**4**). Where there is lateral angulation (**5**) along with posterior angulation (**6**), the hinge should be positioned posterolaterally (**7**).

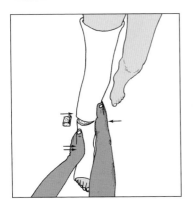
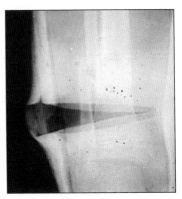

Cut through 7/8 of the circumference of the plaster at the marked level, sparing the hinge; use a plaster saw or a hacksaw with a fine blade. Now spring the plaster 1–2 cm open; maintain the position temporarily by placing a suitably sized piece of previously prepared cork into the mouth of the wedge.

Take check radiographs, and if necessary make any adjustment. The limit of acceptability is 15° of residual angulation in mid-third fractures, and 10° in proximal and distal third fractures. If a satisfactory correction has been obtained (**right**), wool should be packed lightly into the gap on either side of the cork and the plaster reconstituted locally with a 15 cm (6″) plaster bandage. General anaesthesia is not required for wedging, but mild sedation is desirable.

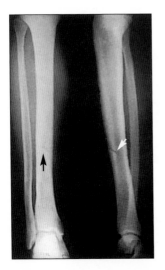

TIBIAL FRACTURES IN THE ADULT

In the adult, many tibial fractures may be treated conservatively, and where good results with few complications are the rule it is unwise to advocate surgery with its additional risks. Conservative treatment may with good reason always be advised for stress, isolated (**left**) and undisplaced fractures, and for slightly displaced stable fractures. A long leg plaster is applied, check radiographs are taken and the limb elevated for 3–7 days until swelling subsides. The plaster is checked for slackness and changed if required. As soon as the patient has mastered crutches he may be allowed home. A walking heel is applied usually after 3–6 weeks (depending on your assessment of stability), and the plaster retained till union.

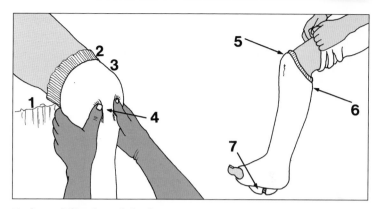

Early mobilisation of the knee

Sarmiento plaster. Instead of maintaining a long leg cast until union has occurred, a Sarmiento cast may be applied at 4–6 weeks post-injury. The patient sits on the edge of the plaster table (1), the foot being steadied by the lap of the operator. Stockingette (2) and wool roll are applied, and the plaster extended over the knee (3). Before it sets, it is firmly moulded round the patellar ligament (4). The plaster is then trimmed from the upper pole of the patella (5) round to the upper part of the calf (6); check that knee movement is free before turning down the stockingette and finishing in the usual way. A rocker sole may then be applied (7), and weight bearing and knee flexion commenced. The plaster is retained until union is sound.

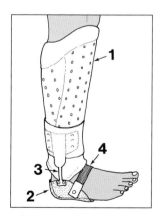

Functional bracing with a gaiter. In the later stages of fixation, or even as early as 4 weeks when instability is not a problem, a supporting gaiter may be used instead of plaster. The type illustrated may be fashioned from perforated Orthoplast (Johnson & Johnson) thermoplastic sheet (1). For additional support, a plastic heel seat (2) may be secured to the brace with polyethylene hinges (3) and a strap (4).

After-care. Intervals between hospital attendances should not exceed 4 weeks, and the fixation (plaster or brace) changed if it becomes unduly slack. Tibial fractures take on average 16 weeks to unite, but union may be sought in 8–12 weeks in the case of a hairline crack, and after 12 weeks in a transverse fracture. It is preferable that check radiographs should be taken out of plaster.

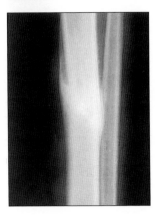

Apparent radiological union **(left)** should be confirmed by clinical examination. If union is judged sound, a crepe bandage support is prescribed for the ankle, leg and knee, and full unsupported weight bearing commenced. Walking sticks or crutches may be required to give confidence over the first few weeks, but the patient should be encouraged to discard these as soon as possible (although the elderly patient may have difficulty in this respect).

The patient should be reviewed 2 weeks after plaster has been discarded, when the following problems may be encountered:

- *The knee.* Pain or discomfort in the knee at the beginning of mobilisation is normal. A small to moderate effusion is common. If the period of immobilisation is under 16 weeks, return of flexion is usually rapid.
- Physiotherapy is nevertheless advisable in the majority of cases to encourage knee flexion, to develop the quadriceps and to help restore the gait to normal.
- *The ankle.* Slight swelling and oedema of the foot and ankle are usual for several months after tibial fractures. A crepe bandage or circular woven support is advised until this swelling subsides. Gross swelling with marked stiffness and pain in the foot and ankle should suggest Sudeck's atrophy. Swelling which is maximal over the fracture calls for re-assessment of union. Slight restriction of ankle movements is common after tibial fractures, but is seldom incapacitating.
- *Athletic activities.* Swimming may be permitted almost as soon as the plaster has been discarded and should be encouraged. Cycling can be allowed as soon as knee flexion will allow (*c.* 110°). Golf may be permitted as soon as limb swelling is no longer a problem. Rugby, football and gymnastics should be forbidden until endosteal callus is sound, till knee flexion is nearly normal (say 130°) and muscle power is restored.
- *Return to work.* The patient should be encouraged to return to work as soon as possible, and in sedentary work the patient may do so while in plaster. Factors which may delay return are severe persistent oedema in jobs involving prolonged standing; lack of knee flexion in work involving kneeling; muscle and functional weakness in jobs involving work at heights.

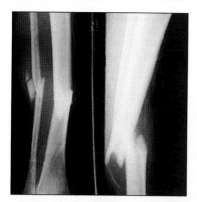

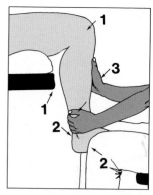

Displaced but potentially stable fractures

Transverse fractures of the tibia in particular are potentially stable (**above left**) if good bony apposition can be obtained. While the tendency is to treat injuries of this pattern by closed intramedullary nailing, some reserve surgery only for cases where closed reduction fails or cannot be maintained.

Reduction techniques.   The fracture may be manipulated as in the case of a child, but it is often helpful, especially if assistance is limited, to let gravity work to your advantage. The patient's knee is flexed over the end of the table (**1**). Use your own knees to steady or to apply traction to the foot (**2**). Both hands are then free to manipulate the fracture (**3**).

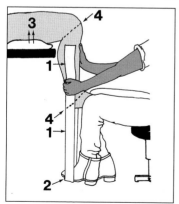

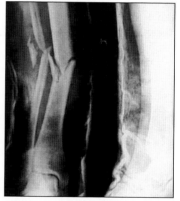

Alternatively, it is sometimes possible to apply temporary traction using skin traction tapes (**1**). The traction may be controlled by the operator's foot on the spreader bar (**2**) and by elevating the table (**3**). After manipulation, a padded plaster is applied over the tapes from the heel to the knee (**4**). The tapes are cut, and the foot of the plaster completed. Once the leg and foot have been encased in plaster, the knee is gently extended to 15° and the thigh cuff completed. Residual angulation (**above right**, which shows the fracture at the top of the page after manipulation) may be treated by wedging.

Unstable fractures with minimal displacement

Oblique and spiral fractures are potentially unstable. Although they may be managed conservatively along the lines indicated, meticulous supervision is necessary during the first 6 weeks. Deal promptly with plaster slackness; accept slight slipping of the fracture, but consider internal fixation if evidence of substantial displacement is found.

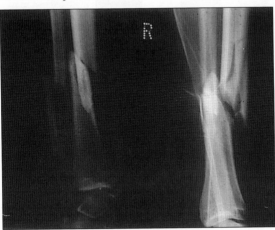 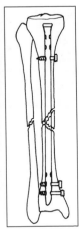

Displaced, unstable fractures

Although these (**above left**) may be managed conservatively, they are as a rule best dealt with by internal fixation.

Fixation by intramedullary nailing. This is the most popular form of fixation, and with the additional use of transverse locking screws (**above right**), gives a high level of support in all planes. The operation is performed as soon as the patient's condition will allow, under image intensifier control, and often with prophylactic antibiotic cover.

After-care. Mobilisation of the knee and ankle may be commenced immediately, and as a result complete recovery of movements in these joints is the rule. As regards weight-bearing, advice on when this should be permitted is dependent on the nature of the fracture and the quality of fixation. Absence of pain at the fracture site on weight-bearing has been said to be a valuable guide as to when full unsupported weight may be taken through the limb. The fracture should be followed up until soundly united, when a decision, based on the usual criteria, should be made regarding removal of the fixation device. Return to work and athletic activities follow along the lines discussed.

Complications. *Knee pain* occurs in about 40% of cases and generally settles on removal of the nail. *Delayed union* may be treated by converting from static to dynamic fixation by removal of the appropriate locking screws, sometimes with an osteotomy of the fibula if it has united. *Hypertrophic non-union* may be dealt with by exchange nailing (removal of the existing nail, re-reaming to a greater diameter and using a larger nail). *Infection* is uncommon, and should be dealt with along the usual lines, preferably retaining the nail until union has occurred. *Compartment syndromes* are also uncommon, but occasionally require treatment by decompression.

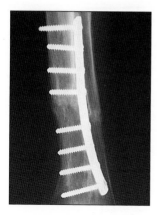

Fixation by plating. Many tibial fractures are amenable to treatment by plating: a well-contoured dynamic compression plate can often provide a high quality of rigid internal fixation, and butterfly and other separate fragments may be secured with interfragmentary screws. Image intensification and the use of an orthopaedic table are of course not required. Plating may be used (with bone grafting) to deal with non-union in fractures which have been previously treated by conservative methods.

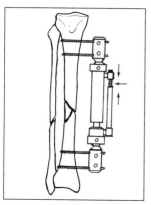

Use of external fixators. These are of particular value in open fractures. Good support is provided with 2–3 threaded cantilever pins on each side of the fracture, with a rigid connector which can give axial compression. The most rigid systems use a total of 12 pins, inserted in pairs at right angles to one another, with two linking bars. At the other end of the scale, tibial length may be preserved in conservatively treated fractures with two Steinman pins incorporated in the plaster.

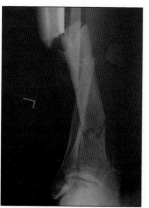

Special situations
Double (segmental) fractures.
Plaster fixation gives poor support, and the incidence of non-union at one level in fractures treated conservatively is high. (Nevertheless, if this occurs and if alignment is satisfactory, success may follow internal fixation and grafting.) The most useful primary treatment is *closed* intramedullary nailing with the insertion of proximal and distal locking screws. *Open reduction* and plating carries the risk of further devitalisation of the intermediate segment.

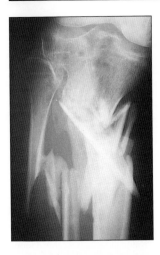

Gross fragmentation. Where the bone is highly fragmented (as may occur in high energy dissipation situations), the multiplicity of small, detached avascular bone fragments **(left)** will prevent any meaningful reduction. Alignment should be restored by manipulation; thereafter, length and position may be maintained by Steinman pins incorporated in a plaster cast, by the use of an external fixator, or using Ilizarov wires and frames. Although generally undesirable, it may be necessary to bridge the knee in order to maintain length.

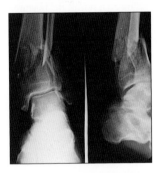

Fractures of the distal shaft. Many of these fractures can be treated conservatively by reduction and plaster fixation, with or without a Steinman pin through the heel to help maintain alignment. Some permanent restriction of ankle joint movements is common. Alternatively, some can be internally fixed so that early movements can be permitted (e.g. by using a buttress plate with proximal cortical and distal cancellous screws); or an external fixator can be applied which can later be hinged to permit early ankle joint movements.

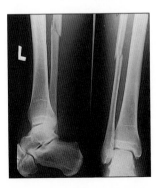

Isolated fractures of the fibula. The fibula may be fractured by direct violence; symptomatic treatment only is required (e.g. a below-knee walking plaster for 6 weeks). Always ensure, however, that the tibia is not fractured at another level, or that the fibular fracture does not represent part of a more complex injury to the ankle joint.

Open fractures. Gustilo's classification of open fractures and the general principles of treatment have been dealt with (Chs 14 & 17).

With specific reference to fractures of the tibia, primary closure of the skin is generally to be avoided (although good results have been claimed in children where contamination has been minimal). In the absence of established infection, small wounds close spontaneously; larger wounds should only be dealt with by secondary suture if this can be performed without tension; and granulating surfaces may readily be covered by split skin grafts.

The importance of the thoroughness of initial and subsequent debridements has been stressed, along with the necessity of obtaining early soft-tissue cover of bone; a number of plastic surgical techniques to this end have been described.

There has been much controversy over the use of internal fixation in the treatment of open fractures, but in many cases the fears expressed of increasing the risks of infection have been shown to be unjustified. In open fractures of types 1 & 2 (Gustilo), the infection rate following intramedullary nailing using the closed technique has been shown to be low and no greater than in closed injuries of a similar pattern.

In Grade 3 open fracture, it has been suggested that reaming of the medullary cavity is undesirable, and for this reason the AO Group recommend the use in these circumstances of a solid intramedullary nail. This pattern of nail is angled and of sufficiently small profile to allow it to negotiate most tibiae without any reaming. Others have shown that in the majority of grade 3 open fractures, the results of nailing (with the use of locking screws) after reaming are comparable in terms of infection with those obtained when external fixators have been employed; and that they are better in terms of joint stiffness, malunion, access for plastic reconstructions and patient preference. Nevertheless, where there has been gross tissue contamination, many would still prefer to use external fixation or where applicable, simple plaster cast support until the situation regarding wound infection has been resolved.

Note:

- If there is a pin track infection following the use of an external fixator, reaming of the medullary canal is contraindicated; reaming carries the almost certain risk of disseminating infection throughout the bone.
- If there is a bone defect involving more than 50% of the circumference of the bone and more than 2 cm long, then bone grafting will ultimately be required in all cases; where the bone defect is smaller, healing may occur without grafting.
- Be alert to possibility of the development of a compartment syndrome with the associated risks of muscle necrosis and nerve palsy, and take appropriate action without delay.

COMPARTMENT SYNDROMES

Diagnosis

The first symptoms are of severe or increasing pain, even if the fracture is well supported. It is relentless in character and not well relieved by opiates. The limb is tense and swollen, and sometimes indurated. Tenderness is diffuse and there is pain on passive stretching of the muscles in the affected compartment (e.g. by flexing the toes in the case of the anterior compartment). There may be muscle paralysis, sensory disturbance and early loss of vibration sense. The distal pulses may be reduced or absent. The intercompartmental pressures may be monitored, and a differential pressure below 30 mmHg is an indication for surgery.

Treatment

Prophylaxis. Where there is an open fracture with extensive muscle damage, the compartment involved should be widely decompressed at the time of the initial exploration.

Established cases. Prompt decompression of all four compartments is advised. This can generally be done through two separate incisions.

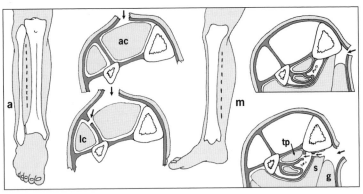

To decompress the compartments two 'safe' incisions which avoid the perforating arteries are recommended; they may also be employed to extend existing wounds. A 15 cm *anterolateral incision* (**a**), placed 2 cm lateral to the shin, may be used to divide the investing fascia and open the anterior compartment (**ac**). (The fascia is grasped with forceps and split extensively in a vertical direction with dissecting scissors.) By retracting the lateral skin flap, the lateral compartment (**lc**) can then be opened by dividing the anterior peroneal septum. Through a safe 15 cm *medial incision* (**m**), placed 2 cm behind the medial tibial border, the superficial posterior compartment may also be opened. By reflecting the gastrocnemius (**g**) and detaching the soleus (**s**) from its bony attachment, the roof of the deep posterior compartment may be split, along with the fascial coverings of tibialis posterior (**tp**) and the two other bi-pennate muscles.

After-care. Often one of the two wounds can be closed immediately, and the other dealt with by controlled tension sutures or split-skin grafting. If the swelling is marked, both should be left open, and closed 3–5 days later.

Classification of ankle
    fractures 480
Diagnosis of ankle injuries
    485
Principles of treatment of
    ankle injuries 486
Complications of ankle
    injuries 495

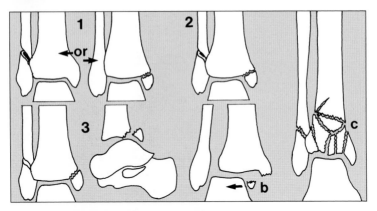

CLASSIFICATION OF ANKLE FRACTURES
Pott's classification
This venerable classification, although long declared obsolete, has not yet disappeared from common usage as it has the merit of simplicity and a certain relevance to decisions regarding treatment.

First degree Pott's fracture (**1**): fracture of a single malleolus (medial or lateral).

Second degree Pott's fracture (**2**): fracture of both the medial and lateral malleoli.

Third degree Pott's fracture (**3**): medial, lateral and posterior malleoli are affected.

The usefulness of this classification may be improved by accepting a fracture of the lateral malleolus associated with a tear of the deltoid ligament as a second degree injury; and adding to the description the presence of diastasis (**b**) or vertical compression of the inferior articular surface of the tibia (**c**).

Weber's classification
This is based on the level of the fibular fracture, once thought to be the key to all ankle fractures.

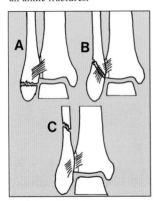

Type A fractures occur distal to the syndesmosis.

Type B fractures start at the level of the tibial plafond; they often spiral in a proximal direction and usually involve the syndesmosis.

Type C fractures start proximal to the syndesmosis which is subject to a variable amount of damage.

While this classification is simple it does not take into account injuries to related structures (e.g. an isolated fracture of the fibula is not distinguished from one accompanied by a fracture of the medial malleolus).

The AO classification:

This follows the lines of the Weber classification (it is sometimes referred to as the AO Weber classification) but takes into account damage to other structures. The Groups within each type tend to follow the Pott's classification.

(44-)A1= isolated infrasyndesmotic injuries
- **A1.1** = rupture of the lateral ligament
- **A1.2** = avulsion of the tip of the lateral malleolus
- **A1.3** = transverse fracture of the lateral malleolus.

(44-)A2 = infrasyndesmotic lesion with a fracture of the medial malleolus
- **A2.1** = rupture of the lateral ligament
- **A2.2** = avulsion of the tip of the lateral malleolus
- **A2.3** = transverse fracture of the lateral malleolus.

(44-)A3 = infrasyndesmotic lesion with a posteromedial fracture
- **A3.1** = rupture of the lateral ligament
- **A3.2** = with avulsion of the tip of the lateral malleolus
- **A3.3** = with transverse fracture of the lateral malleolus.

(44-)B1=isolated transsyndesmotic fibular fractures
- **B1.1** = non-comminuted
- **B1.2** = with rupture of the anterior syndesmosis
- **B1.3** = comminuted (multifragmentary).

(44-)B2 = transsyndesmotic fibular fracture with a medial lesion
- **B2.1** = non-comminuted, with rupture of the medial ligament and of the anterior syndesmosis
- **B2.2** = non-comminuted, with fracture of the medial malleolus and rupture of the anterior syndesmosis
- **B2.3** = comminuted (multifragmentary) fibular fracture.

(44-)B3 = transsyndesmotic fibular fracture, with medial lesion and posterior malleolar fracture
- **B3.1** = non-comminuted fracture of fibula with rupture of the medial ligament
- **B3.2** = non-comminuted fracture of the fibula with fracture of the medial malleolus (illustrated in two planes with Tillaux fracture)
- **B3.3** = comminuted (multifragmentary) fracture of the lateral malleolus with fracture of the medial malleolus.

(44-)C1 = suprasyndesmotic lesion, with non-comminuted fracture of the fibular shaft
- **C1.1** = with rupture of the medial collateral ligament
- **C1.2** = with fracture of the medial malleolus
- **C1.3** = with fractures of the medial and posterior malleoli.

(44-)C2 = suprasyndesmotic lesion with comminuted fracture of the fibular shaft
- **C2.1** = with rupture of the medial ligament
- **C2.2** = with fracture of the medial malleolus
- **C2.3** = with fractures of the medial and posterior malleoli.

(44-)C3 = proximal fibular suprasyndesmotic fracture
- **C3.1** = without shortening or a posterior malleolar fracture
- **C3.2** = with shortening, but no posterior malleolar fracture
- **C3.3** = with a medial lesion and a posterior malleolar fracture.

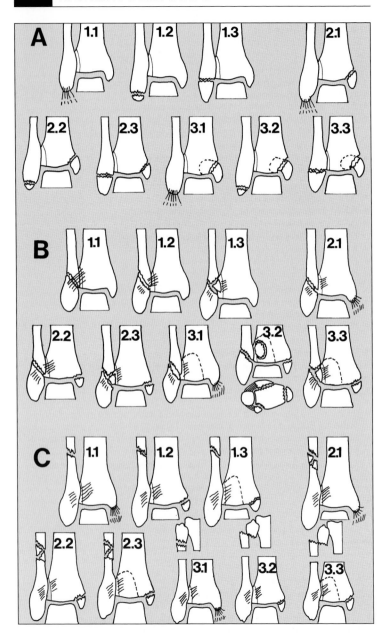

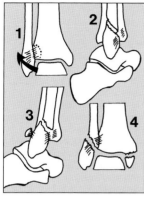

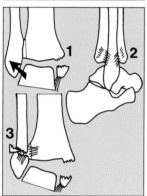

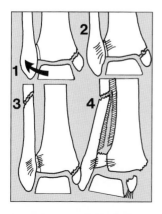

Lauge–Hansen classification

This is based on the position of the foot at the time of injury and the direction in which the causal force is applied.

Supination/lateral rotation injuries (external rotation injury without diastasis). The talus externally rotates, and the structures fail in regular sequence: **Stage 1:** rupture of the anterior (inferior) tibiofibular ligament (or a Tillaux fracture). **Stage 2:** the fibula fractures in an oblique or spiral fashion. **Stage 3:** the fibular fragment drags off the posterior malleolus, or the posterior tibiofibular ligament tears. **Stage 4:** the medial malleolus fractures, or the deltoid ligament tears.

Pronation/abduction injuries (abduction injuries). The foot everts and the talus swings into abduction. **Stage 1:** either the deltoid ligament ruptures or there is a (horizontal) avulsion fracture of the medial malleolus. **Stage 2:** both the anterior and posterior tibiofibular ligaments rupture (or their bony attachments are avulsed). **Stage 3:** the fibula fractures, often close to the level of the joint. The fracture line is often horizontal, comminution may occur and the distal fibular fragment is tilted laterally.

Pronation/lateral rotation injuries (external rotation injuries with diastasis). **Stage 1:** the rotating talus produces an oblique fracture of the medial malleolus, or ruptures the deltoid ligament. **Stage 2:** the anterior tibiofibular ligament ruptures or avulses its attachment (Tillaux fracture). **Stage 3:** there is a spiral or oblique fracture of the fibula which may be as proximal as its neck (Maisonneuve fracture). **Stage 4:** the posterior tibiofibular ligament ruptures or pulls off its bony attachment. The interosseous membrane rips and gross diastasis results (Dupuytren fracture–dislocation of the ankle).

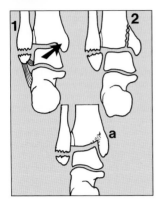

Supination/adduction injuries (adduction injuries). The talus adducts within the ankle mortise. **Stage 1:** there is a complete tear of the lateral ligament or an avulsion fracture of the tip of the lateral malleolus. If the forces are slight, a partial tear of the lateral ligament results (sprain of ankle). **Stage 2:** the adducting talus strikes the medial malleolus causing a *vertical* or *high oblique fracture*. Instead of the medial malleolus being pushed off, there may be a compression fracture of the angle (**a**), and occasionally the medial malleolus may be broken off without damage first occurring to the lateral ligament.

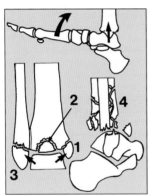

Pronation/dorsiflexion (compression injuries). Dorsiflexion of the ankle combined with a vertical compression force most commonly occurs in falls from a height. **Stage 1:** the wide anterior part of the talus is forced between the malleoli, shearing off the medial malleolus. **Stage 2:** the anterior tibial margin is fractured. **Stage 3:** the lateral malleolus fractures. The talus may sublux anteriorly, carrying the anterior marginal fracture with it. **Stage 4:** with still greater violence, the inferior articular surface of the tibia (tibial plafond) fractures in an irregular fashion, often with great comminution.

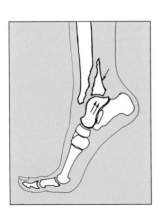

Other compression injuries. If a fall occurs on to the plantar-flexed foot, the posterior articular surface of the tibia may be fractured. In addition, fractures of both malleoli (as in typical pronation/dorsiflexion injuries) may occur when the broad anterior portion of the talus is driven between them.

Be astonished, but not alarmed at the bewildering complexity of these classifications of ankle fractures. *In practice*, a description of the structures involved and any displacement will usually suffice (e.g. 'an undisplaced spiral fracture of the lateral malleolus beneath the syndesmosis').

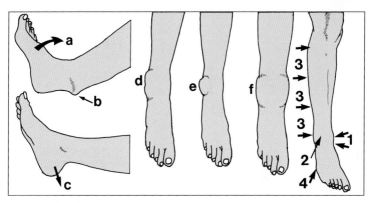

DIAGNOSIS OF ANKLE INJURIES

Is there any deformity? Look in particular for external rotation of the foot relative to the leg (**a**). If the medial malleolus is fractured and laterally displaced, the distal end of the tibia may become quite prominent under the skin (**b**). Posterior displacement of the foot (**c**) is a common feature in posterior malleolar fractures.

Is there any swelling? Note if any is present, if it is accompanied by bruising, and its site and distribution. Diffuse swelling occurs in front of the lateral malleolus (**d**) in many ankle injuries. Egg-shaped swelling (**e**) occurs over the lateral malleolus shortly after complete lateral ligament tears or lateral malleolar fractures. Gross swelling (**f**) and bruising is found in many trimalleolar and compression fractures.

If tenderness is present, where is it situated? In particular, check: (**1**) the medial malleolus and deltoid ligament; (**2**) the area of the anterior tibiofibular ligament; (**3**) the whole length of the fibula; (**4**) the base of the fifth metatarsal. (Avulsion fractures of the base of the fifth metatarsal following inversion injuries are often confused with ankle fractures.)

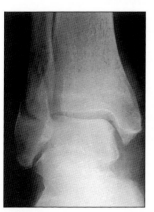

Interpreting the radiographs
If there is a fibular fracture, note its level, pattern and any displacement. The radiograph shows the commonest of fibular fractures, a spiral fracture at the level of the syndesmosis. There is no talar shift. This would be classified as a first degree Pott's fracture, or a Weber type-B, fracture. In the AO system it would be classified as 44-B, and in the Lauge–Hansen system as an S/L injury (external rotation without diastasis).

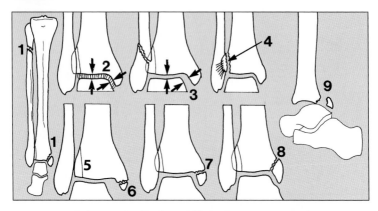

Be sure to exclude a proximally situated fibular fracture—e.g. a Maisonneuve fracture (**1**). Look for fibular tenderness proximal to the ankle joint, and if this is present the whole length of the fibula must be visualised. Look for radiological evidence of talar shift. Normally the joint space between the talus and the medial malleolus should be the same as between the talus and the inferior articular surface of the tibia (**2**). An increase of the so-called medial clear space of more the 4 mm is regarded as being evidence of talar shift (**3**). Look for signs of disruption of the syndesmosis, such as a Tillaux fracture (caused by avulsion of the attachments of the inferior tibiofibular ligaments, (**4**), or an increase of the tibiofibular clear space (**5**).

If the medial malleolus is fractured, note the level, pattern and any displacement. Avulsion fractures are usually transverse and may be near the tip (**6**); fractures due to rotation or abduction of the talus in the mortise are often at the level of the plafond (**7**) and may be oblique (**8**). Note the presence of any fracture of the posterior malleolus (**9**). In doubtful cases, an additional oblique (Cobb) projection may be helpful.

PRINCIPLES OF TREATMENT OF ANKLE INJURIES

The aims of treatment are:

1. The restoration and maintenance of the normal alignment of the talus with the tibia.
2. The provision of conditions favourable to the union of any fracture or the healing of any torn ligaments, so that there is no problem in the future with instability.
3. The optimum restoration of articulating surfaces to lessen the chances of secondary osteoarthritis.

Excellent results can be obtained by conservative methods in the majority of ankle fractures; they are universally good in certain types, and in these surgery would not normally be considered. The unstable bimalleolar or trimalleolar fracture, however, requires precision in reduction, great care in the techniques of plaster fixation and skilled surveillance for many weeks following injury. Many surgeons prefer to avoid these uncertainties by routine accurate open reduction and internal fixation. In a number of fractures, especially where there has been soft-tissue interposition, reduction can only be achieved by open methods.

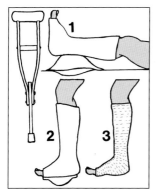

Isolated fracture of the fibula distal to the syndesmosis (A1).

If stable and undisplaced, with no evidence of any significant medial injury, these injuries may be successfully treated conservatively. A below knee cast for six weeks is generally preferred. The limb should be elevated and crutches used until swelling subsides (1), when a walking heel may be fitted (2). While some forego fixation (using bandage supports only in order to facilitate mobilisation (3)), this has not been shown to confer any benefit.

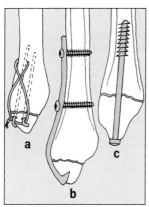

If the fracture is *displaced* or if there is evidence of instability, internal fixation is generally advised. Where the fibular fragment is small and particularly if the bone is porotic and of poor quality, two K-wires with tension band wiring (a) generally give the best results. Alternatively, a hook-plate (e.g. Zuelzer plate, (b)) may be used; this has the advantage of preserving the integrity of the fibular fragment. Where the fragment is larger, a lag screw may be used to engage in the medullary canal (c), although care must be taken to see that it does not lead to angulation of the fragment.

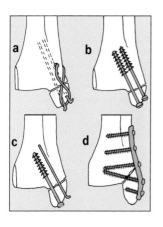

Fracture of the fibula distal to the syndesmosis with an associated medial injury (A2).

There will be medial tenderness indicating fracture of the medial malleolus or detachment of the deltoid ligament. These injuries are unstable, and in addition there may be infolding of the periosteum on the medial side, preventing reduction of the malleolus. As a rule, the medial malleolus should be secured, using, for example, two K-wires and a tension band (a), two cancellous screws (b), a cancellous screw and a single K-wire (c), or a small plate and screws (d). While any of these procedures usually restores stability, many prefer to continue and fix the lateral malleolus as well, using any of the methods previously described.

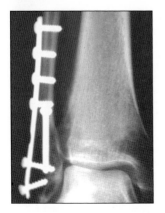

Fracture of the fibula at the level of the syndesmosis (B1).

Isolated spiral fractures of the fibula without significant displacement are the commonest type of ankle fracture and should be treated conservatively, in the same way as already described for stable fractures of the fibula distal to the syndesmosis. Where there is significant displacement, generally indicative of associated ligament injuries or fracture of the medial malleolus (**B2**), internal fixation is ususally advised, e.g. with an interfragmentary screw and a small contoured plate and screws (**left**). Any accompanying medial malleolar fracture should be fixed.

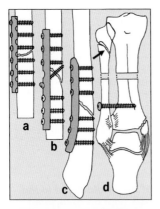

Fracture of the fibula above the level of the syndesmosis (C).

These fractures involve the anterior interosseous ligament, and the fibula may fracture at any level. The rare stable injury may be treated in a cast, but the majority of these injuries require internal fixation. Methods include a low contact dynamic compression plate (**a**), interfragmentary screws and a neutralising plate (**b**), and, if distally situated, by a tubular plate (**c**). Exposure of very proximal fractures (**d**) puts the common peroneal nerve at risk, and these are best stabilised using a transverse syndesmotic screw, taking care to avoid undue compression.

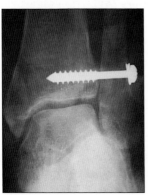

In most fibular shaft fractures, careful reduction (to correct any rotational deformity) followed by secure fixation are generally followed by closure of the syndesmosis. Failure may be due to problems with the tendon of tibialis posterior or other local causes at the ankle, requiring exploration; otherwise a cross screw (**left**) may be used. As this prevents axial rotation and the other movements of the fibula which normally occur when the ankle is dorsiflexed, such a screw should be removed before the ankle is mobilised.

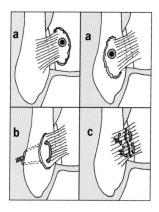

Other considerations
Tillaux fractures and tears of the anterior tibiofibular ligament. If
possible, any accessible large bone fragments forming the tibial or fibular attachments of the anterior tibiofibular ligament should be reduced and held with a small lag screw (a). If the fragment is very small it may be wired in position (b). If the ligament itself is involved it should be sutured (c). The repair may be supported with a syndesmosis screw which should be removed at 8 weeks prior to mobilisation of the ankle.

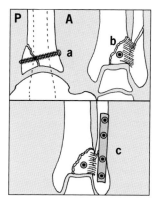

Posterior malleolar fractures. The
pathology of these fragments should be determined with a CAT scan. Sometimes these are in continuity with the medial malleolus, in which case they may fall into position when the malleolus is reduced. This may then be held by any of the methods already described for that fragment. If the fragment has been pulled off by the posterior tibiofibular ligament and is small it may be left: otherwise it may be held with a screw passed into it from the front (retrograde fixation) (a). If it lacks body and is shell-like, it may be fixed with a screw from behind (b) using a posterior approach. An associated fibular fracture may be dealt with through the same incision (c).

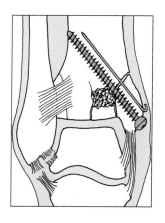

'Corner' fractures. Some adduction or
abduction injuries may result in damage to the articular surface of the tibia (or talus) due to impingement of the 'corners' of the talus. As a general rule, small fragments of bone and cartilage should be removed, but large pieces of bone covered with articular cartilage should be retained. Illustrated is a complete tear of the lateral ligament and a fracture of the medial malleolus (A2.1) accompanied by a 'corner' fracture of the inferior articular surface of the tibia. The malleolus has been held with a screw and a K-wire (to prevent rotation). The articular fragment has been replaced and the defect packed with bone chips.

Conservative treatment of bimalleolar and trimalleolar fractures

In both sexes, conservative treatment should be considered if the patient is frail, a bad anaesthetic risk or the skin and peripheral circulation are poor. In women over the age of 50 years, conservative treatment is said to give results which are comparable with surgery, and this is largely due to the technical difficulty of securing small malleolar fragments which are often osteoporotic and subject to high levels of stress. Nevertheless, for success, conservatively treated cases must be most carefully supervised for the early detection of late displacement.

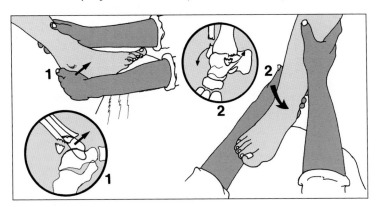

Method. The patient's knee is flexed over the edge of the table, with a sandbag behind the thigh. The table should be adjusted until the surgeon can steady the foot with his knee. *Carry out a reduction rehearsal.* The malleoli preserve their relationship with the talus and the foot, so that *in essence it is a case of re-aligning the foot with the tibia*. First, correct any posterior subluxation by lifting the heel anteriorly **(1)**; then, still grasping the hindfoot, correct any external rotation **(2)**. It should be noted that little force is required for all this: re-alignment often occurs with sensations similar to the reduction of a dislocation.

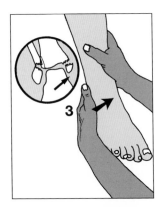

Finally, still grasping the hindfoot, correct any abduction deformity **(3)**.
Note:

- The appearance of the ankle should be restored to normal.
- Overcorrection is difficult or impossible.
- Repeat the procedure until you can remember the movements and the force required for reduction.

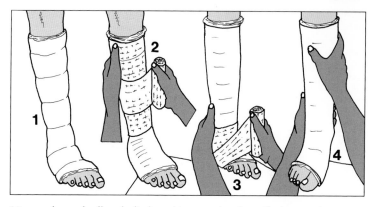

Now apply wool roll to the limb, making sure that the malleolar prominences are well covered (1). Without hurry, follow this with two to three 15 cm (6″) plaster bandages from the level of the tibial tubercle to just above the ankle (2).

Smooth the plaster well down and then quickly apply two 15 cm plaster bandages to the foot and ankle (3). The toes may be steadied with your knee. On completion, you should be left with a plaster which is setting at the calf, but is quite soft and mouldable at the foot and ankle. Now repeat the reduction manoeuvre and hold the limb in the reduced position until the plaster has set (4). Steady the forefoot with the knee (to keep the ankle at right angles) and ease the hands slightly upwards and downwards to prevent local indentation of the plaster. *Extend the cast above the knee if the fracture is very unstable.* Check the position of the fracture with radiographs before the anaesthetic is discontinued, and if necessary, repeat the procedure. Take precautions to avoid swelling and its effects—e.g. by elevation of the limb and perhaps splitting of the plaster.

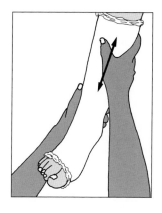

The plaster should be examined for slackness (**left**) as swelling subsides. If it becomes slack, it must be changed with care to prevent slipping of the fracture, and general anaesthesia may be necessary. Radiographs should be taken weekly; remanipulation under anaesthesia or internal fixation may have to be considered if there is any slip. A *walking heel* should not be applied before 6 weeks; prior to that the patient may be mobilised (non-weight bearing) with crutches. Plaster fixation should be maintained until union (usually 9–10 weeks); confirm this clinically and with X-rays. Thereafter, bandage supports should be worn till any swelling subsides. Physiotherapy is often required.

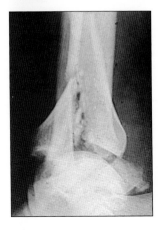

Multifragmented compression (or pilon) fractures

Surgery is difficult but may be considered if there is one substantial intact articular fragment. The steps are: • reduction and fixation of the fibula to obtain length • reconstruction of the articular surface by placing the fragments over the talar dome • packing defects with bone grafts • fixing the main fragments with a buttress plate (and if required, cannulated screws). Where there is substantial skin and soft-tissue damage, an external fixator may be used. In all cases it is highly desirable to commence ankle joint movements as soon as the quality of fixation will allow.

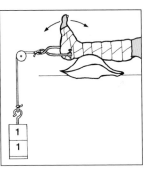

If the fragmentation of the distal tibia is so gross that no substantial articular fragment remains intact, conservative treatment may become necessary. Apply 2 kg of traction through a calcaneal pin to maintain alignment and commence active exercises as soon as pain will permit. Alternatively, a hinged external fixator may be used. Weight-bearing must be deferred until union is quite sound in order to avoid further deformity from compression. If at a later stage secondary osteoarthritis becomes a problem, an ankle joint fusion may have to be considered.

Lateral ligament injuries

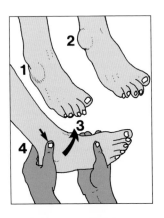

A soft tissue injury is diagnosed where there is a history of trauma, and the radiographs are normal. A history of an inversion injury is obtainable in most lateral ligament injuries. In sprains, swelling and tenderness follow the fasciculi of the lateral ligament (1). In complete tears of the lateral ligament, swelling at first lies over the lateral malleolus (2). If the findings suggest a substantial injury, grasp the foot and gently adduct the talus in the ankle mortise (3), feeling for any gap opening up at the outer corner of the joint (4). Compare with the other side. Excess movement of the talus suggests a complete lateral ligament tear.

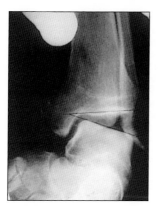

If the manoeuvre cannot be performed adequately because of pain, infiltrate the fasciculi of the lateral ligament with local anaesthetic (e.g. 20 ml of 0.5% lignocaine) or administer a general anaesthetic. Repeat the manoeuvre, and for further confirmation, take AP radiographs under stress **(left)**. Tilting in excess of 15° is pathological; with lesser degrees take comparison films of the other side.

Treatment

Simple sprains resolve in a few days with local supportive measures (adhesive strapping, crepe bandaging, etc.) rest and elevation.

Complete (acute) lateral ligament tears may be treated by either:

- surgical repair (of both anterior tibiofibular *and* calcaneofibular ligaments); this has been claimed to give the best results
- plaster fixation for 6 weeks, followed by a lighter support till free from discomfort, or
- strapping, until the acute symptoms have settled, followed by functional training in the form of range-of-motion exercises and neuromuscular training (e.g. on a tilt board.)

Functional instabilities may be diagnosed if investigation fails to show any obvious ligamentous, muscular or neurological problem, and there is a complaint of pain, swelling, stiffness and instability. These are thought to be due to disorders of muscle coordination or proprioception, and are treated by functional training and sometimes the use of lateral heel and sole wedges.

Chronic lateral ligament instability may be treated by a lateral ligament reconstruction procedure (e.g. Watson–Jones).

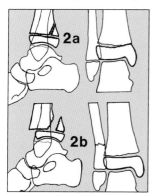

Other injuries about the ankle

Epiphyseal injuries. Salter/Harris *type 1* injuries are rare. *Type 2* injuries, however, are common and are usually a form of supination/lateral rotation injury (external rotation without diastasis). In many, displacement is minimal (e.g. 2a) and can be treated in a below-knee plaster for 4–6 weeks.

Where displacement is appreciable (e.g. 2b), the ankle should be manipulated as previously described.

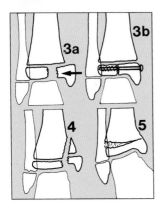

Type 3 (Salter-Harris) injuries may sometimes be reduced by applying firm local pressure (**3a**) under general anaesthesia, but if unsuccessful cross-screwing (**3b**) may have to be considered, taking care to avoid damaging the epiphyseal plate.

Type 4 injuries (**4**) should be treated by open reduction and internal fixation.

Type 5 injuries (**5**) may require late corrective osteotomy.

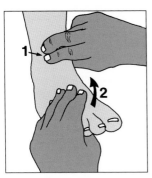

Sprain of inferior tibiofibular ligament. Inversion injuries of the ankle may lead to a first stage supination/lateral rotational tearing of the inferior tibiofibular ligament. Pain may be quite severe, and tenderness is often well localised over the ligament (**1**) and is most marked when the foot is dorsiflexed (**2**). A 6-week period of plaster fixation is advised, although in cases of chronic disability, hydrocortisone injections and even cross-screwing are advocated.

Ankle dislocation without fracture. Rarely, the ankle may dislocate without fracture. Although rupture of both the medial and lateral ligaments must take place, conservative management by closed manipulative reduction and plaster fixation may achieve a good result; some, however, would advocate repair of all the ligamentous structures involved. Avascular necrosis of the talus is a minor risk in this situation.

Recurrent dislocation of peroneal tendons. This is a rare condition in which eversion causes painful clicking sensations as the peroneal tendons repeatedly snap over the lateral malleolus. It is associated with a defect in the superior peroneal retinaculum, and this may be reconstructed surgically.

Footballers' ankle and osteochondritis tali. Tibial and/or talar osteophytes may arise in footballers from repeated anterior capsular tears, and limit dorsiflexion. Excision of these osteophytes in an attempt to improve dorsiflexion is seldom indicated. Pain may follow a fresh capsular tear (and this may be treated symptomatically by a two-week period in a plaster cast) or from early ankle joint osteoarthritis.

Osteochondritis tali. This may give rise to chronic mild ankle pain. It is treated along general lines.

COMPLICATIONS OF ANKLE INJURIES

Swelling. Swelling persisting for weeks or even months after fixation has been discarded is so common as to be an almost normal occurrence. Assuming that the fracture has united in good position, the patient may be reassured, given local supportive measures and advised regarding elevation and activity.

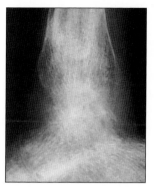

Sudeck's atrophy (complex regional pain syndrome). Where swelling is gross, and especially if the toes are involved, suspect Sudeck's atrophy. There may be glazing of the skin and pain. Radiographs may show typical porotic changes (**left**), and usually confirm union of the fracture. Intensive physiotherapy and continued use of supports will be required. Convalescence may be expected to be slow, with occasionally some permanent functional impairment.

Stiffness, 'weakness' and disturbance of gait. Again, assuming sound union, these symptoms generally respond rapidly to appropriate physiotherapy and occupational therapy. Progress may be assessed by charting the range of ankle and subtalar joint movements.

Instability. Instability due to lateral ligament damage has been described; instability may also follow damage to the medial structures. Non-union of a large medial malleolar fragment should be treated by internal fixation; additional grafting may be necessary. When the tip only is involved, it may be excised and the lateral ligament sutured to the stump.

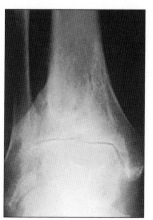

Osteoarthritis. Considering the incidence of ankle fractures, osteoarthritis (**left**) is an uncommon complication. It is most likely to follow compression fractures, and fractures with residual diastasis or talotibial incongruity. If symptoms of pain, swelling, stiffness and disturbance of gait are troublesome, then joint replacement or fusion may occasionally be advised. Late function in the case of the latter is generally good due to persistent midtarsal joint movements.

CHAPTER

28

Regional injuries: the foot

Injuries to the talar neck 498
Other talar lesions 502
Calcaneal fractures 503
Peritalar dislocation 510
Total dislocation of talus 511
Acute rupture of the tendo
    calcaneus 511
Midtarsal dislocations 512
Tarsometatarsal dislocations
    514
Metatarsal fractures 515
Injuries to the toes 518
Crushing injuries of the foot
    without fracture 518

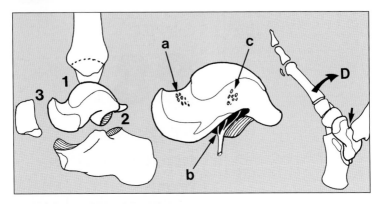

INJURIES TO THE TALAR NECK

Anatomical considerations. The talus plays a key role in no less than three joints: **(1)** the ankle joint, articulating with the tibia and fibula; **(2)** the subtalar joint, articulating with the calcaneus; **(3)** the talonavicular joint, articulating with the navicular; along with the calcaneocuboid joint this forms the *midtarsal joint*. Secondary osteoarthritis may occur as a result of persisting irregularity of the joint surfaces or avascular necrosis which occurs in half of all talar neck fractures. The blood supply of the talus enters at three sites: **(a)** the neck; **(b)** the sinus tarsi area; **(c)** the medial side of the body. The more sources disturbed, the greater the risk to the blood supply. *Mechanisms of injury:* the commonest cause is forced dorsiflexion **(D)** of the ankle, when the talar neck is forced against the inferior margin of the talus. This may occur in drivers involved in road traffic accidents, from contact with the foot pedals. The injury may also follow falls from a height in a crouching position.

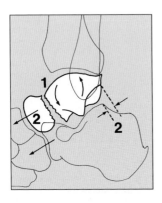

Classification of talar neck fractures. Talar neck fractures have been classified into four types of increasing severity. In *type 1* injuries the talar neck is fractured without displacement. Incomplete hairline cracks are not uncommon. Only the blood supply through the neck is affected, and the incidence of avascular necrosis is under 10%.

In *type 2* injuries **(left)** there is an accompanying subtalar subluxation. The proximal portion of the talus adopts a position of plantar flexion **(1)**. The *head* of the talus maintains its relationship with the navicular and calcaneus (and the rest of the foot) which sublux forwards **(2)**. Avascular necrosis may rise to 50% in severe cases.

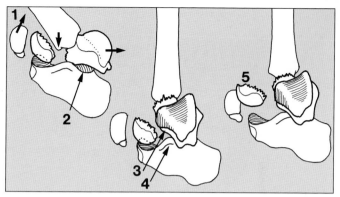

In *type 3* injuries, there is further dorsiflexion (**1**), and the tibia is driven between the two talar fragments. The posterior fragment is extruded backwards, while at the same time the convex posterior articular surface of the calcaneus (**2**) guides it medially. It comes to rest with its medial surface (**3**) caught on the sustentaculum tali (**4**). All three sources of blood supply are disturbed, with the risks of avascular necrosis rising to 85%. In the rare *type 4* injury, the head of the talus dislocates from the navicular (**5**) in association with a type 3 or a type 2 injury. The incidence of avascular necrosis here is also high.

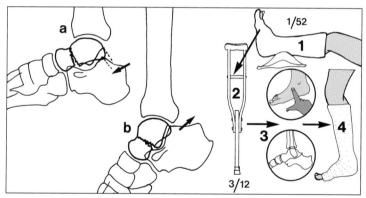

Diagnosis. This is made by X-ray. Differentiate between type 1 and type 2 injuries. If in doubt, laterals taken in dorsiflexion (**a**) and in plantar flexion (**b**) will usually show reduction of any subluxation in the plantar flexion film (type 2 illustrated on left).

Treatment of talar neck fracture

Type 1 injuries. Apply a padded plaster with a toe platform and elevate for about a week (**1**), followed by non-weight-bearing with crutches for 3 months (**2**). Then assess out of plaster for union and absence of avascular necrosis (**3**). If there are no complications, weight-bearing may commence with a light support (**4**). Physiotherapy will be required for the ankle, the subtalar joint and the calf.

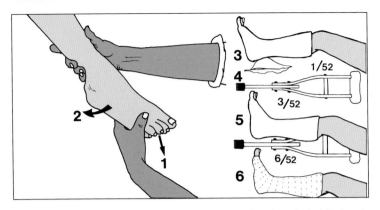

Type 2 injuries. Reduction may be attempted by closed methods: The foot is plantar flexed (1) and everted (2). A padded plaster is applied in this position and check radiographs taken. If a satisfactory reduction has been obtained, then conservative treatment may be continued. The limb is elevated for a week (3) before non-weight-bearing is permitted (4). After 3–4 weeks, the plaster is changed under intensifier control and the foot brought up to a right angle (5). Non-weight-bearing is continued for a further 6 weeks. Thereafter, if the fracture is united and there is no evidence of avascular necrosis, weight-bearing may be allowed with support (6). Physiotherapy will be required.

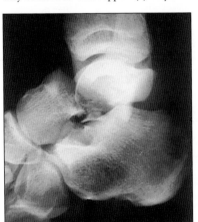

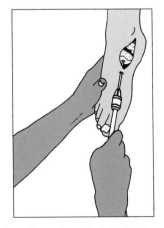

A typical displaced type 2 fracture is shown in the radiographs on the **left**. If such a fracture cannot be reduced by closed methods, open reduction will be required. In many cases, the fracture may then be secured with a Kirschner wire passed backwards from the head of the talus into the body (**right above**). The after-care is as detailed above, with the Kirschner wire being removed at the change of plaster. These injuries may also be internally fixed (e.g. by cancellous screws).

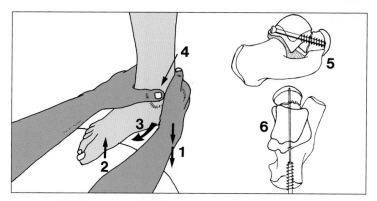

Type 3 injuries. The displaced portion of the talus is situated subcutaneously, and there should be no delay in reducing it as the overlying skin is tightly stretched over the bone and likely to slough. Facilities for open reduction should be available, but closed methods should be attempted first. Begin by gripping the heel and applying traction to it (**1**). Now dorsiflex the foot with your knee (**2**). Maintaining traction, pull the heel slightly forward and evert it to open up the space for the talus (**3**). Apply strong pressure over the displaced body of the talus: press it laterally (**4**) but also slightly anteriorly and downwards. Now plantar flex the foot. If purchase on the heel is poor, a Steinman pin through the heel and a calliper may be used. After reduction, proceed with elevation and gradual mobilisation as previously described. If closed reduction fails (as it often does), open reduction will be necessary. Fixation may be achieved with one or two cortical or cancellous screws, passed from behind through the body of the talus and into the head (**5**). Cannulated screws may also be used; these can be threaded over Kirschner wires which have been inserted temporarily to hold the reduction. (**6**) (The AO group, with an eye to rapid mobilisation, in fact recommend internal fixation along these lines for all talar neck fractures.)

Type 4 injuries. These uncommon fractures are likely to require open reduction. All fragments should be retained, even if completely detached and obviously avascular. On no account should the talus be excised.

Complications of talar neck fractures

Skin necrosis. The skin may become tightly stretched over a displaced talus and undergo necrosis with late sloughing. *Early reduction is imperative to avoid this complication.*

Open fracture. Thorough debridement of the wound is essential, but again every effort must be made to retain the main fragments. Treatment should follow the usual lines established for the management of open fractures. If sepsis occurs *in conjunction with avascular necrosis,* healing may be obtained only after excision of the avascular fragments.

Ankle fracture. Rarely, malleolar fracture may be found complicating talar neck fractures. Closed reduction here is unreliable, and open reduction with internal fixation of the malleolar fracture is desirable.

Avascular necrosis. The diagnosis is by X-ray. *Increased density* is often apparent by 6–12 weeks, but do not be confused by the shadows cast by the overlying malleoli.

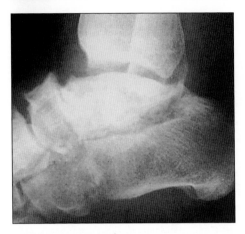

Revascularisation always occurs in closed injuries and is usually advanced by 8 months. *Weight-bearing before revascularisation is complete is likely to cause marked flattening of the talus* (left).

Osteoarthritis. This may occur secondary to avascular necrosis or malunion, and involve the ankle, subtalar or midtarsal joints (or any combination of these), and in severe cases fusion may be indicated.

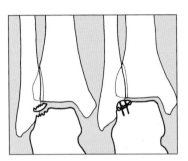 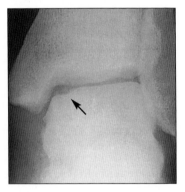

OTHER TALAR LESIONS

Dome fractures (left). A portion of the upper articular surface of the talus may be detached as a result of a shearing injury; occasionally the fragment is inverted, effectively preventing union. If the fragment is substantial, it should be replaced and secured.

Osteochondritis tali (right). This may occur as a sequel to a non-displaced shearing fracture, although frequently there is no history of injury. The defect may be drilled to encourage revascularisation.

Avulsion fractures. Minor avulsion fractures of the talus may result from inversion, eversion, plantar flexion and rarely dorsiflexion strains of the ankle—when flakes of bone are pulled off by ligamentous or capsular attachments. Symptomatic treatment only is required.

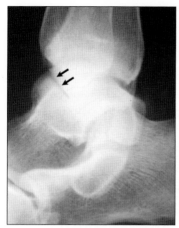

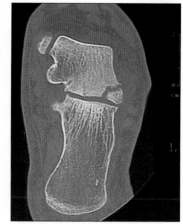

Fractures of the body of the talus. The upper articular surface of the talus may be fractured by the same mechanisms which produce compression fractures of the ankle. Vertical splits (**left**) without significant disturbance of the ankle or subtalar joints may be treated as type 1 talar neck fractures. If displacement has occurred, accurate reduction and cross-screwing should be carried out. If the fracture is highly comminuted, surgical reconstruction may not be possible. Conservative treatment involves pressure bandaging and elevation, with intensive active exercises as soon as pain and swelling will permit. Weight-bearing should be avoided until union is well advanced (about 8–10 weeks). Persistent pain and functional restriction are indications for ankle fusion.

Fracture of the lateral process of the talus. These injuries are uncommon, but may be seen following skateboarding accidents (see CAT scan, **right**). The subtalar joint is involved, and they are best dealt with by open reduction and internal fixation with a cancellous screw.

Compression fractures of the head of the talus. These fractures are uncommon, but are usually highly comminuted and unsuitable for attempts at reconstruction. Treat as for comminuted fractures of the body.

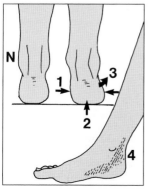

CALCANEAL FRACTURES

The commonest cause is a fall from a height on to the heels. Taking this into account, it is essential that you do not overlook a similar fracture on the other side, or a dorsolumbar junction wedge fracture of the spine.

Clinical appearance. In major fractures, the heel when viewed from behind appears: (**1**) wider, (**2**) shorter and flatter, and (**3**) tilted laterally into valgus. There is often tense swelling of the heel, marked local tenderness and later bruising (**4**), which may spread into the medial side of the sole and proximally to the calf. Weight-bearing is usually impossible.

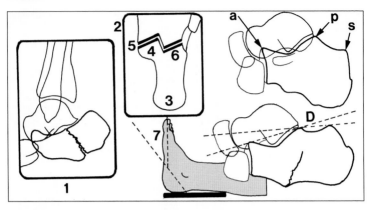

Radiographs. The most important view is a well-centred and well-exposed lateral projection (**1**). An axial projection (**2**) is helpful in visualising the pillar of the heel (**3**), the sustentaculum tali (**4**), the anterior talocalcaneal joint (**5**) and the posterior talocalcaneal joint (**6**). This film is taken with the tube tilted at 40° from the vertical (**7**). A line may be drawn from the anterior articular process of the calcaneus (**a**) through the posterior articular surface (**p**) to intersect with a second line touching the superior angle of the tuberosity (**s**). This is *Bohler's salient angle*, and is normally about 40°. It is decreased (**D**) in fractures which flatten the heel profile. An oblique projection may be helpful if doubt remains. *Note that the key factor in assessing calcaneal fractures is whether or not there is involvement of the subtalar joint.* CAT scans close to the coronal plane are often of great value.

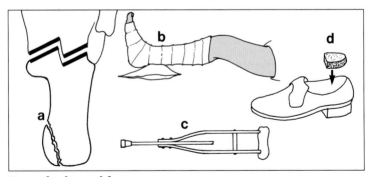

Type of calcaneal fracture
There are seven common patterns of fracture:

1. Vertical fracture of the tuberosity. The subtalar joint is not involved (**a**) and the prognosis is excellent. Swelling may be severe and should be controlled by firm bandaging and elevation of the limb (**b**). Weight bearing will be painful, and crutches will be required for some weeks (**c**); they may be discarded when pain settles. A crepe bandage or similar support may be worn till swelling subsides. Any long-term term heel pain may be controlled with a sorbo rubber heel cushion (**d**).

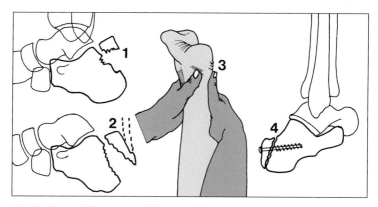

2. Horizontal fractures. These are of two types which must be distinguished. The commoner injury involves the posterior superior angle of the calcaneus without disturbance of the Achilles tendon insertion (1); it is usually caused by local trauma. The second is an avulsion fracture (2). Differentiate between them by noting the level of the fracture on the radiographs, by studying the soft-tissue shadows (looking for proximal retraction of the Achilles tendon) and feeling for a gap between the tendon insertion and the point of the heel.

Treatment. When the fracture is not of the avulsion type, it should be manipulated (3) if severely displaced. Moderate residual displacement can usually be quite safely accepted. Thereafter, a below-knee padded plaster may be applied and crutches used for the first week or so. A further 5 weeks in a below-knee walking plaster is then advised.

If the fracture is of the avulsion type it should be openly reduced and fixed with a screw (4). To remove stress from the screw, a long leg plaster should be applied with the knee flexed and the ankle in plantar flexion. After 4 weeks a below-knee walking plaster may be substituted till union (about 8 weeks).

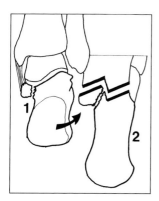

3. Fractures of the sustentaculum tali. These result from eversion injuries (1) and are seen most clearly in axial projections (2). Displacement is generally slight, and persisting disability is rare.

Treatment. Healing of the fracture is generally well advanced by 6 weeks. Prior to this the following treatments may be used: (a) a crepe bandage over wool pressure bandage and non-weight-bearing with crutches for 6 weeks, or (b) a below-knee padded plaster with crutches initially and then a walking heel; after 6 weeks a circular woven support for a further 2 weeks or so.

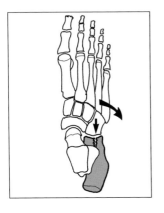

4. Anterior calcaneal fractures.

This fracture affects the anterior part of the calcaneus which articulates with the cuboid. It may result from: • forced abduction of the forefoot in which the cuboid strikes the calcaneus (left) • forced inversion injuries, which have the same effect • forced abduction of the foot in association with a midtarsal dislocation.

Treatment. If there is no significant compression or shortening of the calcaneus, treat conservatively as for a fracture of the sustentaculum tali. If there is evidence of midtarsal instability, treat as for midtarsal dislocation. If there is calcaneal shortening, consider open reduction.

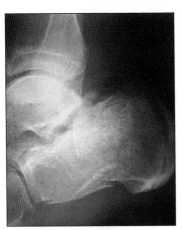

5. Fracture of the body of the calcaneus without involvement of the subtalar joint. The fracture line passes just posterior to the posterior talocalcaneal joint. Frequently, there is a decrease in the salient angle, and if this is the case (left) then flattening of the heel profile may lead to persistent, troublesome localised heel pain.

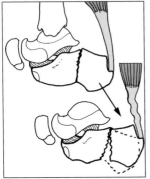

Due to proximal displacement of the portion of the calcaneus carrying the Achilles tendon insertion, there is slackening of the calf muscles, so that there is weakness of plantar flexion at the ankle and loss of spring in the step. This slackness is eventually taken up, but recovery is facilitated by *prolonged, intensive physiotherapy* in the form of calf-resisting exercises.

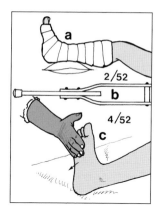

Treatment. If *displacement is slight*, good results may be obtained by conservative treatment along the following lines: (a) pressure bandaging, bed rest, elevation and analgesics for 2 weeks; (b) crutches until gradual weight bearing can be commenced at about 6 weeks; (c) calf resisting exercises as soon as pain will permit, and continued physiotherapy till maximal recovery.

More severely displaced fractures may be treated along similar lines, or an attempt made to reduce the heel fragment. An open reduction may be performed with fixation of the fragments with screws or a plate.

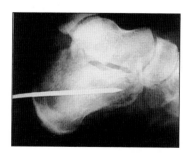

Alternatively, a Gissane spike may be driven into the heel which is then levered distally. The spike is incorporated in a plaster sabot which maintains the reduction while still permitting ankle movements. If a suitable spike is not available, a large diameter Steinman pin may be used. Image intensifier control is helpful.

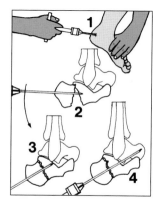

The pin should be inserted a little to the lateral side of the heel (1). The heel fragment is engaged (2) and brought down (3). The pin may, if required, be driven across the sinus tarsi into the head of the talus (following the axis of the subtalar joint) (4). The sabot and spike may be removed after 6 weeks and non-weight-bearing exercises continued for a further 2 weeks before full weight-bearing. Pin-track infection is not uncommon, and at the first sign the pin should be removed and antibiotic treatment commenced. Because of this risk, this treatment should not be employed where there is any doubt about the peripheral circulation.

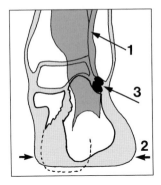

6. Calcaneal fractures with lateral displacement and involvement of the subtalar joint.

Lateral and valgus displacement of the main fragment may cause: (1) calf impairment and local heel pain as previously described; (2) broadening of the heel, which may be unsightly and call for special footwear; (3) impingement symptoms from the lateral malleolus or squashed peroneal tendons. Disruption of the subtalar joint is often most obvious in the tangential projection, and leads to fibrous adhesions, loss of inversion and eversion, and secondary osteoarthritis: this may be associated with pain, poor walking, an acquired fear of heights, and alcoholism.

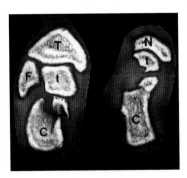

CAT scans may be used to elucidate the extent of any *subtalar joint involvement*. Cuts made far back (left) show the tibia (T), fibula (F), talus (t) and the calcaneus (C). The illustration shows a displaced calcaneal fracture with involvement of the subtalar joint; the sustentaculum tali and the anterior talonavicular joint are also affected. More anteriorly placed cuts show the head of the talus and the navicular (N).

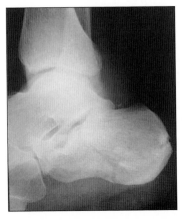

Treatment. If the deformity is *slight* (left), the peripheral circulation poor, or the patient old, the fracture should be treated along conservative lines. With *marked deformity*, morbidity is high but conservative treatment may also be employed. The results of more active treatment are somewhat uncertain. Nevertheless, consider spike reduction of the major fragment with an attempt to elevate any depressed lateral fragments. Depressed articular surfaces may have to be packed up with bone grafts, and the fracture secured with screws and possibly a plate.

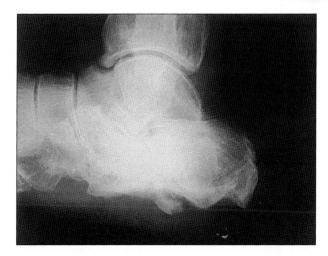

7. Central crushing fractures. In the most severe of calcaneal fracture, the talus drives like a wedge through the central part of the calcaneus, leading to comminution of a severe degree and disruption of the subtalar and calcaneocuboid joints. (The radiograph shows a united fracture of this type, with changes in the calcaneocuboid and subtalar joints.) Surgical reconstruction is generally impossible and complications are common. Nevertheless, a number do well without requiring late fusion if treated wholly conservatively or by spike reduction.

Treatment of calcaneal fractures after union
- Physiotherapy and occupational therapy should be continued until nothing more can be gained.
- Pain under the heel should be treated by a sorbo pad.
- Broadening of the heel may require surgical footwear.
- Impingement symptoms with sharply localised pain and tenderness beneath the lateral malleolus may respond to local surgery (excision of any exostosis and freeing the peroneal tendons).
- Persistent pain and limp, due possibly to secondary subtalar osteoarthritis, require careful assessment. Symptoms should be unremitting, persistent for 6–9 months *at least* after injury and unresponsive to physiotherapy, before surgery may be contemplated. Fresh radiographs should be compared with the original films to confirm subtalar joint involvement, and an assessment made of the state of the calcaneocuboid joint.

If the subtalar joint only is involved, a subtalar fusion is advised. If there is any involvement of the calcaneocuboid joint, a full triple fusion will be necessary (fusion of the subtalar, calcaneocuboid and talonavicular joints).

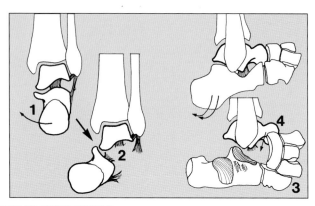

PERITALAR DISLOCATION

Pathology. Forcible inversion (1) of the plantar flexed foot throws stress on the lateral ligament of the ankle and the talocalcaneal ligament. If the strong talocalcaneal ligament ruptures (2), the talus remains in the ankle mortise and a subtalar dislocation results. The forefoot stays with the calcaneus (3), and the talonavicular joint dislocates. As the talus does not displace, this injury is often described as a peritalar dislocation. It may be accompanied by fractures of the malleoli. The talus adopts a position of plantar flexion (4), and this is the position in which the foot must be placed during the initial stage of reduction.

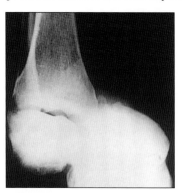

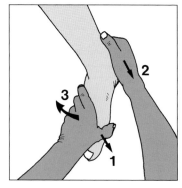

Diagnosis. The diagnosis is confirmed by radiographs (left). Avascular necrosis of the talus does not occur, but late subtalar osteoarthritis is common.

Treatment. Reduction is generally easy under general anaesthesia. Plantar flex the foot (1). Grasp the heel and the forefoot, apply a little traction (2) and swing the foot into eversion (3). Thereafter, apply a padded below-knee plaster with the ankle at right angles and the foot in slight eversion. A walking plaster may be applied after a week and retained for a further 5 weeks. Open reduction is necessary if manipulation fails; difficulty is usually due to button-holing of the talonavicular joint. Instability may be controlled with Kirschner wire.

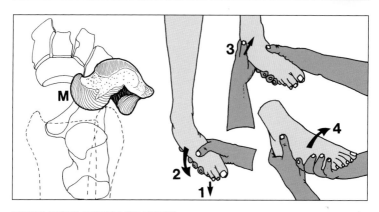

TOTAL DISLOCATION OF TALUS

As a result of severe forced inversion of the plantar flexed foot, there may be complete rupture of the main ligamentous attachments of the talus, which dislocates and comes to lie subcutaneously in front of the ankle and on the lateral side of the foot. The head of the talus points medially (**M**) and its calcaneal surface is directed posteriorly.

Treatment. Manipulative reduction should be attempted under general anaesthesia. It is imperative that delay is avoided, as there is always risk of skin sloughing where it is tightly stretched over the talus. The following technique may be employed: plantar flex the foot (**1**); invert the foot strongly (**2**); push the posterior part of the talus (lying laterally), in a posteromedial direction (**3**); when the talus starts to move into place, evert the foot (**4**). If these measures fail, use a Steinman pin through the calcaneus to apply preliminary traction and control inversion. Occasionally, open reduction may be required. Thereafter, apply a padded plaster. Avascular necrosis is almost inevitable.

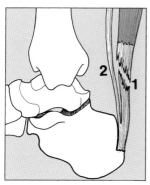

ACUTE RUPTURE OF THE TENDO CALCANEUS

Rupture may follow sudden muscle activity (e.g. jumping or sprinting). It is especially common in the middle-aged, when degenerative changes are appearing in the tendon. It may be precipitated by local steroid injections. Usually the site is 4–8 cm above the insertion; rupture is complete (**1**) and the plantaris is spared (**2**). There is sudden pain with difficulty in walking and standing on the toes. Clinically there may be a visible gap in the tendon, weakness of plantar flexion against resistance, lack of 'firmness' on side-to-side pressure at the site of the rupture, a positive Thomson test, (see p. 182) and a soft-tissue defect on the radiographs or on MRI scans.

Treatment. Both conservative and surgical measures have their advocates, but neither guarantees freedom from complications, which include re-rupture, weakness of plantar flexion, stiffness of the ankle, poor wound healing and deep vein thrombosis.

Conservative treatment. This is often advocated for all cases seen within 48 hours, but is also particularly suitable for the elderly, frail or poor anaesthetic risk patient. The aim of treatment is to hold the foot in plantar flexion in order to approximate the tendon ends, and to keep them there until healing is advanced. A long leg plaster is applied with the knee in about 45° of flexion and the ankle plantar flexed. After 4 weeks, a below-knee plaster is then substituted, with the ankle still in a little plantar flexion. In a further 4 weeks, the plaster can be discarded, weight-bearing permitted and physiotherapy commenced to improve the gait and calf strength. To begin with, an inside shoe lift may be used to reduce dorsiflexion stresses on the healing tendon.

Surgical treatment. This gives the most satisfactory results where there is a delay of a week or more in making the diagnosis or initiating treatment. It is often also advocated for the young athletic patient. The ends of the ruptured tendon are approximated and held with either absorbable, non-absorbable or pull-out sutures. After wound closure, a long leg plaster cast is applied with the knee in flexion and the ankle plantar flexed. At 3 weeks, the skin sutures may be removed and a below-knee plaster applied for a further 3 weeks with the ankle in a more neutral position. Discharging wounds, a common complication, are managed with patience along established lines. The use of small incisions, made possible with the Achillon™ suturing jig, is likely to reduce the incidence of this problem.

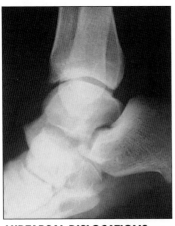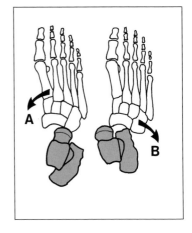

MIDTARSAL DISLOCATIONS

Dislocation of the talonavicular portion of the midtarsal joint may accompany subtalar dislocations. The subtalar joint may reduce spontaneously but incompletely, so that the talonavicular dislocation is the main feature (**left**). The midtarsal joint lies between the talus and calcaneus posteriorly, and the navicular and cuboid anteriorly. *Both* elements of the joint may be disrupted as a result of (**A**) adduction or (**B**) abduction forces applied to the forefoot.

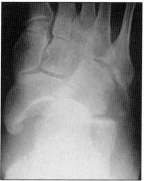

As in any other dislocation, abduction or adduction midtarsal dislocations are associated with ligament rupture or small avulsion fractures, but the talus, calcaneus, navicular and cuboid may escape significant fracture (**left** shows an adduction midtarsal dislocation with small avulsion fracture of cuboid). On the other hand, a midtarsal dislocation may be accompanied by more substantial fractures of any of the components of the joint. The navicular is most frequently involved. When this is the case, reduction is more likely to be unstable, and secondary arthritic changes commoner.

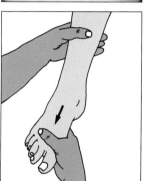

Treatment. Under general anaesthesia, apply traction to the forefoot and realign the forefoot with the hindfoot. If there is instability, stabilise it with percutaneous Kirschner wires. If manipulation fails, open reduction may be required; a large navicular fracture may sometimes need screw fixation, and an external fixator may be required for stabilisation. A padded plaster is applied and split, and the limb elevated. Non-weight-bearing with crutches may start after 1–2 weeks with removal of any wires at 3–4 weeks. Weekly radiographs should be taken to detect late subluxation. The cast may be discarded after 6–8 weeks.

Complications. Stiffness of the foot and ill-localised pain are common and may be followed by secondary osteoarthritis. If this is confined to the calcaneocuboid joint, it may be treated by a local fusion: otherwise, a full triple arthrodesis (arthrodesis of the subtalar and midtarsal joints) may be required. Rarely, medial plantar nerve palsy may be seen, causing intrinsic muscle wasting.

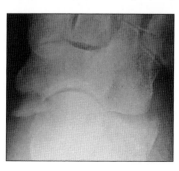

Isolated fractures of the navicular
The tuberosity may be fractured (**left**) by avulsion of the tibialis posterior; this and other undisplaced fractures may be treated conservatively (e.g. by 6 weeks in plaster). Body fractures may be accompanied by dorsal extrusion of a large fragment, which should be accurately reduced and fixed surgically (but do not mistake the common accessory centre of ossification for a fracture).

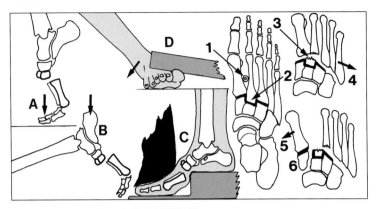

TARSOMETATARSAL DISLOCATIONS

Dislocation of one or more metatarsals may result from **(A)** a fall on the plantar flexed foot, **(B)** a blow on the heel when in the kneeling position (e.g. when a horse falls on top of a thrown rider), **(C)** run-over kerb-side accidents or **(D)** forced inversion, eversion or abduction of the forefoot. *Note:* **(1)** The dorsalis pedis/medial plantar anastomosis may be in jeopardy; **(2)** the metatarsal bases are keyed into the cuneiforms, and fracture of the second metatarsal base **(3)** will allow lateral drift **(4)**. In eversion injuries, the first metatarsal may drift medially **(5)** and may be accompanied by the cuneiform **(6)**.

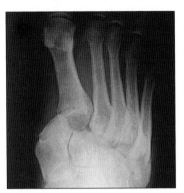
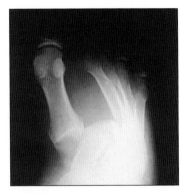

Treatment. Reduction should be attempted promptly because of the risks of oedema and circulatory impairment. If the deformity is unaccompanied by fracture, reduction can often be achieved by applying traction in the line of the metatarsals and pressure over their bases. If stable, a padded plaster is used for 8 weeks before weight-bearing and mobilisation. Where there is lateral drift of all the metatarsals **(left)**, with a fracture of the second metatarsal base, reduction may be difficult and unstable. Open reduction and Kirschner wire fixation are advisable, with a cast for 6 weeks. Where the first ray is displaced medially **(right)**, this should be reduced first. If unstable, hold with Kirschner wires.

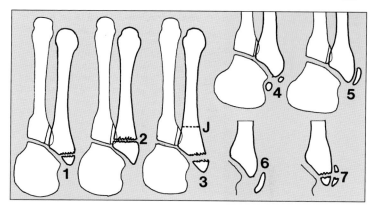

METATARSAL FRACTURES
Fifth metatarsal base

The commonest fracture of the lower limb is an avulsion fracture of the fifth metatarsal base. It follows a sudden inversion strain where in an effort to correct the inversion of the foot, the peroneus brevis avulses its bony attachment.

Diagnosis. Tenderness is well localised over the fracture. As the fracture results from an inversion injury, the patient often complains of having sprained his ankle. If an adequate clinical examination is not carried out, and radiographs taken are of the ankle only, the *fracture line will not be visualised*. Note that the fracture line runs at right angles to the axis of the metatarsal shaft. It involves the joint with the cuboid if the fragment is small (**1**), and with the fourth metatarsal if it is large (**2**). In the former case, separation of the fragments may occur (**3**) . (Note that the classical Jones fracture (**J**) is situated distal to the intermetatarsal joint.) Do not misinterpret the rounded shadows of accessory bones (**4**). In children, the epiphysis (**5**) lying *parallel* to the shaft may also be wrongly taken for a fracture. Nevertheless, separation (**6**) or fracture of the epiphysis (**7**) may occur.

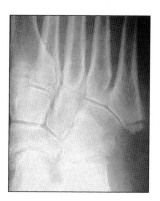

Treatment. Most fractures are undisplaced (**left**) but even marked displacement does not merit reduction. If symptoms are slight, give a crepe or similar support for 2–3 weeks, and if marked a walking plaster for 5–7 weeks. Pain from the occasional non-union may be expected to resolve spontaneously, but *Sudeck's atrophy (complex regional pain syndrome) is a common complication and may require prolonged treatment.*

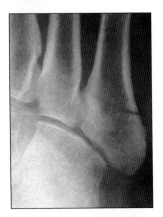

Jones fracture. This fracture is not associated with inversion injuries but tends to occur in athletes during training: it has some of the features of a stress fracture. Non-union is common, and is most often associated with early weight-bearing: because of this, treat with 7 weeks' fixation in a below-knee non-weight-bearing cast. In the professional athlete, internal fixation with an intramedullary AO cancellous bone screw may be considered. Treat delayed or non-union with medullary curettage and bone grafting.

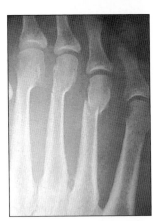

Single or multiple undisplaced fractures of the shaft and neck of the lesser metatarsals. The radiograph shows fractures of the necks of the 2nd, 3rd and 4th metatarsals. These frequently result from crushing accidents, and any associated soft-tissue injury will require careful surveillance. Spiral fractures generally result from forced inversion or eversion of the forefoot. Fractures of this type without much displacement may be treated conservatively by a crepe bandage support, or a walking plaster if pain is severe.

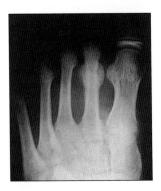

March fracture. Fatigue fractures, usually of the second metatarsal neck or shaft, are not often seen until callus formation has occurred; reassurance, with at most a light support for 2–3 weeks, is all that is indicated. If seen at an early stage, severe pain will occasionally merit treatment in a below-knee walking plaster till union has taken place.

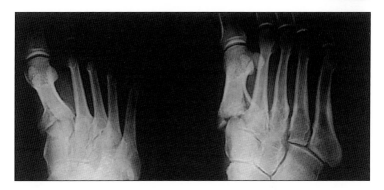

First metatarsal

- AP and oblique projections illustrate a slightly displaced first metatarsal fracture. In this type of injury, damage to the peripheral circulation and post-traumatic oedema may present problems. Admission for a short period of elevation and observation, with the limb supported in a well-padded split plaster is indicated. (Thereafter, a below-knee walking plaster should be employed for 5–6 weeks.)
- If there is marked displacement with off-ending, reduction should be carried out to avoid disturbance of the mechanics of the forefoot. Traction to the toe, with local pressure over the displaced metatarsal may suffice, but open reduction (and sometimes wire fixation) may be necessary, with the after-care being the same as above.
- Hairline fractures without soft-tissue crushing may be treated without preliminary elevation.
- Open injuries will require the appropriate wound treatment.

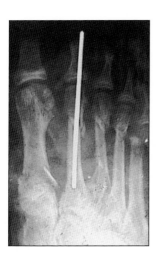

Multiple displaced fractures

Fractures of the four lesser metatarsal shafts are frequently accompanied by lateral drift, an unstable situation. Open reduction and internal fixation are advisable. In many cases, reduction and stabilisation of the second metatarsal will suffice (**left**), as the intermetatarsal alignment is generally preserved. *Displaced neck fractures* may be manipulated, but open reduction and Kirschner wire fixation are often required. Malunion may be treated by local trimming of any metatarsal head prominences in the sole.

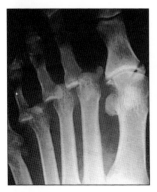

INJURIES TO THE TOES
Toe dislocations. These should be reduced by traction. (The radiograph shows dislocations of the four lateral MP joints, with fractures of all proximal phalanges except the third.) If there is instability, Kirschner wire fixation may be needed. Single dislocations may be reduced under local anaesthesia and supported by strapping to the adjacent toe; multiple dislocations will require general anaesthesia and a walking plaster with a toe platform for 4 weeks.

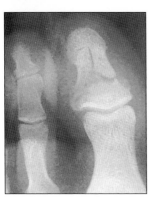

Fractures of the terminal phalanx of the great toe. These usually result from a heavy weight falling on a foot unprotected by industrial footwear. The fracture may involve the distal tuft only, but often runs into the IP joint. Such fractures are often open.

Treatment. All wounds should be cleaned and the edges loosely approximated. The nail should be retained unless virtually separated. Thereafter, the fracture may be supported by:
• adhesive strapping to the adjacent toe
• a light dressing and the wearing of a stout shoe with, if necessary, a cut-out for the toe
• a walking plaster with toe platform—all for 2–4 weeks.

Fractures of the terminal phalanges of the lesser toes. These may be treated in a similar manner.

Fractures of the middle and proximal phalanges. These should be treated by strapping to the adjacent toe for 3–4 weeks, but if there is marked displacement with obvious deformity of the toes, they should be reduced by traction. *In the case of the great toe,* a walking plaster with toe platform for 4 weeks may give greater relief of symptoms. *Note: In all cases the circulation must be carefully assessed and additional precautions taken where necessary* (e.g. admission for elevation).

CRUSHING INJURIES OF THE FOOT WITHOUT FRACTURE
The foot is a resilient structure; it may be run over by a heavy vehicle or be severely crushed without sustaining any obvious fracture. If a history of this type of injury is obtained, admission is nevertheless advisable for light pressure bandaging, elevation and observation of the circulation. Sloughing of the skin over a heart-shaped area on the dorsum is not uncommon, but the area requiring desloughing and skin grafting will be minimised by prompt early care. *Degloving injuries of the foot* are serious, especially when sole skin is involved, and require prompt plastic surgical care.

The fracture clinic

Patient's notes 522

The organisation of fracture clinics varies from hospital to hospital. These differences are often dictated by the layout of the departments involved—records, appointments, secretarial, clinical, treatment, plaster, theatre and X-ray —and also by an established line of practice. Those who work in fracture clinics usually have to do so within a framework imposed upon them, and it would be invidious to suggest a 'best way' of doing things. Nevertheless, it might be helpful for the beginner who is confronted for the first time with a fracture clinic to offer a few guidelines on the handling of the actual consultation.

The newcomer to a fracture clinic is usually impressed by the number of cases dealt with in a short space of time. This speed often conceals the number of rather important decisions that are made about the patients' care. These decisions are of course determined by the basic principles of fracture treatment, but to ensure the smooth running of the clinic, the most professional and kindliest contact with the patient and the avoidance of any error in management, the use of a simple system, at least at the beginning, may be of some help.

Assuming that the usual courtesies of greeting have been made, each consultation should start with asking the two questions, 'what' and 'when', and end with asking 'when' and 'what'. In the middle, there are a number of things to go through which can be conveniently dealt with under three headings, each starting with the letter A—'the three As'.

What

Every decision that is made, and everything that is done, is directly dependent on the diagnosis. *This must be clearly stated at the beginning of the notes on the first fracture clinic attendance*, where it will serve as a guide to everyone who sees the patient subsequently. It is a never-ending source of astonishment how difficult it may be to find this information, the time taken often varying directly in proportion to the size of the records. If there is a problem, a glance at the initial radiographs (they alone are helpful to label) may give the answer. Time spent establishing the diagnosis is essential. Recording it will prevent the effort having to be repeated at the patient's next attendance.

When

The point here is to establish the time that has passed since the patient's injury. It is more professional to establish the primary facts of 'what' and 'when' before confronting the patient, rather than searching through the notes in his presence. When making the appropriate notes, where brevity should not compromise accuracy, the addition of a qualifier in the case of the diagnosis may be helpful: e.g. 'Undisplaced L Colles 2/52 ago'; or '7/52 mid-shaft R femur, I-M locked nail'.

On the solid basis of the knowledge of what you are dealing with, you can proceed to **assessment, action and advice**.

Assessment

• The first step is to establish if the fracture to date has been treated *appropriately* and *adequately*, e.g. if a fracture has been manipulated, then it is necessary to consider whether this was the best method of treatment in the circumstances; the desirability of internal fixation or other methods of dealing with the condition should be reviewed. Then the check radiographs should be studied to assess the quality of the reduction, and an overall assessment made.

- If a plaster cast has been applied, it should be seen to be appropriate for the injury. It should be checked for tightness, slackness or other inadequacy, and if it is only a backslab, a decision should be made as to whether it needs completion. The presence of swelling, the quality of the circulation and any impairment of nerve supply in the limb should be noted.
- If the fracture has been treated surgically, the need for inspection of the wound or removal of sutures should be assessed. If the fracture has been internally fixed, the quality of the fixation should be reviewed so that a decision may be made regarding the degree of mobilisation that may be permitted without the fracture coming adrift.
- If some time has elapsed since the injury, an assessment should be made as to whether a greater degree of freedom may be permitted, e.g. whether a supporting sling may be discarded or whether a cast may be removed to allow joint mobilisation, or whether a walking heel may be applied to a leg plaster.
- A decision when to remove all external splintage is not usually required until an appropriate length of time has elapsed since the injury, and in making the decision, radiographs may be required to check the state of union, and/or the cast may be removed so that a clinical assessment of the fracture may be made.

Action

Having assessed the fracture, the appropriate action should be taken. What should be done generally follows in a clear-cut fashion from the assessment; e.g. if a plaster is too tight it should be split, or if there is complaint of local pressure the plaster should be windowed or trimmed.

The only difficulties that are likely to arise are those associated with the assessment of the treatment that has been carried out. This tends to present less of a problem as experience grows, although with the variety and vagaries of chance and changing opinion, the need for the critical analysis of every case is one of the continuing delights of fracture clinics and one which prevents them ever becoming dull. *The point which it is imperative to note is that if there is any doubt regarding the treatment or progress of a fracture, a more senior opinion should be sought without delay.* Procrastination narrows the available treatment options and will attract the criticism of why an earlier opinion was not sought. It is generally easy and a pleasure for a senior colleague to give timely advice on the treatment of a case, and gives him confidence in the reliability and common sense of his junior. Delay or failure in seeking advice may lead to an undesirable or even tragic outcome.

Advice

The patient should be given clear and appropriate advice. Some of the areas which might be considered include the following:

- He should be told and preferably shown what exercises he should do to encourage or preserve movements in the joints related to his fracture.
- If he has been given an arm sling, he should be advised when and if he may discard it, and how the limb may be exercised with and without it. If he has a leg in plaster, he should be told how much weight (if any) he should take through it.
- If appropriate, he should be given advice on his fitness to drive or work.
- If he is being referred for physiotherapy, he should be advised on what he should do between visits to reinforce the treatment that he will receive.

It is important to explain to the patient, with repetition if necessary, the nature of his injury. It is equally important to keep him informed of his progress and to give, wherever possible, assurance regarding the position of a fracture and the stage of healing. He should be given some idea of when he can reasonably expect to reach the landmarks in his planned line of treatment, e.g. when he can hope to come out of a cast, when he might be able to weight-bear, and when he might be able to return to work.

If a complication arises, this should not be concealed. The proposed line of treatment and what result might be hoped for should be clearly explained. Frankness at all stages lessens the chances of misunderstanding and may avert litigation which in many cases is embarked upon when a patient's anger at a less than perfect result is vented on an imagined lapse in management rather than on the seriousness of an injury which has not been clearly explained to him.

When

The date and time of the next appointment are given, unless the patient is being discharged. In that event it is usually necessary to give a prognosis and advice regarding, for example, return to work or the procedure to follow should any complication arise. It may be necessary to give a recommendation about removal of an implant. It is usual to reinforce these points with the appropriate discharge letter to the patient's own doctor. Do not decide when to see a patient again by guesswork: instead, choose a date when you expect to have to make a further decision about the management of the case, e.g. whether a plaster will have to be changed or when union in a fracture might have to be assessed.

What

The purpose of the patient's next visit should be clearly stated so that the time and trouble that you have spent on assessing and treating the case can be pursued on the next attendance without any waste of precious time—of the patient or the clinic staff. For example, it may be helpful to indicate that on the next visit the patient should have his plaster removed and an X-ray taken to assess union as soon as he arrives at the clinic. Depending, of course, on how the clinic is organised, this may save valuable time by avoiding the patient having to wait and be seen twice.

PATIENTS' NOTES

The smooth running of a clinic is dependent on the clinical notes, but these lose much of their value if they can only be read by the originator; and they become largely pointless if, as is not infrequent, even the writer has difficulty in interpreting them. If there is no facility for having *all* the notes typewritten, it is nevertheless strongly advised the notes should be typed on the first fracture clinic attendance *and* also if there is any significant change in the line of treatment. Otherwise, contractions in *common usage*, printed in upper case letters, may provide oases of understanding appreciated by every reader.

The following example of the commonest condition seen at a fracture clinic is given to illustrate these points:

Colles' fracture

A patient has had a Colles' fracture which was only slightly displaced. The wrist was put in a plaster back shell without manipulation and the arm supported in a sling. Her plaster and the swelling and circulation were checked at a review clinic the following day. She is now attending her first fracture clinic 4 days later.

The post-fracture swelling has subsided and it would seem that the plaster back shell can be safely completed. Review of the initial radiographs indicate that the fracture was only slightly displaced, and the original decision not to manipulate the fracture seems quite correct. No radiographs have been taken to check the fracture, and while the chances of it having slipped are thought to be comparatively slight, it is desirable to have the position confirmed; for if the fracture has slipped and the position is not acceptable, it could be readily manipulated at this stage.

If check films are taken before the plaster is completed, there is the possibility that the position may alter during the course of that procedure. The action taken is therefore to complete the plaster and have check radiographs taken afterwards.

These in fact show that the original position has been maintained and it is thought that the risks of late slipping may now be judged to be slight.

The patient is assured that her fractured wrist is in good position and that it is planned to see if it has joined in 5 weeks' time. She is warned that when she comes out of plaster, her wrist will be rather stiff, but it is anticipated that eventually she will regain a good range of movements and have little handicap. Her sling is removed and she is advised (for what is hoped to be the second time) how she may exercise her shoulder and her fingers.

She is asked to return in 2 weeks' time. The main purpose of that visit is to check her plaster.

Notes to cover this might be made along the following lines:

R Colles 4/7 ago. Circn OK, POP completed. Check X-ray satis. Discard sling. See 2/52 for POP check.

When this next appointment is kept, no search has to be made (because of the content of the note above) for what is wrong or what would normally be expected at this visit. The plaster is checked and not found to be slack. It is decided on the basis of the original radiographs of this impacted fracture that if any slipping of the fracture has occurred, this is likely to be minimal and not requiring correction; so there is no call for further radiographs. There has been some discomfort because of pressure in the region of the metacarpal of the little finger and the plaster is trimmed in this region. The fingers and shoulders are found to have a full range of movements, and the patient is encouraged to continue with the exercises she has been shown. She is told that her plaster will be removed on her next visit to see whether her fracture has joined. She is warned that if it transpires that union is not sufficiently far advanced, she may have to go back into plaster for perhaps a further 2 weeks, although this is not particularly likely.

The note might read:

2/52+. POP trimmed. See 3/52, POP off on arrival.

On removal of her plaster 3 weeks later, no tenderness is found at the fracture site and her fracture involving cancellous bone can be safely judged to have united. (Check radiographs are superfluous and would not be indicated unless any complication were suspected.) There is no swelling, and the use of a Tubigrip or crepe bandage support is not considered necessary. She is advised to continue with her finger exercises and shown what to do to mobilise her wrist. Her good progress is reaffirmed and she is advised to return for review in 2 weeks' time when a decision will be made as to whether she needs to have any physiotherapy.

The note might read:

5/52+. POP off. No tenderness. Mobilise. See 2/52? physio.

Her next visit is her last as she had no complaints of pain and has regained an excellent, if not complete, range of movements. She is told that as she has recovered such a good range of movements at this early stage that physiotherapy is not necessary. She is advised that it is expected she will regain almost full movements in the wrist and that she will recover excellent, if not quite complete, strength, perhaps over the course of the next year. Should she develop any problems with pain, swelling or tingling sensations in the thumb or fingers (anticipating Sudeck's atrophy or carpal tunnel syndrome—now rather unlikely), she should make a review appointment. She should be told how this can be done. A discharge letter would normally be written to her own doctor incorporating the diagnosis, her present state and expected progress. The clinical note may be simply 'See discharge letter' or be made along the following lines:

7/52+. Lacks 20° dorsiflexion and 15° supination. Full finger movements, good grip. Discharged.

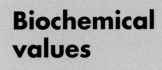

Biochemical values

	Serum calcium	Serum phosphate	Alkaline phosphatase	Total acid phosphatase	Remarks
Normal range	2.12–2.62 mmol/litre 8.5–10.5 mg/100 cc	*Adults* 0.8–1.4 mmol/litre 2.5–4.3 mg/100 cc *Children* 1.3–2.0 mmol/litre 4–6.2 mg/100 cc	*Adults* 21–106 IU/litre *Children* 21–142 IU/litre *Infants* 21–210 IU/litre	2.0–5.5 IU/litre	
Laboratory accuracy	±2%	±2%	±10%	±10%	
Hyperparathyroidism	Raised	Lowered	Raised if bone involved	Normal	
Hypoparathyroidism	Lowered	Raised	Normal	Normal	
Pseudo hypoparathyroidism	Lowered	Raised	Normal	Normal	
Osteoporosis	Normal	Normal	Normal	Normal	
Osteomalacia	Normal to low	Low	Slight increase	Normal	$Ca \times PO_4 < 2.25$ SI units or 28.0 mg/100 cc units
Rickets	Normal to low	Low	Slight increase	Normal	
Paget's disease	Normal, raised in immobilisation	Normal	Raised	Raised	
Uraemic osteodystrophy	Low or normal	Raised	Raised	Normal	
Myelomatosis	Often raised	Normal	Normal	Normal	High ESR
Bone metastases	Normal or raised	Normal or low	Raised	Normal or raised	ESR raised
Sarcoidosis	Often raised	Usually normal	Normal	Normal	ESR raised
Prostatic neoplasm	Normal or raised	Normal or low	Normal or high	Normal or high, raised in 15% of cases without and in 65% with metastases	Prostatic acid phosphatase fraction of total acid phosphatase affected but not in highly malignant undifferentiated tumours

	SI units	mg/100 cc or µg/100 cc
Total serum protein	60–80 g/litre	6.0–8.0 mg/100 cc
Albumin	33–50 g/litre	3.3–5.0 mg/100 cc
Globulin	20–35 g/litre	2.0–3.5 mg/100 cc
Bilirubin	5–20 µmol/litre	0.29–1.17 mg/100 cc
Urea	2.5–7.5 mmol/litre	15–45 mg/100 cc
Serum urate	*Males* 0.13–0.45 mmol/litre	2.2–7.7 mg/100 cc
	Females 0.13–0.35 mmol/litre	2.2–5.9 mg/100 cc
Serum iron	*Males* 14–32 µmol/litre	78–180 µg/100 cc
	Females 10–30 µmol/litre	56–108 µg/100 cc
Total iron binding capacity (TIBC)	45–70 µmol/litre	250–390 µg/100 cc
Fasting blood glucose	3.3–5.6 mmol/litre	60–100 mg/100 cc
Serum cholesterol	3.6–8.5 mmol/litre	140–330 mg/100 cc

Index

Abdominal examination in back pain, 101
Abduction
    femoral shaft fracture, 441
    hip, 121, 126
    shoulder/arm, 45–7
        external rotation in abduction, 46
        external rotation at 90° abduction, 47
        internal rotation in abduction, 46
        pain during, 45
Abduction injuries, ankle, 483
Abductor digiti minimi, tests, 19
Abductor pollicis brevis, tests, 22
Abscess
    Brodie's, 173, 174
    tuberculous of spine, 88
Acetabulum
    fracture, 409–11
        assessment, 409
        classification, 410
        diagnosis, 409
        treatment, 411
    protrusio acetabuli, 129, 135
Achilles tendon (tendo calcaneus), 177, 182
    acute rupture, 511–12
    shortening, 177, 182
    tendinopathy, 176, 181
    tendinosis, 176
Achondroplasia, 75
Acromegaly, 75
Acromioclavicular joint
    injuries, 272–3
        complications, 273
        diagnosis, 272
        radiographs, 273
        treatment, 273
    osteoarthritis, 42
Acute pyogenic arthritis of hip, 114
Acute respiratory distress syndrome, 263
Adduction
    femoral fracture, 441
    hip, 121
Adduction injuries, ankle, 484
Adductor pollicis, tests, 19, 20
Adson's test, 31
Advice to patients, 521
Agee-Wristjack, 334
Airway management, 227
Albumin, 527
Alkaline phosphatase, 526
Anal sphincter, nerves to, 23

Angular kyphosis, 93
Angulation, 216–17
    femoral fracture, 442
    forearm fracture, 318, 321
    thumb fracture, 360
    tibial fracture, 468
Ankle, 10, 175–84
    assessment, 178–82
    common conditions, 176–7
    dislocation without fracture, 494
    footballer's, 176, 184, 494
    fractures (and other injuries), 479–95
        classification, 480–3
        complications, 495
        diagnosis, 485–6
        radiographs, 485
        treatment, 486
        see also Fibular fractures
    inspection, 178
    instability, 179–82
    movements, 179
    painful conditions, 177
    radiographs, 183–4
    sprained see Sprains
    tenderness, 178
    tibial fracture-related problems, 472
Ankylosing spondylitis
    hip, 115
    knee, 143
    spine
        cervical, 37
        thoracic/lumber, 87, 100, 105
Antecubital fossa, palpation, 57
Anterior dislocation of shoulder, 276–80
Anterior drawer test, 155
Anterior leg pain, 170
Anterior metatarsalgia, 188
Anterior shoulder dislocation, 276–80
    late diagnosed, 282
    recurrent, 282–3
Anterior tibial compartment syndrome, 170, 173
Anterior tibiofibular ligament tears, 489
Anterior wedge fracture of cervical spine, 372
Anthrax, 74
Antibiotics, femoral neck fracture, 426
AO Classification, 220–2
    acetabular fractures, 410
    ankle fractures, 481
    femoral fractures, 434

AP tomography, 6
Apical infections, 73
Apley's grinding tests, 162
Apprehension test
    knee, 163
    shoulder, 48
Arches of foot
    examination, 197
    radiographs, 206
Arm *see* Upper limb
Arterial arrest/obstruction *see* Vascular
    problems
Arthritis *see* and inflammatory conditions;
    Osteoarthritis; Rheumatoid arthritis
Arthrography, knee, 145
Arthropathy, rotator cuff, 41
Arthroplasty (hip joint replacement), 428
    conditions associated with, 115–16
    with femoral neck fracture, 447
    radiographs, 133
Arthroscopy, knee, 7, 145
Articular surface
    examination
        ankle, 182
        patella, 164
    fracture involving, 214
        tibial table, 461–3
Aspiration
    elbow, 58
    hip, 124
    knee, 146
    shoulder, 50
    wrist, 70
Athlete's foot, 195
Atlanto-occipital joint, subluxation, 381–6
Atlas
    fractures, 381–2
        radiographs, 382
        treatment, 382
    fusion to axis (C1-C2), 385
    transverse ligament lesions, 382–3
Atrophic non-union, 256, 257
    humeral shaft, 294
    radiographs, 256
    treatment, 257
Atrophy, Sudek's *see* Sudek's atrophy
Avascular necrosis
    femoral head
        with neck fracture, 424, 426
        with slipped upper epiphysis, 422
        with traumatic hip dislocation, 419

humeral head, 259
scaphoid, 347
talus, 501
wrist, 349–50
Avulsion fracture, 214
    carpus, 342
    talus, 502
Avulsion lesions of brachial plexus, 12
Axial rotation, forearm bones
    forces responsible for, 317
    radius, 317
    ulna, 316
Axillary (circumflex) nerve, 50
    examination, 15
    palsy, 261, 277
Axis
    fractures, 385–6
        radiographs, 386
        treatment, 386
    fusion to atlas (C1-C2), 385
    injuries, 384–5

Back pain, 84–5
    causes of, 92
    commoner causes, 92
    mechanical, 91
    see also Thoracolumbar spine
Ballistic injuries, 251–2
Bamboo spine, 105
Bankart lesion, 276, 282, 283
Barlow's provocative test, 125
Barré-Lieou syndrome, 387
Barton's fracture, 342
Beat knee, 143
Bennett's fracture, 226, 355
    treatment, 355
Biceps, long head, assessment, 50
Biceps tendinitis, 49
Biceps tendon
    instability, 49
    rupture, 43
Bigelow's method, 417, 418
Bilirubin, 527
Biochemical values, 526–7
Birth palsy *see* Obstetrical palsy
Bladder
    damage following pelvic fracture, 412
        diagnosis, 413
        treatment, 413
    neurological control, 396
    rupture, 413

Bladder, *continued*
  in spinal injury, 398
Blast injuries, 252
Blood pressure, 229
Blood transfusion, 228–9
Bones
  cysts, pathological fractures, 265
  factors affecting fracture healing, 254
  fracture *see* Fractures
  long, AO Classification *see* AO
    Classification
  metastases, biochemical values, 526
  Paget's disease *see* Paget's disease
  tumours
    hip, 115
    pathological fractures, 265
    secondary *see* Metastases
    tibia, 170, 174
    treatment, 265
Bouchard's nodes, 76
Boutonnière deformity, 72, 75
Bow-leg *see* Genu varum
Bowel injury following pelvic fracture, 414
Brachial plexus, 11
  long-standing lesions, 12
  medial cord, examination of nerves
    arising from, 18–20
  median cord, examination of nerves
    arising from, 20–1
  posterior cord, examination of nerves
    arising from, 15–16
  traumatic lesions, 11, 13–15
    assessment, 13–14
    prognosis, 15
Brachioradialis test, 17
Breathing, 227
Brodie's abscess, 173, 174
Bruising, 4
  femoral neck fracture, 423
  pelvic fracture, 412
Bucket handle fractures, 405
Bullet wounds, 251–2
Bunion *see* Hallux valgus
Bunionette, 192
Bursa, metacarpophalangeal joint, 192
Bursitis
  infrapatellar, 143, 147
  olecranon, 54
  prepatellar, 143
Burst fractures of spine, 369
Butcher's wart, 74

C1 *see* Atlas
C2 *see* Axis
Café-au-lait spots, 94
Calcaneal exostoses, 192
Calcaneal fractures, 503–9
  anterior, 506
  central crushing fractures, 509
  horizontal, 505
  radiographs, 504
  treatment, 509
  vertical fracture of tuberosity, 504
Calcaneonavicular bar/synostosis, 206
  see also Talocalcaneal synostosis
Calcifying supraspinatus tendinitis, 41
Callosities
  foot, 105
  toes, 194
Calvé's disease, 87, 103
Cancer *see* Tumours/neoplasms
Capasso's method, 108
Capitulum (capitellum)
  fracture
    adults, 306–7
    children, 296
Cardiac tamponade, 231
Cardiovascular system *see* Circulation
Carpal tunnel syndrome, 21, 23, 62–3
  Colles' fracture, 338
Carpometacarpal joints, 80
  osteoarthritis, 73
  of thumb
    dislocation, 357
    normal movements, 79
    tests, 79
Carpus *see* Wrist
Carrying angle, 55
Cast
  plaster *see* Plaster casts
  polymer resin, 247–8
Cast syndrome, 262
Cast test, 23
Catterall grading, Perthes' disease, 130
Cauda equina syndrome, 89
Central venous pressure, 229
Cervical curvature, 33
Cervical myelopathy, 28, 36
Cervical rib syndrome, 12, 31
Cervical spine, 28–37
  assessment, 29–31
    in shoulder pain, 50
  common syndromes, 28

congenital abnormalities, 384
injuries/fractures, 370–86
  classification, 372
  diagnosis, 370
  initial management, 371
  treatment, 373–4
movements, 30
neurological examination, 32
radiographs, 33–7
Cervical spondylosis *see* Spondylosis
Chance fracture, 370
Charcot's disease, 143
Child abuse, suspected, 235
Children
  elbow dislocation, 309
  elbow fractures, 296–305
  femoral neck fractures, 430
  foot conditions, 186–7
  humerus fractures, 286, 292
  meniscus injuries, 459
  Monteggia fracture-dislocations, 324
  supracondylar fractures, 447
  tibial fractures, 467–70
Chondrolysis, slipped femoral epiphysis, 422
Chondroma, 73
Chondromalacia patellae, 142
Circulation, 228–30
  see also Vascular problems
Circumflex nerve *see* Axillary nerve
Claudication, 171
Clavicular braces, 271
Clavicular injuries, 270–5
  complications, 274
  dislocation, 270
  fracture, 42, 270, 271, 274
  subluxation, 270
Claw toe, 189, 194
Clergyman's knee, 143, 147
Clonus, 32
Closed fractures, 212
Club foot *see* Talipes equinovarus
Coccydynia, 91
Coccygeal injuries, 408
Collateral ligaments
  knee *see* Lateral ligament; Medial ligament
  ulnar *see* Ulnar collateral ligament
Colles' fracture, 62, 328–38, 522–4
  after-care, 335–6
  complications, 336–8

deformities, 328–9
diagnosis, 329
median nerve palsy, 262
persistent deformity, 337
radiographs, 330, 333
rehabilitation, 336
reversed (Smith's fracture), 341
Sudeck's atrophy following, 259
treatment, 330–4
Comminuted fracture *see*
    Multifragmentary/comminuted
    fracture
Common peroneal nerve, 23
  assessment, 25
  motor distribution, 24
  palsy, 261
  sensory distribution, 24
  sites of involvement, 24
Communication *see* Recording and
    communication
Compartment syndromes, 478
  after-care, 474
  diagnosis, 478
  prophylaxis, 474
  tibial, 474
  treatment, 478
Complex regional pain syndrome *see*
    Sudeck's atrophy
Compound fracture *see* Open fracture
Compression (crush) fracture, 214
  ankle, 484
  calcaneus, 509
  cervical spine, 380–1
  spine, 369
  talus head, 503
  toes, 518
Computed tomography, 6
  back pain, 95
Condyles
  femoral
    bicondylar fractures, 463
    T- and Y-fractures, 449
    tenderness over, 57
    unicondylar fractures, 448, 462–3
  humeral
    injuries, 305
    lateral, 296, 305
    medial, 296
  tibial
    bicondylar fracture, 463
    unicondylar, 448

Congenital conditions
cervical spine, 384
knee
discoid meniscus, 140
patellar dislocation, 456
torticollis, 29
Congenital dislocation of hip *see*
Developmental dislocation of hip
Contracture
Dupuytren's, 72, 76, 195
Volkmann's ischaemic, 76, 297
Cord *see* Brachial plexus; Spinal cord
Corner fracture, 489
Corns, 194
Coronoid fracture, 309
Corrosion, implant, 264
Coxa vara, 117, 129
pertrochanteric fractures, 430
slipped femoral epiphysis, 422
Crepitus
ankle, 182
wrist, 66
Cruciate ligaments
anterior, 140
injuries, 459
radiological analysis, 157
posterior, 140
injuries, 458
radiological examination, 158
tests, 157
Crush fractures/injuries *see* Compression
(crush) fracture
Cubitus valgus and varus, 54
Curly toe, 189, 194
Cysts
bone, 265
implantation dermoid, 73
meniscus, 141, 162, 461
mucous, 73
unicameral bone cyst, 174

De Quervain's tenosynovitis, 62, 64, 65, 66
Debridement, wound, 250
Deformity
fixed flexion, 5
fractures, 215
Colles' fracture, 337
hip flexion, 121
see also specific named deformities
Degloving injuries, 251

Delayed union, 255
treatment, 256
Deltoid muscle, assessment, 50
Dermatomes, 10
Dermoid cysts, implantation, 73
Developmental dislocation of hip, 112–13
adults, 113
aetiology, 112
diagnosis, 112–13
neonate, 132
older child, 113, 132
radiographs, 134
terminology, 112
tests for, 125–6
Diaphragm, rupture, 414
Diffuse idiopathic skeletal hyperostosis, 87
Dinner fork deformity, 328
Disc prolapse, 90–1, 97
Discography, back pain, 85
Discoid meniscus, congenital, 140
Dislocation, 212
ankle/heel/foot, 494
midtarsal, 512–13
peritalar, 510
talar, 511
tarsometatarsal, 514
toes, 518
atlanto-occipital, 381–6
carpometacarpal joint of thumb, 357
cervical spine, 372–3
clavicle, 270
acromioclavicular joint, 272
sternoclavicular joint, 274–5
elbow, 296, 308–11
anterior, 310
associated injuries, 309
complications, 308
isolated, 310
late diagnosed in children, 309
hip, 115–16
after-care, 417
anterior, 418
central, 409
diagnosis, 415
with femoral neck fracture, 446
irreducible, 419
late diagnosed, 420
radiographs, 415, 417
recurrent, 420
reduction, 416–18
traumatic, 415–20

see also Developmental dislocation of hip
interphalangeal joint *see* Interphalangeal joint
knee, 456
metacarpal base (5th), 361
metacarpophalangeal joint, 364
neurological problems *see* Neurological problems
patella, 456
peroneal tendon, 494
scaphoid, 350
shoulder, 42, 276–83
    anterior, 276–80
    late diagnosed anterior, 282
    late diagnosed posterior, 282
    luxation erecta, 281
    neurological complications, 283
    posterior, 280
    recurrent anterior, 282–3
    recurrent posterior, 283
ulna, 310
wrist, 347–50
    complications, 349–50
    hamate, 351
    late diagnosis, 350
    lunate, 70, 348–9, 350
    perilunar, 351
    periscapholunar, 351
    scaphoid, 351
    trans-scapho perilunar, 351
    trapezium, 351
    trapezoid, 351
    treatment, 348–9
see also Fracture-dislocation
Displacement, 216
Dome fracture, 502
Double fracture *see* Segmental fracture
Down's syndrome, 75
Drawer tests
    knee, 155
    shoulder, 48
Duchenne sign, 123
Dupuytren's contracture
    foot, 195
    hand, 72, 76
Dysplasia of hip, 113
    developmental *see* Developmental dislocation of hip

Effusion, knee, 149

Egyptian foot, 193
Ehlers-Danlos syndrome, 63, 67
Elbow, 10, 54–60, 295–314
    assessment, 55–8
    carrying angle, 55
    common pathologies, 54, 60
    dislocation *see* Dislocation
    fracture
        adults, 306–7
        children, 296–305
    injuries, 295–314
    movements, 56
    pulled, 311
    radiographs, 59–60
Electromyography, traumatic lesion of brachial plexus, 14
Elephant's foot appearance, 255
Embolism, fat, 263, 450
Epicondyles of humerus
    detachment, 309
    injuries, 303–4, 306
    lateral, 304, 306
    medial, 303–4, 306, 309
Epiphyseal plate injuries
    growth effects, 257
    treatment, 257
Epiphysis
    femoral *see* Femur
    injuries, 218
        ankle, 493
        classification of, 219
    radial, slipped, 340
Episodic blanching, 72
Erb's palsy, 11, 12
Erysipeloid, 74
ESIN nails, 320
Esses-Lopresti fracture-dislocation, 312
Exostoses
    calcaneal, 192
    foot, 187
    subungual, 189
        fingers, 81
        toes, 189
Explosions, 252
Extension injuries (hyperextension)
    cervical spine, 379–80, 384
    knee *see* Genu recurvatum
Extensor mechanisms/apparatus, knee, 451–4
Extensor pollicis longus tendon, delayed rupture, 338

Extensor tendons of hand
   division, 72
   injury, 81
Extensor tenosynovitis, 62
External plaster fixation *see* Plaster casts
External skeletal fixation
   Colles' fracture, 334
   femoral fracture, 426
   pelvic fracture, 403–4
   tibial fracture, 474–5

Fanconi syndrome, 264
Fasciitis, plantar, 189
Fasting blood glucose, 527
Fat embolism, 263, 450
Fat pad injuries, 142
Felt, 239
Femoral nerve, 23
   motor distribution, 24
   sensory distribution, 24
   sites of involvement, 24
   testing, 24
Femur
   condyles *see* Condyles
   epiphysis
      displaced, 449
      slipped, 114, 131
   head
      avascular necrosis *see* Avascular
         necrosis
      fracture, 419
      radiographic shape, 128
   neck, anteversion, 124
   neck fracture, 423–8
      aetiology, 423
      after-care, 427
      in children, 430
      complications, 426
      diagnosis, 423
      extracapsular, 423
      Garden classification, 424
      with hip dislocation, 446
      intracapsular, 419, 423, 424–5, 428
      investigations, 426
      level of fracture, 423
      radiographs, 425
      treatment, 425, 428
   shaft fracture, 419
      after-care, 442, 445
      causes, 434
      classification, 434

      complications, 450
      conservative treatment, 434–43
      diagnosis, 434
      fluid loss, 434
      intramedullary nailing, 444–5
      metastatic, 446
      non-conservative treatment, 444–5
      open, 446
      radiographs, 440
      segmental (double), 449
      special situations, 446
      support, 440
      treatment, 451
   shortening, 441, 450
   slipped upper epiphysis, 114, 131
      complicating hip dislocation, 419,
         420
      radiographs, 421
      treatment, 422
Fibula, fracture
   above syndesmosis, 487
   at level of syndesmosis, 488
   distal to syndesmosis, 487
      with associated medial injury, 487
   isolated, 476, 487
Fibular collateral ligament *see* Lateral
      ligament
Fingers, 10
   deformities, 75
   hypertrophy, 75
   injuries
      extensor tendon, 81
      flexor tendon, 80
   mallet *see* Mallet finger/thumb
   movements, 78–9
      composite, 78
      individual joints, 78
   phalangeal fractures, 359–63
   ring removal with casts, 244
   stiffness, 362
   trigger, 72
   vibration white finger, 72, 80
   see also specific parts
Fixation, 233–4, 252
   application, 252
   Colles' fracture, 334
   devices and systems, 252
   external plaster *see* Plaster casts
   external skeletal *see* External skeletal
      fixation
   femoral neck fractures, 426

forearm fractures, 320
metacarpal fractures, 354
open fractures, 250
supracondylar fracture, 299–300
thoracolumbar spine fracture, 393
tibial fracture, 474–5
see also Reduction
Fixed flexion deformity, 5
Flat foot *see* Talipes (pes) planus
Flexion contracture, hip, 117–19
Flexion injuries of spine, 372–3, 374–7, 385
causes, 372
treatment, 373
Flexor carpi radialis, tests, 21
Flexor carpi ulnaris, tests, 19, 20
Flexor digitorum profundus, 18, 20, 22
Flexor pollicis longus, tests, 22
Flip test, 99
Fluid displacement test (knee), 149
Foot, 185–207
adolescent conditions, 187
adult conditions, 188–9
childhood conditions, 186–7
club, 191
diagnosis of complaints, 190
examination, 192–200
injuries, 497–518
crushing, 518
talar neck, 498
movements, 201–2
pronation, 201
supination, 201
radiographs, 204–7
see also specific parts
Footballer's ankle, 176, 184, 494
Footprint, 203
Forearm injuries, 319–25
after-care, 321
fractures
adults, 322
angulation, 318, 321
children, 319–21
displaced, 319–20
undisplaced, 319
radiographs, 320
see also Radius; Ulna
Forefoot tenderness, 199
Forestier's disease, 87
Fracture clinic, 519–24
Fracture-dislocation, 226
ankle, 483

Bennett's, 355
cervical spine, 378
Esses-Lopresti, 312
fingers, 365
forearm
Galeazzi, 226, 316, 325, 339
Monteggia, 226, 310, 316, 323–4
humerus, proximal, 284, 285, 291
spine, 370
Fracture(s)
angulation, 216–17
articular, 214
avulsion, 214
axial rotation, 217
causes, 212
classification, 220–2
closed, 212
complications, 255–64
compression *see* Compression (crush)
fracture
definitions, 212
deformity, 215
diagnosis, 224–6
displacement, 216
double *see* Segmental fracture
fixation, 233–4
greenstick *see* Greenstick fracture
hairline, 212
healing, 219
factors affecting, 254
history, 224
impacted, 214
level of, 215
multifragmentary (comminuted) *see*
Multifragmentary/comminuted
fracture
note-taking, 522–4
open *see* Open fracture
pathological, 264–6
radiographic evaluation, 224–6
reduction, 232–3, 238
simple, 213
treatment, 226–35
plaster casts, 239–46
primary aims, 226
priorities, 226–7
resuscitation, 227–30
see also specific bones and types
Freiberg's disease, 188, 207
Froment's test, 19
Frozen shoulder, 41

Functional overlay, 99–100

Gait assessment, 25, 117, 126
Galeazzi fracture-dislocation, 226, 316, 325, 339
  treatment, 325
Gallows traction, 443
Gamekeeper's thumb, 80, 358
Ganglion
  hand, 73
  wrist, 18, 62
Ganz drawer test *see* Drawer tests
Garden classification, femoral neck fracture, 424
Genitofemoral nerve, 23
Genu recurvatum (hyperextension), 143, 151, 162
Genu valgum (knock-knee), 143, 152, 172, 195
Genu varum (bow-leg), 143, 152, 172
Glasgow Coma Scale, 231
Glenohumeral joint
  movement, 40
  osteoarthritis, 42
  stability, 48
Glenohumeral movement, 40
Globulin, 527
Glomus tumours, 73
Gluteal muscle function, 123
Golfer's elbow, 57, 58
Gout, toes, 189
Great toe *see* Toes
Greek foot, 193
Greenstick fracture, 212
  clavicle, 270
  forearm, 318
  radius, 339
  thumb, 357
Grip strength, 82
Gunshot wounds, 251–2
  explosions, 252
  high velocity, 252
  low velocity, 251
  plastic bullets, 251
Gustilo's classification, 477

Haemarthrosis, knee, 138, 146
Haemoglobin, 229
Haemorrhage, 228
  and pelvic fracture, 412
Haglund deformity, 181

Hairline fracture, 212
Hallux
  examination, 192–3
  nail conditions, 189, 193
  tenderness, 200
Hallux rigidus, 188, 193
Hallux valgus, 187, 192
  radiographs, 205
  tenderness, 200
Halo traction, 375–7
Hamate
  dislocation, 351
  hook, fractures, 18, 351
Hamilton-Russell traction, 443
Hammer toe, 189, 194
Hand, 71–82
  assessment, 75–82
    principle functions, 82
  common syndromes, 72–3
  movements *see* Fingers
  myelopathy, 32
  see also Wrist; and parts of hand
Haversian systems, 219
Head injury, 230–1
  Glasgow Coma Scale, 231
Healing of fractures, 219
  factors affecting, 254
Heart, tamponade, 231
Heberden's nodes, 77
Heel
  inspection, 192
  posture, 198
  tenderness, 199
Hemiarthroplasty, 428
Herbert screw, 307
Herring lateral pillar classification, 131
High velocity gunshot wounds, 252
Hip, 10, 111–35
  assessment, 116–26
    in knee pain, 164
  common conditions, 112–15
  dysplastic, 113
  irritable, 113–14
  movements
    abduction, 121, 126
    adduction, 121
    extension, 121
    external rotation, 122
    flexion, 121
    internal rotation, 122
    telescoping, 126

radiographs, 127–35
rare conditions, 115
shortening, 117–19
special tests, 123–6
Hip replacement, 115–16, 133, 428
fractures in, 447
Hip spica, 443
Hippocratic reduction, 279
Histamine test, traumatic lesion of brachial plexus, 14–15
Hoffmann's test, 32
Hook of hamate fracture, 18, 351
Horner's syndrome, 12, 13
Housemaid's knee, 143, 147
Hume fracture, 310
Humerus
    condyles *see* Condyles
    epicondyles *see* Epicondyles
    greater tuberosity fracture
        displaced (group IV), 290
        with shoulder dislocation (group VI), 291
        undisplaced (group I), 286–7
    lesser tuberosity fracture, displaced (group V), 290
    neck fracture
        anatomically displaced (group II), 288
        severely displaced/angled (group III), 289
    proximal fractures, 284–92
        classification, 284–5
        diagnosis, 286
        treatment, 286–92
    shaft fracture, 292–4
        complications, 294
        diagnosis, 292
        treatment, 293–4
Hurler's syndrome, 75
Hyperextension of knee, 143, 151, 162
Hyperhydrosis of foot, 195
Hypermobility, wrist, tests for, 67
Hyperostosis, diffuse idiopathic skeletal, 87
Hyperparathyroidism, 526
Hypertrophic non-union, 255, 356
    humeral shaft, 294
Hypoparathyroidism, 526

Idiopathic adhesive capsulitis, 41
Ileus, paralytic, 414
Iliohypogastric nerve, 23

Ilioinguinal nerve, 23
Iliopsoas test, 24
Imaging *see specific modalities and fractures*
Impacted fractures, 214
Impingement fracture of radius, 342
Impingement syndromes of shoulder, 41
Implant complications, 263–4
    corrosion, 264
    mechanical effects, 263
Implantation dermoid cysts, 73
Index finger, injuries, 361
Infant club foot, 191
Infections
    apical, 73
    elbow, 58
    femoral shaft fracture, 450
    great toe, 189
    hand, 73–4, 81
    hip, 124
    knee, 138, 145, 146
    pulp, 73, 81
    sacrococcygeal joint, 105
    shoulder, 42, 50
    wrist, 70
Inferior gluteal nerve, 23
Inferior tibiofibular ligament, 180
    sprains, 494
Infrapatellar bursitis, 143, 147
Infrapatellar fat pad injuries, 142
Infraspinatus, test, 14
Ingrowing toenail, 189
Insertional tendinitis, Achilles tendon, 176
Inspection, 4
Instability
    ankle, 179–82, 493, 495
    biceps tendon, 49
    knee, 153–60
        anterior, 155
        patellofemoral, 141
        posterior, 157–8
        posterolateral, 159
        rotatory, 140, 158–60
        varus stress, 155
    patellofemoral, 141
    pelvic, 400
    spine, 368
    wrist/carpus, 351
Interossei, tests, 19
Interphalangeal joint
    distal, 78
    movements, 202

Interphalangeal joints, 79
  dislocation, 359, 364
  hand, osteoarthritis, 73
  normal movements, 78, 202
Intertrochanteric basal neck fractures, 428
Intestinal injury, 414
Intoeing (metatarsus varus), 186
Intramedullary nailing
  femoral shaft fracture, 444–5
  tibial fracture, 474
Inverted radial reflex, 32
Irritable hip, 113
Ischaemia
  pelvic fracture, 412
  supracondylar fracture, 301
Ischaemic contracture, Volkmann's, 76,
    297, 466

Jakob's reverse pivot shift test, 160
Jerk test, 49
Joints
  fractures indirectly causing stiffness *see*
    Stiffness
  movements, 4–5
  warmth, 4
  see also individual joints
Jones fracture, 516
Jumper's knee, 139, 163

Kienbock's disease, 70, 350
Kirschner wires, 305, 314, 334, 349, 354
Kissing spines, 103
Klippel-Feil syndrome, 28, 33, 43, 44
Klumpke's palsy, 11, 12
Knee, 137–68
  acceptable functional range, 451
  common pathology, 138–43
  diagnosis of complaints, 144–6
  extensor mechanism
    injuries of, 452–4
    lack of extension, 451
  fractures, 450
  injuries, 419
  instability, 153–60
    anterior, 155
    patellofemoral, 141
    posterior, 157–8
    posterolateral, 159
    rotatory, 140, 158–60

    valgus stress, 153–4
    varus stress, 155
  lack of flexion, 451
  ligaments, 139
    cruciate ligament, 139, 140
    lateral ligament and capsule, 140
    medial ligament and capsule, 139
  locked, 461
  movements, 151–64
    extension, 139, 151
    flexion, 151
    hyperextension, 143, 151, 162
  pain post-tibial fracture, 472, 474
  radiographs, 164–8
  soft-tissue injuries, 456
  stiffness with femoral fracture, 450
  tenderness, 150
  with tibial fracture, mobilisation, 471
  see also Patella
Knock-knee *see* Genu valgum
Kocher's reduction, 278
Kohler's disease, 187
Kyphosis, 86–7, 93
  angular, 93
  juvenile *see* Scheuermann's disease
  senile, 88, 102
  tibial, 171

Lachman test, 156
Lasegue test, reverse, 98
Lateral capsule of knee, 140
Lateral cutaneous nerve of thigh, 23, 26
  assessment, 26
Lateral epicondyle, palpation, 57
Lateral ligament
  ankle, 179–80
    injuries, 492–3
    instability, 493
  knee, 140
    injuries, 458
Lateral tomography, 6
Lauge-Hansen classification of ankle
    fractures, 483
Leg
  straight leg raising test, 98
  see also Lower limb
Levator ani, nerves to, 23
Lhermitte's test, 32
Ligaments
  ankle

injuries, 493, 494
tests, 179–80
knee *see* Cruciate ligaments; Lateral
ligament; Medial ligament; Patellar
ligament
transverse, of atlas, lesions, 382–3
ulnar collateral, rupture, 80, 358
Lightning pains, 170
Locked joint, knee, 461
Long bones, AO fracture classification *see*
AO Classification
Long thoracic nerve, 50
Loose bodies in knee, 142, 166
Looser's zones, 167, 264
Lordosis, 102
Losee pivot shift test, 159
Low velocity gunshot wounds, 251
Lower limb
peripheral nerves, 23–6
shortening
with femoral fracture, 441, 450
with pelvic fracture, 414
telescoping, in congenital hip
dislocation, 126
see also specific parts
Lumbar lordosis, 94
Lumber spine *see* Thoracolumbar spine
Lumbosacral joint, 106
Lumbosacral junction, 106
Lumbosacral trunk, 23
Lunate
dislocation, 70, 348–9, 350
Kienbock's disease, 70, 350
Luxatio erecta, 281

MacIntosh test, 158
McMurray manoeuvre, 161
MacMurray osteotomy, 427
Madelung's deformity, 64
Magnetic resonance imaging, 6
back pain, 95
knee, 145
traumatic lesion of brachial plexus, 14
Maisonneuve fracture, 483, 486
Malignant tumours *see* Tumours/neoplasms
Malleolar fracture
bimalleolar, 490–1
complicating talar neck fracture, 501
posterior, 489
trimalleolar, 490–1

Mallet finger/thumb, 72, 75, 363
treatment, 364
Mallet toe, 189
Malunion, 257
Colles' fracture, 337
phalangeal fracture, 363
shortening as sequela, 257
Manipulation *see* Reduction
March fracture, 516
Marfan's syndrome, 67, 75
Medial arch of foot, 197
Medial capsule of knee, 139
Medial epicondyle, tenderness, 57
Medial ligaments of knee (tibial collateral
ligament), 139
injuries, 457
Medial tibial syndrome, 170
Median nerve
common sites affected, 21
compression *see* Carpal tunnel
syndrome
inspection, 21
motor distribution, 20
motor function tests, 21–3
palsy, 261, 262
wrist dislocation, 350
sensory distribution, 20
tests for impairment, 23
Menisci
cysts, 141, 162, 461
examination, 160–2
injuries, 459
adults, 459–61
children, 459
diagnosis, 460
treatment, 461
McMurray manoeuvre, 161
tears, 141, 161, 461
Meralgia paraesthetica, 26
Metacarpophalangeal joint
fingers
dislocation, 364
movement, 78
thumb
injuries, 357
movements, 79
toes, bursa, 192
Metacarpus, injuries, 352–65
assessment, 352
fifth metacarpal, 359–60
dislocation of base, 361

Metacarpus, injuries, *continued*
  fracture of head, 361
    fracture of shaft and base, 360
  fracture of base of thumb, 357
  index, middle and ring metacarpals, 361
  soft-tissue management, 355
  treatment, 352–3
Metal implant, corrosion, 264
Metastases
  bone, biochemical values, 526
  hand, 73
  spine, 89
Metatarsal fractures, 515–17
  diagnosis, 515
  fifth metatarsal base, 515
  first metatarsal, 517
  Jones fracture, 516
  March fracture, 516
  multiple displaced fractures, 517
  single/multiple undisplaced fractures of
    shaft and neck, 516
  treatment, 515
Metatarsalgia
  anterior, 188
  Morton's, 188
Metatarsophalangeal joint
  movements, 202
  osteoarthritis *see* Hallus rigidus
Metatarsus varus, 186
Midpalmar/thenar space infections, 74
Milch reduction, 279
Mobilisation, knee with tibial fracture, 471
Mobility
  wrist, excessive, 67
  see also Movements
Monteggia fracture–dislocation, 226, 310,
    316, 323–4
  aftercare, 324
  in children, 324
  late diagnosis, 324
  patterns, 323
  treatment, 324
Morquio-Brailsford's disease, 67
Morton's metatarsalgia, 188, 199
Motor distribution
  common peroneal nerve, 24
  femoral nerve, 24
  median nerve, 20
  radial nerve, 17
  sciatic nerve, 26
  tibial nerve, 25

    ulnar nerve, 18
Movements, 4–5
MRC scale, 5
Mucous cysts, 73
Multifragmentary/comminuted fracture,
    213
  ankle, 492
  radius, 314
  tibia, 476
Muscles
  grip strength, 82
  wasting, 4
  see also specific muscles
Myelography
  back pain, 95
  traumatic lesion of brachial plexus, 14
Myelomatosis, biochemical values, 526
Myelopathy
  cervical, 28, 36
  hand, 32
Myositis ossificans, 54, 60
  hip dislocation, 420
  post-fracture
    humerus, 259
    pelvis, 414
Myotomes, 10

Nail disorders
  foot *see* Toenail
  hand, 81
Nailing *see* and various types of nails;
    Intramedullary nailing
Nancy nails, 320
Navicular bone
  of foot, isolated fractures, 513
  of hand *see* Scaphoid
  osteochondritis, 187
  see also Calcaneonavicular
    bar/synostosis
Neck
  acute pain in young adults, 28
  postural pain, 28
  soft-tissue injuries, 386–8
    Barré-Lieou syndrome, 387
    classification, 387
    diagnosis, 387
    further investigation, 387
    MRI scans, 387
    radiographs, 387
    treatment, 387

Necrosis
    avascular *see* Avascular necrosis
    skin, talar neck fractures, 501
Neer's classification, 284–5
Neoplasms *see* Tumours/neoplasms
Nerve root rupture, 12
Nerves
    injuries *see* Neurological problems
    motor *see* Motor distribution
    segmental distribution, 10
    sensory *see* Sensory distribution
    see also specific nerves
Neuritis, ulnar, 54
Neurofibromatosis, 12, 94
Neurological problems
    fractures, 261–2
        delayed, 262
        pelvis, 414
    shoulder dislocation, 283
    spinal injuries, 32, 395–6
        see also Paralysis
Neuroma, plantar, 188, 189
Non-union, 255
    atrophic, 256, 257
    femoral neck fractures, 427
    femoral shaft fracture, 450
    humeral shaft, 294
    hypertrophic, 255, 356
    scaphoid fracture, 347
Note-taking, 522–4

Obstetric difficulties following pelvic
        fracture, 414
Obstetrical palsy, 11, 12
    lower (Klumpke's), 11, 12
    upper (Erb's), 11
Obturator nerve, 23
O'Donoghue's triad, 140, 459
Odontoid fractures, 383–4
    classification, 383
    diagnosis, 384
    mechanisms, 384
    radiographs, 384
Oedema, 4, 248
Olecranon, 296
    bursitis, 54
    fractures, 311–12
        diagnosis, 311
        treatment, 311–12
Oligaemic shock, 450

Ollier's disease, 73
Onychogryphosis, 189, 193
Open fracture, 212, 217, 234, 250–1
    associated vascular/neurological injuries,
        250
    debridement, 250
    fixation, 250
    Gustilo classification, 218
    immediate care, 250
    later treatment, 251
    tibia, 477
Open-book fracture, 402
Ortolani's test, 125
Osgood-Schlatter's disease, 139, 144, 150,
        167, 173, 174, 455
Osteitis
    cervical spine, 28
    pathological fractures, 265
    post-fracture, 260
    pyogenic, of spine, 89
    staphylococcal, 42
    symphysis pubis, 114
    tibia, 170
Osteoarthritis
    ankle/foot, 177, 495, 502
    carpometacarpal joint of thumb, 73
    elbow, 54
    hip, 114–15, 129, 135, 414
        Patrick's test for early disease, 124
        secondary, 420
    interphalangeal joints, 73
    knee, 142, 144
    post-scaphoid fracture, 347
    shoulder, 48
        acromioclavicular joint, 42
        glenohumeral joint, 42
    spine, 89, 103
    wrist, 62
Osteochondritis
    ankle
        navicular, 187
        talus, 176, 178, 494, 502
    metatarsal head (2nd) *see* Freiberg's
        disease
Osteochondritis dissecans, 54, 142, 144,
        167
Osteochondritis tali, 494
Osteochondrosis, spinal *see* Scheuermann's
        disease
Osteogenesis imperfecta, 67
    pathological fractures, 265

Osteoid osteoma
    hand, 73
    tibia, 174
Osteomalacia
    biochemical values, 526
    pathological fractures, 264
Osteoporosis
    biochemical values, 526
    pathological fractures, 264
Oswestry pedicle screw system, 393
Otto's disease, 129, 135
Overlapping fracture of radius, 339–40

Paget's disease, 75
    biochemical values, 526
    hip, 128
    pathological fractures, 264
    spine, 88, 103
    tibia, 174
Palm
    grasp, 82
    mid-palm infection, 74
Palmaris longus, 21
Palpation, 4
Palsy
    axillary (circumflex) nerve, 261, 277
    common peroneal nerve, 261
    Erb's, 11, 12
    with femoral shaft fracture, 446
    Klumpke's, 11, 12
    median nerve, 261, 262
    radial nerve, 261, 294
    Saturday night, 16
    sciatic nerve, 261, 419
    tourniquet, 16
    ulnar nerve, 261
        tardy, 54, 262
    see also Paralysis
Paralysis in spinal injury, 368
    cervical spinal, 381
    treatment, 397–8
Paralytic ileus, 414
Paratendinitis, Achilles tendon, 176
Paronychia, 73, 81
Patella
    alta, 162, 168
    baja (infera), 141
    chondromalacia patellae, 142
    examination, 162–4

    fractures, 419, 446
        undisplaced horizontal, 453
        vertical, 453
    infrapatellar bursitis, 143, 147
    infrapatellar fat pad injuries, 142
    injuries, 452–4
        diagnosis, 452
        mechanisms, 452
        radiographs, 452
        treatment, 453
    radiographs, 165
    tap test, 149
    tenderness, 163
Patellar ligament rupture, 455
Patellofemoral instability, 141
Pathological fractures, 264–6
    investigation, 265–6
Patients' notes, 522–4
Patrick's test, 124
Pauwel's osteotomy, 427
Pelligrini-Stieda disease, 139, 166, 457
Pelvic injuries
    contralateral compression (bucket handle fractures), 405
    fractures, 400–14
        bucket handle, 405
        complications, 412–14
        diagnosis, 400
        general principles, 400
        stable, 400, 401–2
        tile classification, 400
        treatment, 403–4
        unstable, 400
        see also Acetabulum, fracture
    ipsilateral lateral compression, 405
    radiographs, 406
    rotationally unstable, vertically stable, 402, 405
    treatment, 406–8
Pelvic ring
    stable fracture of, 401–2
    stable fracture of pelvis not involving, 401–2
Penile urethra, damage to, 413
Perilunar dislocation, 351
Peripheral nerves, 10
    lower limb, 23–6
    upper limb, 15–23
Periscapholunar dislocation, 351
Peritalar dislocation, 510
Peroneal (spastic) flat foot, 187

Peroneal tendon
  dislocation, 494
  snapping, 176–7
Perthes' disease, 113–14, 128, 130–1, 134
  Catterall grading, 130
  Herring lateral pillar classification, 131
  radiographs, 134
Pertrochanteric fractures, 429–30
  after-care, 430
  complications, 430
  treatment, 429
Pes cavus *see* Talipes (pes) cavus
Pes planus *see* Talipes (pes) planus
Phalanges, injuries, 352–65
  assessment, 352
  fractures
    complications, 362–3
    middle, 362–3
    proximal, 358, 362
    terminal, 359, 363
  treatment, 352–3
Physiotherapy
  femoral shaft fracture, 451
  spinal injuries, 398
Pilonidal sinus, 74
Pivot shaft test of Losee, 159
Plantar (digital) neuroma, 188
Plantar fasciitis, 189
Plantar neuroma, 188, 199
Plantar wart, 189, 195
Plantaris tendon rupture, 171, 173
Plantigrade foot, 196
Plaster casts, 239–46
  complete, 243–4
    application, 243
    elevation, 244
    precautions, 244
    removal, 246
    removal of rings, 244
    size of bandages, 243
    skin protection, 243
    wetting, 243
  patient aftercare, 245–6
  plaster slabs, 239–42
  skin protection, 239
    felt, 239
    stockingette, 239
    wool roll, 239
  see also various fractures
Plaster of Paris *see* Plaster casts
Plaster slabs, 239–42

  applying, 241
  reinforcing, 242
  removal, 246
  securing, 242
  tailoring of, 240
  wetting, 241
Plastic bullets, 251
Plexus
  brachial, 11, 13–15
  lesions, 12
  long-standing lesions, 12
Polymer resin casts, 247–8
  application, 247
  assessment of union, 248
  removal, 248
Positron emission tomography, 7
Post-traumatic osteodystrophy *see* Sudeck's
  atrophy
Posterior leg pain, 171
Posterior shoulder dislocation, 281
  late diagnosed, 282
  recurrent, 283
Postural myelopathy hand, 32
Posture, 4
  heel, 198
Pott's fractures, 480
Prepatellar bursitis, 143, 147
Pressure epiphyses, 218
Pressure sores, 397
Profundus tendon injury, 72, 80
Prolapsed intervertebral disc, 90–1, 97
Pronation/dorsiflexion injuries, ankle, 484
Pronation/lateral rotation injuries, ankle,
  483
Pronator teres, tests, 21
Prostate cancer, biochemical values, 526
Protrusio acetabuli, 129, 135
Proximal interphalangeal joint, 78
Pseudarthrosis of tibia, 171
Pseudo-hypoparathyroidism, 526
Psoriasis, great toe, 189
Pubic symphysis, instability, 414
Pudendal nerve, 23
Pulled elbow, 311
Pulp infections, 73, 81
Pulse absence with supracondylar fracture,
  301
Pyarthrosis, 138
Pyogenic infections
  hip, 114
  spine, 88

Quadriceps, 24
  tethering, 450
  wasting, 139, 148
Quadriceps tendon rupture, 455
Quinti varus deformity, 194

Radial nerve
  examination, 16
  motor distribution, 17
  palsy, 261, 294
  sensory distribution, 16, 17
  sites affected, 16
Radiohumeral joint, 57
Radius
  axial rotation, 317
  Barton's fracture, 342
  greenstick fracture, 339
  head fracture, 312–14
    assessment, 313
    classification, 313
    comminuted, 314
    diagnosis, 313
    radiographs, 313
  impingement fracture, 342
  injuries, 316
  isolated dislocation, 310
  isolated fracture, 325
  neck fracture, 314
  overlapping fracture, 339–40
  slipped epiphysis, 340
  Smith's fracture, 341
  styloid fracture, 342
  see also Forearm
Range of movement, 4–5
Recording and communication, 266–7
Records, 266
Rectangular foot, 193
Reduction, 232–3, 238
  cervical spinal injuries, 377–8
    failure of, 378
  Colles' fracture, 330–3
  femoral shaft fracture, 438
  hip dislocation, 416–18
  supracondylar fracture, 298–9
  tibial fractures, 473
  see also Fixation
Reiter's syndrome
  hip, 115
  knee, 143
Remanipulation, supracondylar fracture,
  301

Resin casts see Polymer resin casts
Resuscitation, 227–30
  airway, 227
  breathing, 227
  circulation, 228–30
Retropatellar pain syndromes, 142
Retrospondylolisthesis, 394
Reverse Lasegue test, 98
Rheumatoid arthritis
  ankle, 177
  cervical spine, 28, 37, 366
  elbow, 54
  foot, 189
  hand, 72
  hip, 115
  knee, 142, 144, 145
  shoulder, 42
  spine, 89
  wrist, 62
Rhomboids, nerve to, 13
Ribs, cervical see Cervical rib syndrome
Rickets, 152, 172
  adult, 264
  biochemical values, 526
Risser's sign, 108
Rolando fracture, 355
Roos test, 31
Rotation
  axial see Axial rotation
  see also Flexion injuries of spine
Rotator cuff, 40
  arthropathy, 41
  tears, 41, 283
  tests, 47
Rupture
  bladder, 413
  diaphragm, 414
  ligaments
    patellar, 455
    ulnar collateral, 80, 358
  nerve root, 12
  tendons
    Achilles, 511–12
    biceps, 43
    delayed, 262
    extensor pollicis longus, 338
    plantaris, 171, 173
    quadriceps, 455
  urethra, 413

Sacrococcygeal joint

infections, 105
tests, 101
Sacroiliac joint, 101, 105
persistent pain, 414
Sacrum, fracture, 408
Sarcoidosis, biochemical values, 526
Sarmiento plaster, 471
Saturday night palsy, 16
Scaphoid (navicular bone of hand)
avascular necrosis, 70
dislocation see Dislocation
fracture, 70, 338, 343–7
aftercare, 347
complications, 347
diagnosis, 343
displaced, 346
features, 343
fracture patterns, 343
mechanisms of injury, 343
plaster cast, 345
radiographs, 344
treatment, 344
undisplaced, 345–6
fractures, tuberosity, 344
Scapula
high, 42
snapping, 42
winged, 43
Scapular injuries, fractures, 275
Scapulothoracic joint, movement, 40
Scheuermann's disease, 87, 93, 102, 109
Schmorl's nodes, 103, 109
Sciatic nerve, 23
assessment, 26
motor distribution, 26
palsy, 261, 419
sensory distribution, 26
sites involved, 26
Scoliosis, 86, 94–5, 108
Seat belt injuries, 370
Sedimentation rate, 101
Segmental fracture
femoral shaft, 449
tibia, 475
Segmental nerve distribution, 10
Segments, long bones in AO Classification
see AO Classification
Senile kyphosis, 88, 102
Sensory distribution
common peroneal nerve, 24
femoral nerve, 24
median nerve, 20
radial nerve, 16, 17
sciatic nerve, 26
tibial nerve, 25
ulnar nerve, 18
Serratus anterior, nerve to, 13
Serum calcium, 526
Serum cholesterol, 527
Serum iron, 527
Serum phosphate, 526
Serum urate, 527
Sesamoiditis, 200
Sesamoids, radiograph, 206
Sever's disease, 187
Shenton's line, 129
Shield fracture, 284, 285
Shin splints, 170
Shoes, examination of, 203
Shortening
Achilles tendon (tendo calcaneus), 177,
182
femoral shaft fracture, 441, 450
in fracture healing, 257
hip, 117–19
leg, following pelvic fracture, 414
Shoulder, 10, 40–52
aspiration, 50
assessment, 44–50
basic features, 40
common pathologies, 41–2
dislocation see Dislocation
radiographs, 51–2
Shoulder cuff see Rotator cuff
Sinding-Larsen-Johansson syndrome, 139,
150, 163
Single-photon emission computed
tomography, 7
back pain, 95
Skeletal hyperostosis, diffuse idiopathic, 87
Skeletal traction see Traction
Skew foot, 188
Skin appearance
back pain, 94
knee, 147
neurofibromatosis, 197
spina bifida, 197
spinal paralysis, 397
Skin necrosis, 501
Skin protection, plaster casts, 239, 243
Skull tongs, 376
Slabs see Plaster slabs

Slings, 233
    clavicular fracture, 270
    elbow dislocation, 308
    forearm fractures, 318
    humeral neck fractures, 287
    radial head fracture, 313
    shoulder dislocation, 280
    supracondylar fracture, 300
Slow union, 255
    treatment, 256
Smillie pins, 307
Smith's fracture, 341
Snapping hip, 115
Snapping peroneal tendons, 176–7
Snapping scapula, 42
Soft-tissue injuries
    knee, 456
    neck, 386–8
Sole of foot *see* Plantar
Special tests, 5
Speed test, 49
Spina bifida, 90, 104
Spinal concussion, 395
Spinal cord
    compression
        cervical, 28
        radiographs, 32
    special features, 396
Spinal injuries, 368–70, 394
    assessment, 368–9
    fracture-Dislocation *see* Fracture-
        Dislocation
    fractures
        burst, 369
        compression, 369
        transverse process, 394
    neurological assessment, 395–6
    neurological lesion, 395
    occupational therapy, 398
    physiotherapy, 398
    retrospondylolisthesis, 394
    seatbelt type, 370
    see also Cervical spine; Thoracic and
        lumber spine
Spinal nerves, 10
Spinal osteochondrosis *see* Scheuermann's
    disease
Spinal stenosis, 90, 107
Spinous process, isolated fractures, 386
Splay foot, 188
Splints

plaster *see* Plaster casts
    Thomas, 436–7
Spondylitis, ankylosing *see* Ankylosing
    spondylitis
Spondylolisthesis, 89, 94, 107
Spondylolysis, 89
Spondylosis
    cervical, 12, 28
        radiographs, 37
Sprains, 212
    acromioclavicular joint, 272
    ankle, 493, 494
    fingers, 365
Sprengel shoulder, 42
Staphylococcal osteitis, 42
Sternoclavicular dislocation, 274–5
Stiffness of joints with fractures, 258, 338,
    362
    femoral fracture (knee), 450
    fingers, 362
Stimson reduction
    hip, 418
    shoulder, 279
Stockingette, 239
Straight leg raising test, 98
Stress fracture, tibia, 170
Stress tests, ankle instability, 179, 180
Stryker frame, 392
Styloid fracture, 342
Sublimis tendon injury, 80
Subluxations, 212
    acromioclavicular joint, 272
    atlanto-occipital, 381–6
    clavicle, 270
    fingers, 365
Subtalar joint *see* Talocalcaneal joint;
    Talocalcaneal synostosis
Subtrochanteric fractures, 430
Subungual exostoses
    finger, 81
    toe, 189
Sudeck's atrophy, 64, 65, 70, 258–9
    aetiology, 258
    ankle, 495
    bone scan, 7
    Colles' fracture, 338
    diagnosis, 259
    scaphoid fracture, 347
    treatment, 259
    wrist dislocation, 350
Sulcus sign, 49

Superficial peroneal nerve compression
        syndrome, 200
Superior gluteal nerve, 23
Supination/adduction injuries, ankle, 484
Supinator test, 17
Supracondylar fracture
        adults, 448
        children, 447
        humerus
                adults, 306
                anterior (reversed), 302–4
                children, 296–301
                diagnosis, 296
                radiographs, 296–7, 300
                vascular complications, 297
        manipulation/remanipulation, 298–9,
                301
Suprascapular nerve, 14, 50
Supraspinatus
        calcifying tendinitis, 41
        test, 14
Sustentaculum tali fracture, 505
Swan-neck deformity, 75
Sweating test, 23
Swelling, 4
        ankle, 176, 485, 495
        knee, 138
        plaster cast-related, 245
        supracondylar fracture, 297
Symphysis pubis, osteitis, 114
Synostosis
        calcaneonavicular, 206
        talocalcaneal, 206
Synovitis
        hip, 113
        knee, 138
Syphilis, 74
        see also Tabes dorsalis
Syringomyelia, 86

T-fracture, femur, 449
Tabes dorsalis, 170
Talipes (pes) calcaneus, 186
Talipes (pes) cavus, 186
        assessment, 190
Talipes (pes) equinovarus, 186
        infant, 191
Talipes (pes) planus, 186, 197
        adult, 188
        assessment, 190
        peroneal (spastic), 187

Talocalcaneal joint
        involvement in calcaneal fracture, 508
        movements, 201
        non-involvement in calcaneal fracture,
                506–7
Talocalcaneal synostosis, 206
Talus
        avulsion fractures, 502
        body fractures, 503
        dome fracture, 502
        head, compression fractures, 503
        lateral process fractures, 503
        neck fractures, 498–9
                complications, 501
                diagnosis, 499
                open, 501
                treatment, 499–501
        osteochondritis, 176, 178, 502
Tardy ulnar nerve palsy, 54, 262
Tarsal tunnel syndrome, 25, 189, 200
Tarsometatarsal joint
        dislocations, 514
        movements, 202
Tears
        anterior tibiofibular, 489
        cruciate ligaments
                anterior, 459
                posterior, 458
        meniscal, 141, 161, 461
        rotator cuff, 41, 283
        urethra, 413
Technetium bone scan, 6–7
Telephone calls, 266–7
Temperature
        foot, 198
        joints, 4
        knee, 147
Tenderness, 4, 248
        ankle, 178, 485
        femoral neck fractures, 423
        forefoot, 199
        great toe, 200
        heel, 199
        knee, 150, 163
        medial epicondyle, 57
        tibia, 173
        wrist, 329, 330
Tendinitis
        Achilles tendon, 176
        biceps, 49
        calcifying supraspinatus, 41

Tendinopathy, ankle, 176, 181
Tendinosis, Achilles tendon, 176
Tendo calcaneus *see* Achilles tendon
Tendon rupture, delayed, 262
Tendon sheath infections, 74, 81
Tennis elbow, 54, 58
Tenosynovitis
    ankle, 176, 181
    de Quervain's, 62, 64, 65, 66
    extensor, 62
Terrible triad, 314
Thomas splint, 436–7
Thoracic outlet syndrome, 28, 31
Thoracic spine *see* Thoracolumbar spine
Thoracolumbar spine, 83–110
    assessment, 93–5
    common syndromes, 84–91
    fractures, 388–94
        diagnosis, 388
        mechanisms of injury, 388
        radiographs, 389, 390
        stable, 389, 392
        treatment, 392–4
        unstable, 390–2, 392–3
        wedge, 389
    functional overlay, 99–100
    inspection, 94–5
    movements, 95–101
        extension, 96
        flexion, 95–6
        lateral flexion, 97
        rotation, 97
    radiographs, 102–10
    see also Back pain
Thrombophlebitis, 171
Thumb
    carpometacarpal joint, osteoarthritis, 73
    dislocation *see* Dislocations
    fractures
        base of metacarpal, 357
        Bennett's, 226, 355
        proximal phalanx, 358
        terminal phalanx, 359
        treatment, 356
    gamekeeper's, 80, 358
    injuries to base of thumb, 355–9
    mallet *see* Mallet finger/thumb
    movements, 79
    trigger, 72
    ulnar collateral ligament, tests of, 80
    see also Carpometacarpal joints;

    Metacarpophalangeal joints
Tibia, 169–74
    assessment, 172–3
    bowing, 171
    condyles *see* Condyles
    deformities, 171
    fractures, 170, 173, 465–78
        adults, 470–8
        after-care, 471–2
        in children, 467–70
        displaced but potentially stable, 473
        displaced unstable, 474–5
        distal shaft, 476
        double (segmental), 475
        early mobilisation of knee, 471
        gross fragmentation, 476
        mechanism of injury, 466
        open, 477
        unstable with minimal displacement,
        474
    pain
        anterior, 170
        posterior, 171
    pseudarthrosis, 171
    radiographs, 174–5
    screening tests, 173
    shape, 172
    stress fracture, 170
    tenderness, 173
    torsion, 171, 172
Tibial collateral ligament *see* Medial
        ligaments of knee
Tibial kyphosis, 171
Tibial nerve, 23
    assessment, 25
    motor distribution, 25
    sensory distribution, 25
    sites of involvement, 25
Tibial table fractures, 461–3
    diagnosis, 462
    lateral, 461
    medial, 461
    treatment, 462
Tile classification of pelvic injuries, 400
Tillaux fracture, 483, 486
Tinel's sign
    carpal tunnel syndrome, 23
    tarsal tunnel syndrome, 200
    traumatic lesion of brachial plexus, 14
Toenail
    disorders of, 189, 193

ingrowing, 189
Toes, 189
    callosities, 194
    claw, 189, 194
    curly, 189, 194
    fractures, 518
    great *see* Hallux
    hammer, 189, 194
    injuries, 518
    mallet, 189, 194
    nails, 189
    quinti varus deformity, 194
    see also Foot; Intoeing
Torsion, tibial, 171
Torticollis, 29
Total acid phosphatase, 526
Total iron binding capacity, 527
Total serum protein, 527
Tourniquet palsy, 16
Tourniquet test, 23
Traction
    cervical spinal injuries, 378
    femoral shaft fracture, 434–6
        fixed traction, 439
        gallows traction, 443
        Hamilton-Russell traction, 443
        hip spica, 443
        skeletal traction, 434, 435–6
        skin traction, 434, 435
Traction epiphyses, 218
Trans-scapho perilunar dislocation, 351
Transverse ligament lesions, 382–3
    diagnosis, 382
    radiographs, 382
    treatment, 382
Transverse process fracture, 394
Trapezium dislocation, 351
Trapezoid dislocation, 351
Traumatic epiphyseal arrest, 257
Trendelenberg's test, 123
Triangle of Marcille, 23
Triceps, 17
Trigger finger/thumb, 72, 76
Trochanteric fractures, 431
Tuberculosis
    ankle, 177
    elbow, 54
    hand, 74
    hip, 114
    knee, 145, 167
    shoulder, 42

    spine, 88, 105
    wrist, 63
Tumours/neoplasms
    bone
        hip, 115
        pathological fractures, 265
        tibia, 170, 174
        treatment, 265
    cervical spine, 28
    hand, 73
    see also Metastases
Turner's syndrome, 75

Ulna
    axial rotation, 316
    fracture, 322
        see also Monteggia fracture–
        dislocation
    injuries, 316
    isolated dislocation, 310
    see also Forearm
Ulnar collateral ligament rupture, 80, 358
Ulnar nerve
    associated deformities, 18
    common sites affected, 18
    inspection, 19–20
    motor distribution, 18
    palpation, 19–20, 57
    palsy, 261
    sensory distribution, 18
    tardy ulnar nerve palsy, 54
Ulnar neuritis, 54
Ulnar tunnel syndrome, 54, 63
Ultrasound, 6–7
Unicameral bone cyst, 174
Union
    assessment, 248
        Colles' fracture, 336
    delayed, 255, 256
    slow, 255, 256
Upper limb
    peripheral nerves, 15–23
    see also specific bones and parts
Uraemic osteodystrophy, biochemical
    values, 526
Urea, 527
Urethral injury, 402
    following pelvic fracture, 412
        diagnosis, 413
        treatment, 413
    rupture, 413

Urinary output, 229

Valgus deformity
  elbow, 54
  knee, 153–4
  toes, hallux *see* Hallus valgus
Varus deformity
  elbow, 54
  knee, 155
Vascular problems
  arterial arrest, 260–1
  with fractures
    post-fracture, 260
    supracondylar fracture (elbow), 297,
      301
Verruca pedis, 189, 195
Vertebral bodies, 33–4
Vibration syndromes, 72, 80
Visceral complications of fracture, 262
Volkmann's ischaemic contracture, 76, 297,
  466

Wart, plantar, 189, 195
Web space infections, 74, 81
Weber's classification of ankle fractures,
  480

Wedge fractures
  cervical spine, 372
  thoracolumbar spine, 389
Whiplash injuries, 386–8
Wool roll, 239
Wrist/carpus, 10, 62–70
  assessment, 64–7
  common syndromes, 62–3
  crepitus, 66
  dislocation *see* Dislocations
  fractures
    avulsion, 342
    chip fractures, 351
    Colles' fracture *see* Colles' fracture
    hook of hamate, 18, 351
    radius *see* Radius, fractures
    Smith's fracture, 341
  hypermobility tests, 67
  instability, 351
  movements, 65–6
  radiographs, 68–70
  see also specific parts

Y-fracture, femur, 449

Z-deformity, 75